WW 400   1060

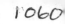
WITHDRAWN

Duke-Elder's Practice of Refraction

For Churchill Livingstone
Publisher: Mike Parkinson
Project Editor: Dilys Jones
Copy Editor: Helen Macdonald
Sales Promotion Executive: Douglas MacNaughton

Duke-Elder's Practice of Refraction

Revised by

David Abrams DM FRCS FCOphth
Consultant Ophthalmic Surgeon to the Royal Free Hospital
and the Hospital of St John and St Elizabeth, London

TENTH EDITION

CHURCHILL LIVINGSTONE
EDINBURGH LONDON MADRID MELBOURNE NEW YORK AND TOKYO 1993

CHURCHILL LIVINGSTONE
Medical Division of Longman Group UK Limited

Distributed in the United States of America by Churchill
Livingstone Inc., 650 Avenue of the Americas, New York,
N.Y. 10011, and by associated companies, branches and
representatives throughout the world.

© Longman Group UK Limited 1993

First edition 1928
Second edition 1935
Third edition 1938
Fourth edition 1943
Fifth edition 1949
Sixth edition 1954
Seventh edition 1963
Eighth edition 1969
Ninth edition 1978
Tenth edition 1993

ISBN 0-443-03856-2

British Library Cataloguing in Publication Data
A catalogue record for this book is available from the
British Library.

Library of Congress Cataloging in Publication Data
Abrams, David.
    Duke-Elder's practice of refraction. — 10th ed. /
revised by David Abrams.
      p. cm.
    Includes index.
    ISBN 0-443-03856-2
    1. Eye — Accommodation and refraction.
2. Eyeglasses. I. Duke-Elder, Stewart, Sir, 1898–1978.
Duke-Elder's practice of refraction. II. Title. III. Title:
Practice of refraction.
    [DNLM: 1. Refraction, Ocular.   WW 300 A161d]
RE925.D8   1993
617.7'55 — dc20
DNLM/DLC
for Library of Congress   92–49141

Printed in Great Britain by The Bath Press, Avon

Preface

The purpose of this book is to present in a manner suitable for the student and the practitioner the essential principles of the theory and practice of the correction of defects in the optical system of the eyes and their associated muscles. A simple and essentially non-mathematical form of presentation has been adopted wherein all that is necessary for the clinical routine of refraction is described and explained without burdening the reader with innumerable mathematical proofs. The book is thus clinical rather than theoretical, and its object is essentially practical; and, while theoretical matters are dealt with sufficiently to make their application to actual problems understandable and are explained in words rather than formulae, no attempt has been made to enter into the mathematical foundations of the subject.

Basic *Clinical Optics* is nicely dealt with in a short text by Elkington and Frank. Reference to a deeper mathematical approach may be obtained from the updating of Fincham's *Optics* by M. H Freeman. For a more extensive review of practical dispensing Bennett and Blumlein's *Ophthalmic Prescription Work* will be found helpful.

Whatever the type of book the would-be refractionist uses, it cannot be insisted upon too strongly that the art of refraction cannot in any sense be learned by reading. There is only one way of attaining efficiency therein, and that is by assiduous and painstaking practice in the clinic of a hospital, where large numbers of cases of all kinds are available, where the findings can be supervised and corroborated, and where long practice makes the interpretation of results instantaneous. If these pages serve as a guide in this they will have achieved their aim.

This edition, approaching 15 years since the last, surveys several new topics. Whilst some of these might at first glance appear to be remote from the daily practice of refraction they have been included with the prime purpose of putting the refractionist in the picture as regards some directions which clinical optics is taking, even though the requirement for him or her to put them into their own routine may seem remote. They should at least allow for sensible answers to be given to enquiring patients as, for example, about the prospects of corrective surgery for refractive errors.

Inevitably the most difficult task has been the updating of the section on contact lenses and perhaps the greatest problem has been to decide the extent of the contribution on this topic to a work of this nature. It is to be hoped that enough has been included to see the tyro on his way into contact lens practice, to acquaint those always outside actual contact lens work with problems which might present in general ophthalmic consultation, and at the same time to confine the subject to basics. Recherché details of specialised fitting techniques are beyond the scope of this section. For this reason the reader developing a particular interest in the subject should go to one of the larger texts. Contact lens literature is every bit as prolific as contact lens type but the following are recommended. The *CLAO Guide to Basic Science and Clinical Practice* is probably the 'bible' of the contact lens literature. *Contact Lenses* by Philip Stone will be found helpful, as will Ruben's *A Colour Atlas of Contact Lenses and Prosthetics*.

I am extremely indebted to a number of

colleagues and associates who have offered advice or made available material and illustrations, and particular thanks are due to Stephen Bailey and Kenneth Pullum for contact lens illustrations, to David Harrisberg for his critical review of the contact lens text, to Jeffrey Hillman for help with the 'IOL' calculations section, to John Parker and the Association of Contact Lens Manufacturers for permission to abstract from Mr Parker's work on the classification of contact lens material, to Mr Michael Pater of The British Standards Institution who has been of great help in relation to special types of spectacle and contact lenses, to Mr Dowie, Mr Paul Cooper and Mr Colin West of Keelers, and to Elizabeth Chambers and Clare Kirkpatrick of Clement Clarke International.

My thanks finally to my secretarial helpers, Jill Basten and Daphne Morgan, whose sanity has probably been saved by word processing.

London 1993   David Abrams

Contents

SECTION 1
Introduction

1. The clinical importance of the refraction 3

SECTION 2
Refraction and its application to the eye

2. The principles of refraction — general optics 11

3. The refraction of the eye — physiological optics 29

SECTION 3
Clinical anomalies

PART 1
Refractive errors

4. Hypermetropia 45

5. Myopia 53

6. Astigmatism 65

7. Aphakia and pseudophakia 71

8. Changes in refraction 79

PART 2
Accommodation and its disturbances

9. Accommodation 85

10. Presbyopia 91

11. Anomalies of accommodation 95

PART 3
Binocular vision and its anomalies

12. Binocular optical defects — anisometropia 105

13. Binocular optical defects — aniseikonia 109

14. Binocular muscular co-ordination — orthophoria 115

15. Binocular muscular anomalies — heterophoria 119

16. Binocular muscular anomalies — heterotropia 125

17. Binocular muscular co-ordination — convergence 131

18. Binocular muscular anomalies — anomalies of convergence and other reading difficulties 137

SECTION 4
Clinical investigation

19. The place of refraction in general ophthalmological examination 143

20. Visual acuity 145

21. Objective methods of refraction 155

22. Subjective verification of the refraction, and testing of muscle balance 181

23. The prescription of spectacles 195

SECTION 5
Optical appliances

24. The making and fitting of
spectacles   199

25. Contact lenses   233

26. Visual aids   273

Appendices   283

Index   295

Colour Plates

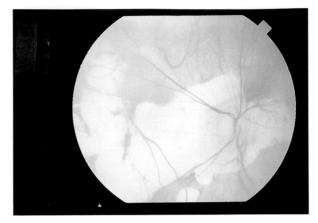

Plate 1 The fundus in myopia, showing widespread peripapillary and macular degeneration (see p. 56).

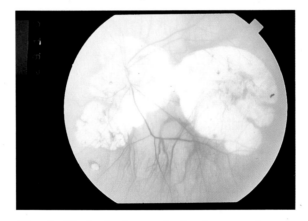

Plate 2 The fundus in myopia, showing a complete annular crescent and the remains of a Förster–Fuchs fleck at the macula (see p. 56).

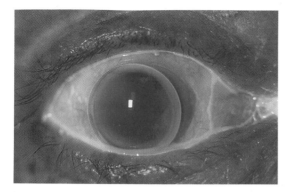

Plate 3 Minimal apex clearance (see p. 245).

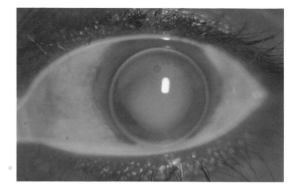

Plate 4 Steep fitting lens (see p. 245).

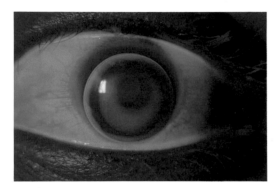

Plate 5 Flat fitting lens (see p. 245).

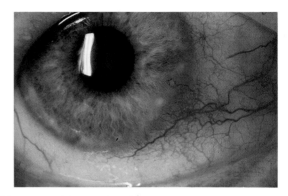

Plate 6 3 o'clock and 9 o'clock pathology (see p. 249).

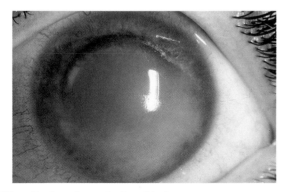

Plate 7 Acanthamoeba keratitis (see p. 256).

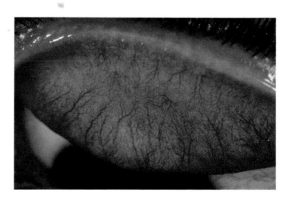

Plate 9 Normal upper tarsal plate (see p. 257).

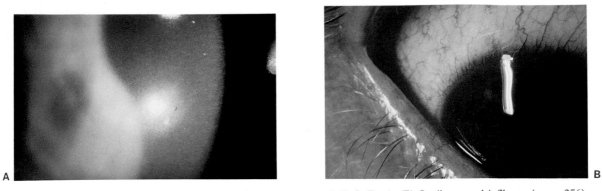

Plate 8 (A) Staphylococcal corneal infiltration in a soft lens wearer (J. K. S. Dart). (B) Sterile corneal infiltrate (see p. 256).

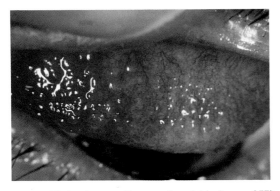

Plate 10 Early giant papillary conjunctivitis (see p. 257).

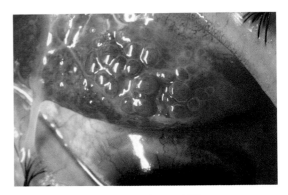

Plate 11 An advanced case (see p. 257).

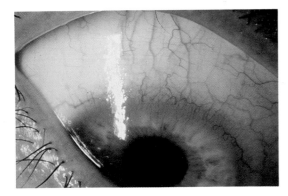

Plate 12 Early Thiomersal toxicity (see p. 257).

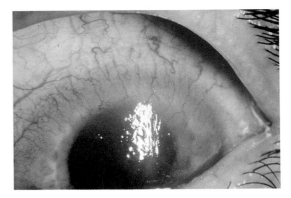

Plate 13 Established Thiomersal keratopathy (see p. 257).

Introduction

1. The clinical importance of the refraction

The methods of evaluating the optical state of the eye, *the refraction*, and the means employed to correct it when abnormal, play an important part in the management of many ophthalmic conditions. As an introduction to the description of these techniques, it is therefore pertinent to review the clinical circumstances in which it is important to estimate the refraction.

VISUAL FAILURE

Anomalies of the optical state of the eye, *refractive errors*, are by far the commonest cause of defective vision; they must be looked for in any patient complaining of inability to see clearly. The various types of refractive error and the distinctive ways in which they affect the vision will be considered in subsequent chapters.

While the short-sighted child unable to see the blackboard clearly at school or the presbyope finding it difficult to read a telephone directory in poor light may make direct complaint of their disability, refractive errors may be discovered in other ways. Thus, reviews of vision at schools and places of work or parental observation of visual inadequacy may also prompt an examination of the optical state of the eyes.

Apart from an initial examination, defective vision may occur in subjects known to have refractive errors who may already be using an optical correction, whether spectacles or contact lenses. Again, such a defect may be noticed by the patient or simply be brought to light during routine re-examination of the eyes. Myopia increasing in degree during adolescence and undercorrected hypermetropia of middle age are examples of this.

Indeed, not only may a spectacle correction be inadequate, it may be wrong, giving rise to poor vision on its own account. Thus, in all who wear spectacles, the complaint of blurred vision is an indication for a re-examination of the refraction. The same considerations apply to the wearers of contact lenses; here, however, the additional possibility of some corneal upset must be borne in mind as a possible cause of visual disturbance.

It is also important to remember that the refraction of the patient may be of great significance when visual failure is *not* due primarily to a refractive error. No assessment of visual capacity is possible without an estimation of the visual acuity in optimal optical conditions.

The interaction between optical anomalies and ocular disease has both diagnostic and therapeutic implications. Thus the ophthalmoscopic view may give rise to doubt as to the health of the macula; such a situation may be regarded less seriously if the examination of the refraction shows the corrected vision to be normal. Again, the decision to advise surgery in a case of cataract will always be influenced by the acuity obtained with the best optical correction. Finally, we may note the importance of the examination of the refraction after ophthalmic surgery.

DISTURBANCES OF THE MUSCLE BALANCE

The co-ordination of the ocular movements and the ocular refraction are inter-related. This relationship derives from a flexible but far from haphazard association between accommodation — the alteration in focus from far to near, and convergence — the movement in which each eye turns nasally to look at some close object. We will examine the implications of this situation in later chapters. Suffice it to point out here that this association between accommodation and convergence may be put in jeopardy if the optical state of the eyes requires an abnormal degree of accommodation in order to obtain clear vision. For this reason hypermetropic refraction is often accompanied by a tendency to an excess of convergence; indeed, hypermetropia is frequently found in children with concomitant convergent strabismus.

It is clear that in any ophthalmic problem which involves the muscle balance, an examination of the refraction is mandatory and may indicate both the pathogenesis of the condition and its proper treatment.

EYE-STRAIN, HEADACHE AND PSYCHOLOGICAL FACTORS

In the grosser degrees of refractive error, visual failure is the cardinal presenting symptom. In lesser degrees, however, visual failure may be only one of a number of complaints a patient may make. Indeed, the symptom of inability to see clearly may be a negligible part of the symptomatology. Other symptoms arise as a result of the effort made to overcome or compensate for the visual defect. Conditions of sustained excessive accommodation, as may be found in some hypermetropes, or attempts to stimulate accommodation when it is becoming a physiological impossibility in presbyopes, are circumstances typically productive of non-visual symptoms with or without visual complaints. Similarly, anomalies of the binocular state may also give rise to symptoms which are not primarily visual. Examples of this are disturbance of the accommodation–convergence association and disparities between the refractive states of the two eyes.

The notion of effort and the fact that the pathological basis of the symptoms may depend on the ocular musculature, internal and external, has led to the mechanical concept of strain, hence *eye-strain*.

The symptoms which this term embraces are diverse, and as some are neither visual nor ocular the condition may go unsuspected. The difficulty which this presents is aggravated by the fact that the symptoms do not by any means appear in proportion to the gravity of the causal defect. They vary from individual to individual to the most surprising degree without any apparent cause, this one showing no sign of trouble, and that one, with apparently equal cause and seemingly equally constituted, complaining bitterly; but as a general rule two types of case are strikingly common. The first of these are subjects of a neurotic disposition or even normal people during a period of prolonged mental worry and anxiety. To many of these, spectacles are a help since they remove one cause of irritation from a personality under stress. The second group comprises the debilitated and those convalescing from an acute illness, women after a confinement and during lactation or children taking exams; fatigue which in normal circumstances would be barely appreciated readily manifests itself, and an optical error which would give rise to no symptoms of discomfort were they in robust health may become acutely felt, and may necessitate the use of spectacles which may frequently be discarded at a later date in happier circumstances. Indeed, in some such cases the ciliary muscle may not be able to perform a normal amount of work without showing signs of distress, and symptoms of eye-strain may make themselves evident in the absence of any appreciable error in the optical system.

The symptoms themselves are conveniently considered in the following groups:

1. Visual symptoms

The characteristic feature of these is their intermittent nature. It may thus be taken that in the case of small refractive errors the actual visual acuity forms little or no reliable guide to the ocular condition, for the defect may be compensated more or less completely by the patient at the time it is assessed and indeed at many other times. In fact, it is sometimes true that the symptoms are most marked in those cases wherein for this reason the vision remains good. One person will live placidly and comfortably with a small degree of astigmatism and considerably reduced vision, while another more highly organised, suffering the same disability, will attain normal or supernormal sight — and pay for it. There frequently comes a time, however, either in periods of unusual strain or during a temporary deterioration of the general health or vitality, when fatigue comes on and the visual acuity fails. This is especially seen in those who use the eyes much for reading or the study of small objects over long periods of time, while fine sewing, the cinema, motor driving in the distractions of confusing traffic, or any relaxation or employment which calls for a high degree of visual acuity combined with attention or anxiety, is frequently the cause of such a breakdown. A sense of confusion and a temporary blurring of vision are experienced, the letters when reading, for example, appearing to run together. Here the ciliary muscle gives up any attempt to focus and the image becomes indistinct, or the ocular muscles slip back into their condition of rest and diplopia results. This may be momentary and pass off, to recur again at more frequent intervals, the eyes gradually becoming tired and the lids heavy, while a sensation of weariness or drowsiness makes itself progressively felt and renders continued attention difficult or impossible. A relaxation of attention brings relief, but a resumption of the matter at hand induces a repetition of the trouble, until ultimately the individual is tempted to give up from annoyance or exhaustion.

2. Ocular symptoms

The symptoms which affect the eye itself are sometimes spoken of collectively as *asthenopia*.

The ocular symptoms associated with eye-strain are directly due to the increased muscular work which the defect invokes and the discomfort of the resultant muscular fatigue, to which may be added the effects of a condition of vascular engorgement determined by this state of sustained and forced activity. Subjectively, especially after long periods of close application to work, the eyes feel tired, hot and uncomfortable; temporary relief is obtained by resting or by rubbing them, but if the work is continued the vague discomfort gives place to a feeling of actual strain, and this may develop into pain. Pain in the eyes unconnected with inflammation is generally due to eye-strain and rarely to any deep-seated disease. It is usually mild and aching, but may on occasion be severe and acute; it may be situated in the eyes themselves or be located more deeply in the orbits, or spreading therefrom become referred as a general headache.

Objectively, the eyes frequently have a typical appearance. The continued state of irritability and congestion brings about an unhealthy condition of the lids and conjunctivae with a characteristic look, watery, suffused and bleary. This is especially notable in children, in whom an intractable blepharitis or conjunctivitis should always suggest an examination of the refraction. Such low-grade infections are probably accentuated and prolonged by the child constantly rubbing his eyes with his fingers; the eyes feel strained and sore, and a child's hands are rarely clean.

Eye-strain has at one time or another been credited with a share in the aetiology of almost every ophthalmic disease. Frequent mention is made of it in association with iritis and iridocyclitis, with glaucoma, and even with cataract. The factors determining the incidence of these diseases are usually complex and often not a little obscure; but to ascribe to eye-strain an important or determining share in the aetiology of any of them seems to be laying undue stress on what should more reasonably be regarded as coincidence.

3. Referred symptoms

The commonest symptom associated with eye-strain is *headache*. This occurs in a multitude of varieties. It is most commonly localised around the region of the eyes; it may be frontal or temporal but it may occasionally be vertical or occipital.

Eye-strain is traditionally thought to embrace every imaginable type of headache, of whatever distribution. Its nature is said to be dull, aching, boring, superficial, deep-seated or migrainous; its time of occurrence as constant, intermittent, related or unrelated to the use of the eyes. Aggravating factors such as fatigue or poor illumination are said to be common.

It is only reasonable to conclude that the headache of eye-strain is difficult to diagnose with certainty; the rational course to adopt is to examine the eyes as a matter of routine in all cases wherein such an origin might be suspected. No case of obscure headache should be treated on general medical lines without first eliminating the possibility of eye-strain as being at least one of the factors in its aetiology.

The mechanism of the headache is not fully understood, but presumably it rests upon the same basis as other referred pain of visceral origin. It is now generally accepted that visceral pain is referred to the area which shares a common segmental origin with the viscus concerned, and in the same way as overstrain of the cardiac muscle produces angina which spreads over the shoulder, down the arm and up the neck, so ciliary pain is referred to the areas associated with the cervical segments which connect with the superior cervical ganglion, the somatic outflow from which is represented by the bulbo-spinal root of the trigeminal and the upper cervical nerves. It will be remembered that the early metameric arrangement of the fifth nerve is maintained whereby the ophthalmic division is represented most caudally, so that ciliary pain is primarily frontal and occipital in distribution.

The other general symptoms of eye-strain are of more uncertain status. Digestive upsets such as dyspepsia and nausea, vague 'nervous' disorders such as dizziness, insomnia and depression, and many other symptoms have all in the past been variously attributed to eye-strain. The aggravation of neurological or mental disorders and the causation of general debility have been explained on this or a similar basis.

While there is little doubt that these attributions are to be considered exaggerated, eye-strain does probably have some effect on the general health and mental well-being of those who, from instability of temperament or from overwork, are living too freely upon the margin of their reserves. It is not only in the neurotically inclined that it makes its influence felt, but also in those highly organised individuals who enrich more particularly the intellectual spheres of life and find happiness only when they are lavishly spending themselves. In these the wasteful expenditure of energy in the continuous attempt at correction may act as the final straw in bringing about a condition of nervous exhaustion. Even in those not so highly strung, eye-strain may have a similar result in circumstances of mental or physical stress.

Nevertheless it is probably true to say that ophthalmologists and others have in the past attributed to eye-strain more evils than can reasonably be laid to its account. We have seen that neurotic temperament is frequently associated with the condition, and we have noted that anomalies in the optical mechanism may well be the means of the aggravation and prolongation of such psychopathological states. But it happens, perhaps more commonly in women, that functional troubles which are without any reasonable organic basis are often referred persistently to the eyes. Such patients will insist that they cannot use their eyes for any length of time, or that when they attempt to do so they cannot see at all. Frequently they see spots floating about in front of them. Sensitivity to light is especially marked, and they are quite unable to bear illumination of any unusual intensity; even in diffuse daylight they prefer to go about in dark glasses. Headache is the most frequent symptom, and its neurotic origin can frequently be recognised from the sensations they describe. A patient with a true organic headache rarely hesitates to describe his sensations as those of pain, pure and simple; they, on the other hand, with no evidence of emotion, will describe a sense of pressure, of emptiness, of the head opening or shutting, or of its being bored through by a nail, or being constricted by a band. These, and many more: but whatever it is, the impression is given that it is horribly unpleasant. There may be an optical anomaly, or there may not; but in either case, producing a host of spectacles obtained from as many surgeons and opticians — each of which they have worn punctiliously — they will declare in a firm and quiet voice that none of them is of any use. Usually some muscular imbalance is present, and reading presents the greatest difficulty, intense discomfort coming on so that near work has to be discontinued after a few minutes' application. The real trouble is a pathological attitude of mind, none the less real, it is to be noted, because it is so, and treatment should be directed thereto with all sympathetic consideration and forbearance.

Indeed, as a final comment on the place of eye-strain in the symptomatology of refractive errors, we should remind ourselves that the abolition of symptoms by therapy directed at any supposed cause is *not* proof of causation. Many headaches and other vague ocular complaints may be relieved in whole or in part by the wearing of a weak spectacle correction. But here the treatment could well be exerting the well-recognised placebo effect, and the cause of the symptoms may lie quite elsewhere than in the ocular or refractive state. An important part of the clinician's role will therefore always be the decision as to the relevance of optical treatment. Admittedly it may act as a beneficial prop to the mentally ill, deferring or preventing a serious breakdown. But its effect in organic disease arising elsewhere in the body could be to delay appropriate investigation and treatment.

The taking of the correct decision clearly involves the consideration by the clinician of the whole patient, his general and mental health, his life-style as well as his optical and ocular states. It is evident that the art of refraction is acquired only with long experience, and what this implies in the developing climate of electronic instrumentation is that it will continue to be inadequate to prescribe a correction solely on the basis of a computer printout. The art will lie in judging its appropriateness.

THE NATURE OF THE VISUAL TASK AND EYE-STRAIN

Some degree of close work is called for in a high proportion of occupational and leisure activities. Failure properly to attend to clarity of vision at all working distances has always been an important cause of eye-strain. Even before the explosion of information technology it was necessary to take into account, for example, the varying near requirements of the typist, the many intermediate distances of documents being read at a large desk, of pictures in an art gallery or books on library shelves.

These tasks call for a constantly altering accommodative requirement as well as the necessity to maintain binocular co-ordination in many, some perhaps unusual, directions of gaze.

One modern visual task which encompasses many of these possible visual difficulties and perhaps new ones as well is the now widespread use of the visual display unit (VDU). Since their introduction within the last 25 years, a host of optical and ophthalmological complaints have been attributed particularly to their use. In fact one has seen almost a repetition of the most bizarre symptoms supposedly part of the eye-strain complex (see above) being attributed to them. It appears that at least some of these generalised 'somatic' complaints are not visually related at all but arise from truly non-ocular ergonomic factors such as posture at work, working heights of desk and seating, position of material to be copied, siting of satisfactory illumination, etc. Added to these are other considerations of working conditions such as temperature and humidity, perhaps more relevant to complaints of dry eyes.

There are reports which suggest that VDU employment may bring out eye-strain symptoms related to minor refractive errors, accommodative inadequacy, perhaps aggravated by a monochromatic screen, and latent anomalies of binocular co-ordination. It is certainly claimed that in some cases these symptoms may be relieved by appropriate attention to these faults. In organisations where the use of VDUs is widespread, modern practice may include the routine assessment of such factors before VDU work commences and at intervals during employment. Agreement is likely to be required between employers and workforce with regard to specific features of the VDUs such as acceptable degrees of screen glare and luminosity, character size and clarity and keyboard pressure, as well as on the optimal periods of VDU work before a rest is advisable.

Hard evidence of permanent deleterious effects from VDU work is still lacking. Temporary anomalies of colour vision have been reported in VDU workers; achromatic patterns may seem faintly coloured some hours after the VDU has been used (the McCollough effect). How or whether this has any relationship to other visual effects of the VDU is uncertain. The possibility that subjects prone to epilepsy or migraine are at risk of having attacks precipitated, although not well established, calls for some caution when considering that they should use VDUs.

Considerable publicity has been given to the possibility that the use of VDUs by pregnant women leads to an increased number of birth defects; this again is not proven. Controversy also continues as to whether general more minor effects such as headache, colds, sore throats, aches and pains are more prevalent in VDU operators; it is now accepted that the occurrence of facial dermatitis previously attributed to VDUs is perhaps more likely to be related to static electricity in office carpets and in circumstances of low humidity.

Refraction and its application to the eye

2. The principles of refraction — general optics

THE NATURE OF REFRACTION

It may be said, in general terms, that light travels through space in straight lines. It is true that recent advances in physical science have shown that this is not strictly accurate; but, for the purposes of the optical problems which we propose to consider, it may be taken to be the case. If, however, a ray of light meets a body in its passage through space, one of three things may happen to it. Some substances, for example black bodies, *absorb* the light which falls on them; these are called opaque. Others, such as mirror surfaces, *reflect* the light backwards; while others, such as glass, which are described as transparent, *transmit* the light, or at any rate a considerable proportion of it, allowing it to pass through them. Many substances combine these effects to some degree.

In space, light maintains a constant speed of about 186 000 miles per second, but as it travels through the substance of such a transparent body it is obvious that it will encounter more resistance than previously, and, as we would expect, this retards its progress.

In such a case, if a beam of light enters a transparent body perpendicularly to its surface, its progress will be retarded. The condition of affairs may be gathered from Figure 2.1. But, on the other hand, if the beam strikes the body obliquely, one edge of the advancing beam will enter the body before the other, and consequently will be retarded earlier. The condition of affairs in this case will best be understood from Figure 2.2. At the position AB the entering beam is beginning to meet with the resistance offered by the transparent body at A, and for the next part

of its course the part of the beam which is within the body will necessarily travel more slowly than that which, being outside, is still unimpeded. The distances travelled in the same interval of time

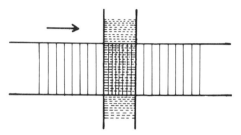

Fig. 2.1 Passage of light through a glass plate. When a beam of light strikes a glass plate with parallel sides normally, it is retarded while traversing the plate, and then travels on unaffected.

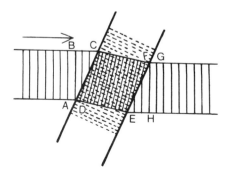

Fig. 2.2 Refraction of light through a glass plate. When a beam of light strikes a glass plate obliquely, the portion which enters first at A meets with resistance. The beam is therefore bent during its course AD, BC. After the position DC is reached it travels as a parallel beam through the substance of the plate. At EF an opposite process takes place, involving an equal amount of refraction, with the result that at GH the beam travels on in the same direction as before, but displaced from its original path.

are therefore unequal, AD being less than BC, and consequently the front of the beam is swung round and its direction is changed. This phenomenon of the bending of light as it passes from one transparent medium to another of different density is known as *refraction*.

The amount by which the beam of light is bent depends on three factors. In the first place, since the bending is dependent upon the retardation of the light, the more resistance the body offers, the more slowly will the light be made to travel and consequently the more acutely will the rays of light be bent. This property of offering resistance to light is known as *optical density*, and it varies within wide limits between different substances. For practical purposes the universal medium through which light travels is the air, and so the optical densities of different substances are usually compared with that of air taken as a standard. The refractive power of a substance in comparison with that of air is spoken of as its *refractive index*: thus the refractive index of air is 1, that of water 1.33, that of crown glass is 1.5, and so on (see Table 1 — Appendix I).

The refractive index is worked out from the relationship of the angle of incidence to the angle of refraction (*i* and *r* respectively in Fig. 2.3). We know that sin *i*/sin *r* is constant for all angles of incidence (Snell's law), and this constant factor is the refractive index when the first medium is air.

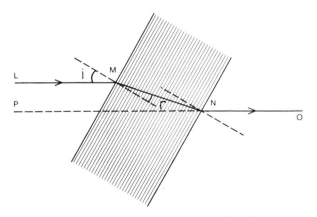

Fig. 2.3 Refraction of a ray of light by a glass plate. The ray of light LMNO is refracted at M as it passes from air to glass, and N as it passes from glass to air. When an eye is situated at O, the source of light, L, appears to come from P. For *i* and *r* see text.

Because of this relationship, it follows that a second important factor affecting the amount of bending is the angle at which the rays strike the surface between the two media; the more oblique this is, the greater will be the bending.

The third factor influencing the degree of bending is the wavelength of the light, blue light for example is more bent in the conditions of Figure 2.2 than red. The differences, however, are small and we can simply speak of 'light' being the composite white light of common experience. We shall see, later, that we cannot completely ignore this factor.

By making use of refraction light can be manipulated to a considerable extent, and instead of travelling, as it ordinarily does, in defined straight lines, its directions can be made to alter into well-defined paths. It is the essential function of all optical systems to turn the course of rays of light from their original indiscriminate directions into definitely determined paths, and we will proceed to study the methods used for this purpose by the refractive system of the eye.

REFRACTION BY A PLATE WITH PARALLEL SIDES

When parallel rays of light fall perpendicularly upon a glass plate, the front of the beam will be equally retarded throughout its extent; no deviation therefore occurs, and consequently when it leaves the plate on the other side the beam proceeds unaffected (Fig. 2.1).

But when parallel rays fall obliquely upon a glass plate, we have seen that their direction is changed on account of the retardation of one edge of the beam (A, Fig. 2.2) before the other (B). When the entire width of the beam has entered the substance of the glass at CD, all rays will be equally retarded throughout, and consequently, travelling at a uniform though lessened speed, they will once more proceed as a parallel beam, running, however, in a different direction through the thickness of the plate until the other surface is reached. Here exactly the opposite process takes place. At the position EF the edge of the beam at E, on entering the air, at once regains its original velocity, while at F the resistance of the glass is still felt. This inequality of speed obtains until the position GH is reached, when the entire beam once more travels on as before. Since the processes at either side are exactly the reciprocals of each other, the beam is bent to an equal and opposite degree, and therefore, although its path has been changed, the emergent light is parallel to the incident light.

If we consider the course of a single ray (Fig. 2.3), and draw perpendiculars at the two points M and N where it cuts the surfaces of the plate, it becomes evident that when light passes obliquely from a medium of less density to one of greater density it will be refracted towards the perpendicular; if it passes from one of greater to one of less density it will be refracted away from the perpendicular, the amount of refraction depending on the difference between the densities of the two media. Since the degree of refraction in passing between the same two media is always the same, the emergent ray, although it is displaced, runs parallel with the incident ray. Now the phenomena of refraction enter but little into our everyday experience, and so we tend to ignore the optical effects to which they give rise, and are accustomed to project objects visually along the direction of the rays of light as they enter the eye. Consequently, if L be a luminous object and O the observer's eye, the object will appear to be situated at P.

REFRACTION BY PRISMS

We have seen that when light passes through a medium with parallel sides the incident rays and the emergent rays are parallel; but if the sides of the medium are not parallel the direction of the rays must also change. Thus in Figure 2.4 the incident beam of light is retarded at A so that AD is shorter than BC; it is therefore bent round and runs through the substance of the glass until it reaches the position EF. Here the upper part of the beam (FG) accelerates on entering the air, while the lower part (EH) is still retarded; consequently the beam is bent round further in the same sense and is deviated out of its original path altogether.

Such a medium is typified in the *prism* (Fig. 2.5). It is made up of two sides, AB and

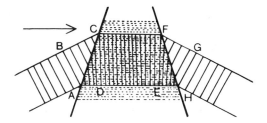

Fig. 2.4 Refraction by a glass plate with non-parallel sides. The two sides AC and HF are not parallel. The beam is therefore bent from the position AB to DC on entering the plate, and from the direction EF to HG on leaving the plate. Its original direction is thus completely changed.

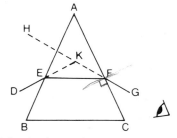

Fig. 2.5 Refraction by a prism.
ABC is a prism with the apex at A, the base BC, and the sides AB and AC. The angle of the prism is BAC. A ray of light DEFG is refracted at E and F as in Figure 2.4. The total amount of refraction, that is the difference in direction between DE and FG, is represented by the angle DKH (the angle of deviation). If the eye is at G, the source of light, D, will appear to be at H. The angles made by the incident ray (DE) and the emergent ray (FG) with the normals to the surfaces at E and F are called the angles of incidence and emergence; and when these are equal the deviation produced by the prism is minimal. A ray suffering *minimal deviation* in this way is said to traverse the prism *symmetrically*.

AC, meeting at an apex, A, joined by a base, BC. The angle between the two sides at A, which denotes the angle at which the two refracting surfaces are inclined, is called the *angle of refraction*. Since a ray of light is bent towards the perpendicular on entering a dense medium (glass) from a rare one (air), the incident ray will be bent towards the base as it enters the prism, as is seen in the figure, and, since refraction away from the perpendicular occurs on re-entering the rarer medium, the emergent ray will be further bent towards the base as it leaves the prism. The path of the ray is thus seen as DEFG, where it

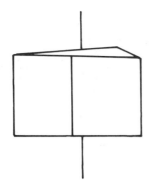

Fig. 2.6 The deviation produced by a prism. An object viewed through a prism is always deviated towards the apex of the prism.

is evident that the entire deviation is towards the base. The total amount of the deviation between the incident ray (DE) and the emergent ray (FG) is called the *angle of deviation*, and is represented by the angle DKH. If an observer is at G and a luminous body is placed at D, it will appear to be in the position H; thus while the light is deviated towards the base, the image is displaced towards the apex of the prism (Fig. 2.6).

The detection and measurement of prisms

By utilising this phenomenon we are able to detect the presence of a prism in an optical system. We hold the glass up between the eye and any object which forms a straight line, and if the continuity of the straight line is broken, as is seen in Figure 2.6, we know that a prism is present; and since the line appears to be deviated towards the apex, we know in which direction the apex of the prism lies. The amount of displacement which is produced is an index of the strength of the prism, and this can be measured by neutralising the unknown prism with which we are dealing by placing in contact with it other prisms of known strengths facing the opposite direction.

This principle is seen in the effects produced by *rotating prisms*. If two equal prisms are placed base to apex, a plate with parallel sides is formed with no prismatic action; if now these be rotated upon each other in reverse directions they produce the effect of a single prism of gradually increasing

strength, until eventually, when they are apex to apex, a maximum effect is obtained equal to the sum of the single prisms.

The nomenclature of prisms

From our consideration of the principles of refraction it follows that the amount of deviation produced by any prism depends on the refractive index of the substance of which the prism is made, the manner in which the light strikes the prism, and the size of the refracting angle. In ophthalmological practice, prisms are usually made of crown glass, and we assume that the rays fall upon the prism symmetrically (see Fig. 2.5); consequently the amount of deviation usually depends on the size of the refracting angle. In these circumstances the deviation produced is minimal, and where the angle is as small as it is possible to use for clinical purposes (i.e. less than 10 degrees) it is found that this deviation is equal to half the refracting angle of the prism.

It is unfortunate that the nomenclature of prisms is not uniformly standardised, for four different methods of standardisation have been suggested and were employed at various times. The terminology now most frequently used is based on the *prism dioptre* (Δ). A prism of 1 Δ gives an apparent displacement of 1 cm to an object situated 1 metre away (Fig. 2.7).

REFRACTION AT A CURVED SURFACE

When parallel rays of light strike a spherical surface, each individual ray will be bent to a different degree and the rays may then all meet at a focus. The distance of this focus from the surface depends on the curvature of the latter and the optical density of the two media concerned, and again on the wavelength of the light. (See Fig. 2.32 p. 23.)

Refraction by lenses

When *two* smooth curved surfaces are aligned and enclose a uniform optical medium, we have a lens. The first surface of such a system tends to

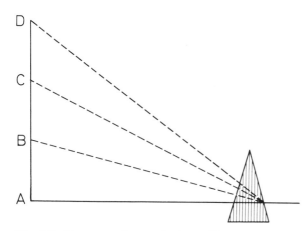

Fig. 2.7 The nomenclature of prisms. The prism dioptre. A straight line passing through a prism appears to be deviated towards the apex. If the distance from the prism to A is 1 metre, the amount of deviation may be measured in prism dioptres along the line ABCD. When the distances AB, BC, etc., are each 1 cm, the dotted lines represent prism dioptres. It is to be noted that the figure indicates not the actual deviation of the light but the apparent deviation, which is considerably exaggerated.

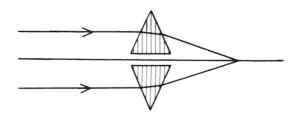

Fig. 2.8 Refraction to a focus by two prisms. Two prisms placed base to base can bring two rays of light, originally parallel, to a focus.

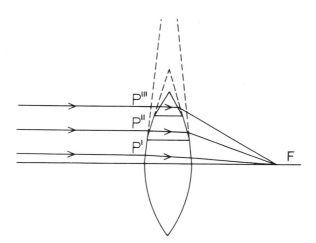

Fig. 2.9 Refraction of light to a focus by a system of prisms. A system of prisms arranged base to base, as shown in the figure, refracts light to a focus at F. Such a system constitutes a convex lens. P′, P″, P‴ may be taken as the prism elements in the lens.

focus parallel incident rays and then again at the second surface a further focusing occurs.

Another simple way of considering the focusing effect of lenses is to think of a lens as a series of prisms.

Since light after passing through a prism travels on in a parallel beam, it is never brought to a focus and no image is formed, but since it can be deviated by a controlled amount we have ready to hand the essential factor necessary to bring this about. Suppose, for example, that two prisms are placed base to base (Fig. 2.8); it is evident that two rays which were originally parallel can be brought to a focus. If this effect is multiplied several times (Fig. 2.9), several such rays are similarly focused; and if we continue the process indefinitely, and combine an infinite number of prisms in a similar arrangement, the sides of the individual prisms become infinitely small, until eventually they merge into one another and form one uniform curve. At this ultimate stage all parallel rays of light will be focused at a point; here the formation of an image occurs, and the arrangement of prism elements becomes a *lens*, in this case a *convex lens* which converges the incident light to a point. A

diverging effect is produced (Fig. 2.10) by a *concave lens* (Fig. 2.11). Although the incident light is not converged to a point in this way, it will be seen later that such a diverging action is a necessity in many optical systems. Lenses are of many varieties, and the ones most commonly used in ophthalmic practice are spherical and cylindrical with either convex or concave surfaces or combinations of these. They are illustrated in Figure 2.12.

Refraction by spherical lenses

The theory of lenses is simple, if we neglect their thickness, this we can do in most cases for ophthalmological purposes. A spherical lens has one or both of its surfaces curved in the form of

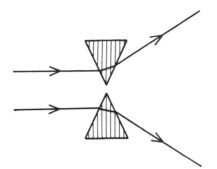

Fig. 2.10 The refraction of light by two prisms. Two prisms placed apex to apex refract light in a diverging manner.

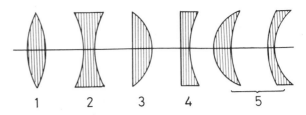

Fig. 2.12 Types of spherical lenses.
1. Biconvex lens, with both sides convex.
2. Biconcave lens, with both sides concave.
3. Plano-convex lens, with one side plane, the other convex.
4. Plano-concave lens, with one side plane, the other concave.
5. Meniscus lenses:
    Convex meniscus; meniscus-shaped with the greater curvature convex.
    Concave meniscus; meniscus-shaped with the greater curvature concave.

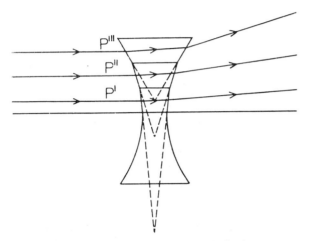

Fig. 2.11 Refraction of light by a system of prisms. A system of prisms arranged apex to apex, as shown in the figure, refracts light in a diverging manner. Such a system constitutes a concave lens. P′, P″, P‴ may be taken as the prism elements in the lens.

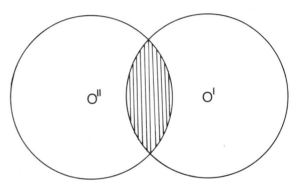

Fig. 2.13 The formation of convex lenses. A biconvex lens may be considered as formed by the intersection of two spheres whose centres are O″ and O′.

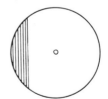

Fig. 2.14 The formation of convex lenses. A plano-convex lens is formed by the intersection of a sphere by a plane surface.

a sphere. The formation of a biconvex lens may be understood from Figure 2.13, of a plano-convex lens from Figure 2.14, of a biconcave lens from Figure 2.15, and of a plano-concave lens from Figure 2.16. The centre of the sphere, of which the surface forms a part, is called the *centre of curvature* (O), and the radius of the sphere is called the *radius of curvature*.

In discussing the theory of lenses we shall take the liberty of assuming certain theoretical postulates. Thus in the following pages we shall imagine that rays of light emanating from a point can be reassembled at another point, whereas, as

will be pointed out later, this assumption cannot be reconciled with the actual facts. We shall see that aberrations or errors occur in natural conditions which render such a purely mathematical concept impossible. Further, for

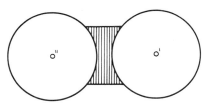

Fig. 2.15 The formation of concave lenses.
A biconcave lens may be considered to be formed by the
approximation of two spheres whose centres are O″ and O′.

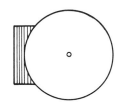

Fig. 2.16 The formation of concave lenses.
A plano-concave lens, is formed by the approximation of a
sphere and a plane surface.

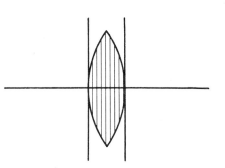

Fig. 2.17 The principal axis.
The central part of the lens through which the principal
axis travels may be considered to be a plate with parallel
sides. The ray of light traversing this is therefore not
deviated (cf. Fig. 2.1).

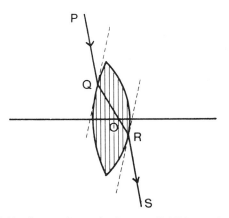

Fig. 2.18 A secondary axis. Any ray (PQRS) passing
through the optical centre (O) may be considered as
traversing a plate with parallel sides. PQ is thus parallel to
RS. QR is a secondary axis (cf. Fig. 2.2).

the moment we shall assume that the lenses with
which we are dealing are infinitely thin; but such
a lens, of course, is never realised in practice.
Although we are in this way inventing a system
of mathematical imagery, the liberties which we
are taking are largely extenuated by the fact that,
in the first place, a point image would be useless
for physiological purposes, while, in the second,
the lenses which are used in ophthalmological
practice are all relatively thin and of low power.
When thick lenses of high power are used, the
errors and aberrations introduced make their
applicability extremely limited. This matter will
be dealt with at a later stage.

In the case of a *convex lens*, we have seen that
parallel rays falling upon it are rendered
convergent. There is one small element in the
centre which may be considered to have parallel
sides (Fig. 2.17); it thus acts as a parallel plate,
and the central ray which passes through it is
therefore not refracted and emerges undeviated.
The line of this ray is called the *principal axis* of
the lens. If the beam strikes the lens not
transversely, but obliquely, there is again one
central ray which again emerges undeviated
(Fig. 2.18). PQRS represents such a ray, since
from the figure it will be seen that parallel

tangents can be drawn at the points where it
meets the two surfaces, Q and R, showing that
this element of the lens can be considered to act
as a plate with parallel sides. Although it is
slightly refracted, as in traversing a plate
obliquely, this ray therefore leaves the lens
parallel to its original direction; and, if the lens
is thin, this slight refraction may be neglected,
and it may be considered to proceed in a
direction continuous with that of the incident ray.
Such a ray is spoken of as occupying a *secondary
axis*, and the point O which forms the centre of
the optical system of the lens, where all the
secondary axes meet the principal axis, is called

the *optical centre*; all rays which pass through it may thus be considered to be undeviated.

It is to be noted that the optical centre does not always correspond to the geometrical centre of the lens; it need not, indeed, be inside the lens at all. It is so in a biconvex or biconcave lens; it is situated on the convex or concave side of a plano-convex or plano-concave lens; and in a meniscus it lies outside of the lens altogether.

Apart from the rays forming these axes, all the rays of light incident upon the lens are deviated, and consequently they must meet (theoretically) somewhere. Rays from a luminous point are thus brought to a *focus*, and a collection of foci corresponding to all the luminous points of an extended object comprises an *image*. It is of great importance to be able to determine the position and nature of the images formed by lenses in various conditions.

Images formed by convex lenses

If the incident rays are parallel, that is if they come from an infinite distance, they will be converged upon a single point on the other side of the lens; at this point the image will be formed (F, Fig. 2.19). This point is known as the *principal focus*, and its distance from the lens is called the *focal distance* or *focal length*.

Rays coming from a point nearer than infinity (A, Fig. 2.20) are divergent when they reach the lens, and these will therefore be brought to a focus at a point (B) beyond the principal focus. It is evident that if the direction of the light be reversed, it will traverse the same path. The points A and B can therefore act reciprocally as object and image, and they are consequently

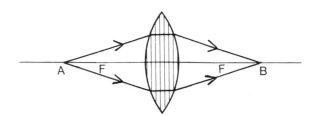

Fig. 2.20 The source of light (A) is between infinity and F; the focus is at a point, B, a corresponding distance on the other side of the lens. A and B are conjugate foci.

called *conjugate foci*. This will hold good until the source of light reaches the principal focus itself, when the converse condition shown in Figure 2.19 will be established. Here it is evident that rays issuing from the principal focus will emerge from the lens as parallel rays on the opposite side, and the image will be formed (theoretically) at infinity. If the luminous source is brought nearer to the lens, the rays will still be divergent when they issue from the opposite side, and consequently they will only meet 'beyond infinity'. In this case no real image is therefore formed, but a *virtual image* appears behind the luminous point on the same side of the lens (Fig. 2.21). Such an image cannot be cast upon a screen, but it can be seen by an observer on the opposite side of the lens.

The size and position of an image can be reconstructed pictorially in all these cases. To locate the position of the image of any point in an object it is sufficient to know the direction of any two rays, for where these two cross there the image must be. We know that rays passing through the optical centre are not deviated, and that parallel rays pass through the principal focus. By drawing lines representing these rays the two typical figures represented in Figures 2.22 and 2.23 are obtained. From then it is apparent that when the object is beyond the focal distance the image is inverted; when it is nearer than the focal distance it is erect and magnified.

In practice, an object which is a considerable distance away, say 6 metres or more, may be considered to be at infinity, and the rays of light issuing from it may be taken as parallel. In this case a real image is formed by the lens at the principal focus: it is very small and inverted. If the object is gradually brought nearer to the lens,

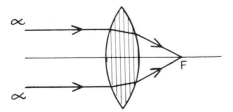

Figs 2.19, 2.20 and 2.21 The focus of a convex lens. **Fig. 2.19** The incident rays are parallel, coming from infinity; the focus (F) is called the principal focus.

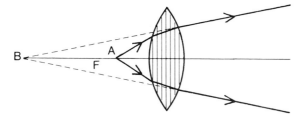

Fig. 2.21 The source of light (A) is between F and the lens; the focus is at a point, B, behind the source of light. B is a virtual focus.

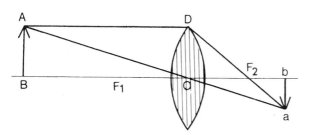

Fig. 2.22 The image formed by a convex lens. The object (AB) is beyond the principal focus (F₁). The image (*ab*) is smaller, inverted, and also beyond the principal focus (F₂) on the other side of the lens. In this case the image is real.

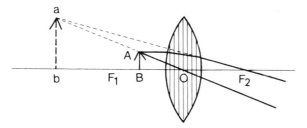

Fig. 2.23 The image formed by a convex lens. The object (AB) is within the principal focus (F₁). The image (*ab*) is larger, erect, and behind the principal focus on the same side of the lens. In this case the image is virtual.

the image recedes further and becomes larger, still remaining inverted, until, when the object reaches the principal focus, the image is infinitely far away and infinitely large, that is nothing determinate is seen. If the object is brought still closer to the lens, a virtual image can be appreciated by looking through the lens, and it will be found to be erect and the object will seem to be magnified.

Images formed by concave lenses

The construction of images formed by concave lenses depends on the application of the same principles as we have just considered. It is to be remembered that these diverge the rays of light so that they never form a real image but always a virtual one. If the incident rays are parallel they will be diverged, but if they are produced backwards they will all cross the principal axis in a single point on the same side of the lens from which they come (Fig. 2.24): this is the principal focus. When the object is in any position, it will be found that the image is virtual, erect, and smaller than the object (Fig. 2.25).

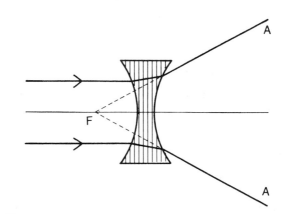

Fig. 2.24 The principal focus of a concave lens. When the incident rays are parallel, coming from infinity, they are diverged in the direction AA. They thus appear to come from a point F (the principal focus) on the other side of the lens.

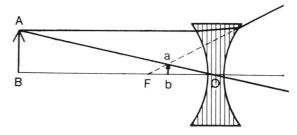

Fig. 2.25 The image formed by a concave lens. If AB is the object, the image *ab* is diminished and erect and, being formed on the same side of the lens as that from which the incident light comes, is virtual.

The concept of a *virtual image* may be difficult to understand. Emerging from a concave lens the rays of light diverge further and further apart from each other, and therefore no point of union, or focus, can exist. We have noted, however, that in our mental experience we ignore the effect of refraction and project an object visually along the direction of the rays of light as they enter the eye. Consequently, an observer stationed at A (Fig. 2.24), receiving the diverging rays into his eye, will neglect their refraction and will get the impression that they come from the point F, where they would meet if they were prolonged backwards. Although there is no image formed at this spot, or, indeed, at any point at all, the observer will believe that he does see the image of the object emitting the rays here. This apparent image is called *virtual*.

Refraction by cylindrical lenses

We have seen that spherical lenses may be looked upon as composed of a refractive medium (usually glass), one or both of the surfaces of which are in the shape of a sphere; and that a plano-spherical lens, for example, may be imagined as formed by the cutting off of a portion of a solid sphere by a plane (see Figs 2.14 and 2.16). Similarly, a cylindrical lens as used in ophthalmology is a piece of glass, one of the surfaces of which is cylindrical; and it may be regarded as formed by the intersection of a solid cylinder ABCD (Figs 2.26 and 2.27), by a vertical plane EFGH in the line of the axis XY. It is thus curved in the horizontal meridian (LM), in which it acts as a spherical lens, and not in

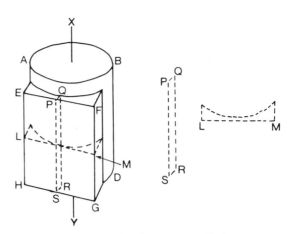

Fig. 2.27 The formation of a concave cylinder. ABCD is a solid cylinder with an axis XY. It is cut by a plane EFGH which runs parallel to the axis, and the segment so delimited forms a cylinder. In the plane parallel to the axis XY the cylinder may be considered as a glass plate with parallel sides, PQRS. No refraction therefore occurs in this meridian. In the plane perpendicular to the axis, the cylinder may be considered as a lens, LM. Refraction therefore occurs in this meridian.

the vertical (PQRS), in which it acts as a plate with parallel sides; this latter meridian is called the *axis*. Consequently it does not refract light falling perpendicularly upon it in the plane corresponding to the line of the axis. Since, as we have seen, a lens can be considered to act optically as a series of prisms, a cylinder can be considered as acting as if it were composed of many series of prisms arranged in superimposed rows.

The action of a *convex cylinder* is thus demonstrated in Figure 2.28. Rays falling upon it in a direction at right angles to the axis are refracted just as in the case of a convex spherical lens; thus one section of parallel rays will be brought to a principal focus at F', while rays which are in the plane of the axis of the cylinder will proceed undeviated. This will occur down the entire length of the cylinder, and thus in place of a point of convergence we will have a *line of convergence* running in the same direction as the axis of the cylinder: in the figure, where the incident rays are parallel, each segment of which the cylinder may be regarded as being composed will have a principal focus at a corresponding point, and the line F'F″, which is made up of the

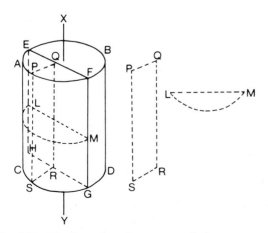

Fig. 2.26 The formation of a convex cylinder.

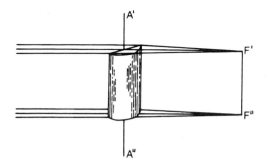

Fig. 2.28 The action of a convex cylinder. Rays of light striking the cylinder perpendicularly to the axis A'A" are brought to a focus in the focal line F'F".

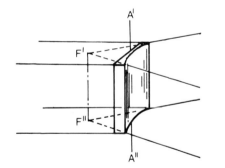

Fig. 2.29 Refraction by a convex cylinder.
A point of light is brought to a focus as a line after refraction through a cylinder.

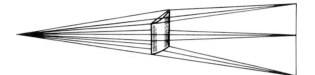

Fig. 2.30 Refraction of light by a concave cylinder. Rays of light striking the cylinder perpendicularly to the axis A'A" are diverged, and appear to be brought to a virtual focal line F'F".

sum of these individual foci, will be the *focal line*. Consequently, if a point of light is placed in front of the cylinder, no sharp image as a point can be formed on a screen, but a bright line may be obtained (Fig. 2.29). Conversely in the case of a *concave cylinder*, rays falling perpendicular to the axis are diverged (Fig. 2.30) according to the same principles as we have discussed when

considering the refractive properties of concave lenses.

Refraction by astigmatic lenses

We have seen that with a spherical lens where all meridians have the same curvature the rays coming from a point can be focused as a point; further, in a cylindrical lens where one meridian is curved and the one at right angles has no curvature at all, the image formed of a point object is a straight line. This therefore is the simplest form of an *astigmatic lens* (α, privative; $\sigma\tau\acute{\iota}\gamma\mu\alpha$, a point). We can now imagine a more complicated system where both meridians are curved but to a different degree; such an astigmatic surface is exemplified in the bowl of a spoon, the curve from side to side being greater than that from handle to tip. It can therefore be appreciated that an astigmatic lens, because of the different curvature of its meridian, can never produce a point focus of a point object. Where the two meridians in question are at right angles to each other, the condition is termed *regular astigmatism*. With this alone we need concern ourselves here.

The refractive properties of such a complicated lens may be gathered from a consideration of Figure 2.31, where a lens is represented as having different curvatures in two meridians, the vertical meridian (VV) being more curved than the horizontal (HH). It is evident that the more

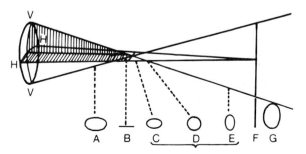

Fig. 2.31 Refraction by an astigmatic lens: Sturm's conoid. VV, the vertical meridian of the refracting body, is more curved than HH, the horizontal meridian. A, B, C, D, E, F, G show different sections of the beam after refraction. At B the vertical rays are brought to a focus: at F the horizontal rays are brought to a focus. From B to F is the focal interval of Sturm. D shows the circle of least diffusion.

curved meridian will refract the rays incident upon it to a greater degree than the less curved, and consequently, if parallel rays fall upon it, the vertical rays will come to a focus before the horizontal rays. There are thus two foci, the distance between which is termed the *focal interval*. No definite image is therefore ever formed, but merely the blurred effect produced by a diffused bundle of rays, from the astigmatic lens to F, known as Sturm's conoid.

The appearance of the bundle of rays at different points is illustrated in the figure. At A, where the vertical rays are converging more rapidly than the horizontal, a section of the bundle will be in the form of a horizontal oval ellipse. At B, the vertical rays have now come to a focus while the horizontal rays are still converging; here the section will be a horizontal straight line. Beyond B the vertical rays are now diverging while the horizontal rays are still converging; at first the section (C) of the bundle will be a horizontal oval ellipse, but when the point D is reached, where the two opposing tendencies are equal and opposite, the section becomes a circle: this is called the *circle of least diffusion or confusion* where the least amount of distortion takes place. Beyond this point the divergence of the vertical rays becomes preponderant, and an ellipse is again formed, this time with its long axis vertical (E), until at F, where the horizontal rays come to a focus, the section will become a vertical straight line. Beyond this point, as at G, where both sets of rays are always diverging, the section will take the form of a gradually increasing vertical oval.

THE NOTATION OF LENSES

The more a lens is able to refract light the more powerful we consider it to be. The power of a lens is measured by reference to its focal length, and this depends on the curvature of its surfaces, the distance between them and the refractive index of the substance of which it is made. For all practical purposes therefore, the power of thin glass lenses is related to the surface curvature.

The focal length of a lens, we may recall, is the distance from it of the focus which it forms of rays of light parallel to the principal axis. This distance forms a convenient standard by which to measure the refractive power. A focal distance of 1 metre is taken as the unit, and a lens with a focal distance 1 metre away is spoken of as having a refractive power of 1 *dioptre* (1 D), a term introduced by Monoyer. Since a stronger lens has a greater refractive power, the focal distance will be shorter: it therefore follows that a lens of a refractive power of 2 D will have a focal distance of 0.5 metre, while a lens of 0.5 D will have a focal distance of 2 metres. The strength in dioptres is therefore the reciprocal of the focal length expressed in metres.

A means of differentiation is required to indicate whether the light falling upon the lens is converged or diverged, and for this purpose the symbols + and − are employed. A convex lens which brings parallel light to a focus 1 metre away has therefore a refractive power of +1 D, while a concave lens which in similar circumstances has a virtual focus 1 metre on the same side as the incident light has a refractive power of −1 D.

We may also consider a thin lens as being the optical combination of two curved surfaces very close to one another. For this purpose we should mention that the power of a single spherical refracting surface can be considered in a similar way and here it is given by the reciprocal of the focal length expressed in metres multiplied by the refractive index relating to the change of optical medium.

The position is not quite as simple as it appears because a single refracting surface has two differing focal lengths according to the side from which the parallel ray strikes it. Thus in Figure 2.32 if the medium on the right has a refractive index of n then the surface power is the reciprocal of the distance CQ, in metres, multiplied by n.

The advantages of the dioptric notation — vergence

The concept of dioptric power can be usefully extended to a general statement about the optical effect of lenses and surfaces. This brings in the notion of vergence of rays. The interposition of a lens at a certain point in the path of converging rays has an effect depending on its strength and

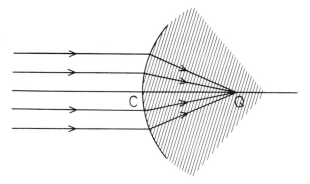

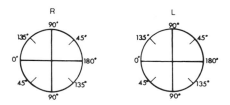

Fig. 2.33 The standard notation for recording the orientation of cylinder axes from the observer's view facing the patient.

Fig. 2.32 Refraction by and power of a single spherical surface.

on the vergence of the rays. Suppose that the converging rays are 'due' to focus at a certain distance from where the lens is to be interposed, we speak of them as having a vergence which is the reciprocal of that distance in metres. Where they actually do focus after the lens is interposed is then simply calculated by adding to the vergence of the original rays the power of the lens (each in dioptres). Thus if the rays have +2 D of vergence (the plus means convergence) then a −4 D lens interposed will mean that the vergence of the emerging rays will be −2 D and that a virtual point image is formed 50 cm in front of the lens. It is to be remembered that the vergence of a system of rays is not a fixed entity but relates only to a certain position in its path. (In the above example, the position is that at which the lens is to be interposed.) Parallel rays, of course, have no vergence.

This simple additive system arises from the well-known thin-lens formula relating object to image distances (*u* and *v* respectively) with focal length (*f*)

$$\frac{1}{v} - \frac{1}{u} = \frac{1}{f}$$

All distances are measured from the lens and are regarded as positive if in the direction of the incident light and negative if in the opposite direction.

The notation of cylinders

Exactly the same principles are applied to the case of cylinders. It is obvious that the effect of a cylinder upon a beam of light passing through it depends not only on the dioptric power of the cylinder, but also upon the position of its axis. The notation now universally adopted in determining the orientation of cylinders in relation to the patient's eyes, is illustrated in Figure 2.33. In this system a similar notation is used for each eye: the observer is facing the patient, the zero is at the observer's left, and the scale is read below the horizontal with 90 degrees at the bottom and 180 degrees at the right side.

Conventional abbreviations widely employed are sph. for sphere, cyl. for cylinder, ax. for axis or, alternatively, simply an arrow or line marking cylinder orientation on a printed dial as, for example, in Figure 2.33.

The detection and measurement of lenses

Spherical lenses

As we saw in the case of prisms, this is done by examining the image formed by the lens. Thus if a convex lens is held up before the eye and a distant object is regarded through it, when the lens is moved a little from side to side the image is seen to move in the opposite direction (Fig. 2.34). This reverse movement is due to the fact that the image formed by such a lens is inverted. With a concave lens, on the other hand, the image is erect, and therefore moves in the same direction. From the direction of this movement we can tell at once the nature of the lens with which we are dealing. A lens of known refractive power and of the opposite kind is now placed in apposition to the first, and when the combination is moved the displacement is noted; by a process of trial and error a combination is

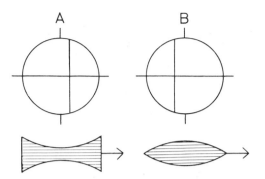

Fig. 2.34 The measurement of the strength of lenses. A straight line is viewed through the lens and the latter is moved in the direction of the arrow. In the case of a concave lens (A) the line appears to be displaced in the direction of movement. In a convex lens (B) the line appears to be displaced in the opposite direction.

found which gives no displacement at all, and the strength of this lens is equal and opposite to that of the unknown lens.

Cylindrical lenses

By a similar method the presence of a cylinder may be detected. When such a lens is moved in front of the eye, an object looked at through it appears to be unequally displaced in different directions. When the cylinder is moved in the line of its axis, since there is no refraction in this plane, no displacement is produced, but when the cylinder is moved in any other plane a gradually increasing degree of displacement is evident, which becomes maximal when the plane at right angles to the first is reached. This gives us the direction of the axis of the cylinder. The direction of the displacement, whether in the same or the opposite sense, gives us information as to the nature of the cylinder, whether concave or convex; and by neutralising the displacement by combining it with another cylinder of the opposite kind with a refractive power already known, we can determine its strength. The presence of a cylinder in a lens system is thus most easily determined by rotating it while viewing a linear object, if a cylinder is present, the difference in refraction in the two meridians will produce an apparent rotation of the object, in the reverse direction if the cylinder is convex,

in the same direction if the cylinder is concave, an effect which is absent if a spherical element only is present. It is important to remember that in such a test the lenses should be held closely together and their optical centres should be in line.

OPTICAL SYSTEMS

Refraction by combinations of lenses

We have already demonstrated that when two lenses are placed in apposition to one another the effect of the combination is additive. This may be expressed more accurately by saying that in a system of lenses, provided these are infinitely thin, are infinitely near and are accurately centred on the same optic axis, the total refracting power of the system is equal to the algebraic summation of the refracting power of each component lens. Thus if a +2 D be combined with a −3 D lens, the combination will have a refracting power of −1 D; and so on.

A similar result will be obtained by combining cylindrical lenses. If they are in contact with their axes parallel, their combined power will be the sum of the power of each. If, however, they are held with their axes at right angles, there will be two focal lines perpendicular to one another, and, since all rays must pass through both of these they must meet at the point where these lines intersect. If the component lenses are of the same strength the combination thus acts as a spherical lens, the refracting power of which is equal to the refracting power of the cylinders. Thus a +2 Dcyl. axis horizontal combined with a +2 D cyl. axis vertical will combine to form a +2 D sphere, which may be represented thus:

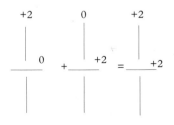

In the same way, combinations of spheres and cylinders are additive. When the two are of the same sign the matter is simple; when they are of opposite sign the same principles hold although their application may appear superficially to be somewhat confusing. Thus if a +2 D sphere is combined with a −2 D cyl. axis horizontal the two curvatures in the vertical meridian will neutralise each other, leaving those elements of the sphere the curvatures of which are horizontal to act as a +2 D cyl. with its axis vertical. Thus:

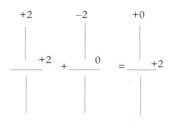

These simple relations hold when the lenses which compose the system are so thin and so close together that their thicknesses and their distances apart can be neglected. Where this cannot be done, however, the determination of the nature and the position of the resultant image becomes more complicated; it involves the construction of the image formed by the first element in the system, its consideration as the object presented to the second element and the construction of the image by this, and so on through all the component parts of the system. This may be relatively easy when the refractive elements are few and we confine ourselves to cases wherein the component lenses are centred on a common optic axis (that is, if the system is *homocentric*); thus the refraction by two convex lenses is illustrated in Figure 2.35 and that by a system of a convex and a concave lens in Figure 2.36. In a complex system, however, such as the

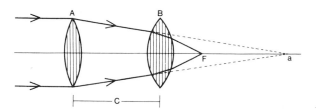

Fig. 2.35 Refraction by a system of lenses.

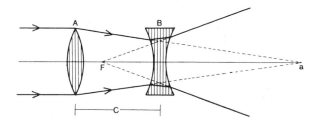

Fig. 2.36 Refraction by a system of lenses. If the system consists of two lenses, A and B, separated by a distance C, the image after refraction by the first lens would be formed at *a*, but on meeting B, the rays are further converged (or diverged), and brought to a final focus at F.

eye, or more particularly the eye in combination with a spectacle lens, such a process would obviously be very tedious. Fortunately, the matter has been much simplified in its mathematical treatment by Gauss and Listing. From their calculations we can construct the image formed by any lens system, the elements of which are centred on the same optic axis, provided we know the relative position of three pairs of *cardinal points*, which are usually easily determined.

Compound homocentric systems

No matter how complex a homocentric system of refractive elements may be, it is obvious that there will always be a ray (AP, Fig. 2.37) originating from the object running parallel to the axis before it reaches the first refracting surface of the system; after it emerges from the last refracting surface this ray will be refracted towards the axis and will cut it at some point. Such a ray corresponds to the rays shown in Fig. 2.19. The point where this ray cuts the axis is called the *second principal focus* (F″, Fig. 2.37). If we neglect the refractive elements of the system entirely and prolong the (initial) incident and (final) refractive paths of this ray, they will meet at a point Q. It is obvious that the total refracting power can be represented by a single imaginary refractive element at Q; the plane passing through Q (that is the plane of the theoretical equivalent lens) is called the *second principal* (or *equivalent*) *plane* and it cuts the axis at the *second principal* (or *equivalent*) *point* (H″). Again, in conformity

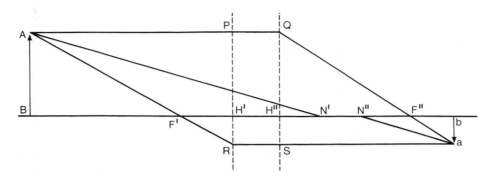

Fig. 2.37 The cardinal points of a compound homocentric system.
AB, the object; *ab*, the image; *Bb*, the line upon which the system is centred; F′ and F″ are the two principal foci; H′ and H″, the two principal points; N′ and N″ the two nodal points; PR and QS are the two principal planes.

with the focus of a simple lens (Fig. 2.19), the distance of this point from the second principal focus, that is the focal distance of the imaginary equivalent lens, is called the *second principal (or equivalent) focal distance* of the system.

Similarly, there must be a ray emanating from A which enters the system and is refracted to emerge parallel to the axis. The point whereat this ray (AR) crosses the principal axis in front of the first refracting element is called the *first principal focus* (F′), and the point whereat its incident and emergent directions theoretically meet (R) may be considered as the site of a single theoretical equivalent lens. R is therefore said to lie in the *first principal (or equivalent) plane* of the system; this plane cuts the principal axis at the

first principal (or equivalent) point (H′). Again, the distance from the first principal plane to the first principal point is the *first equivalent focal distance* of the system. This is the same as the second focal distance if the light emerges from the system into a medium identical to that from which it enters. The two principal foci (F′, F″), thus correspond in the complex system to the two principal foci of a simple lens (Fig. 2.20), and it is obvious that if an object is situated at the first its image will be at infinity; if an object is at infinity, its image will be at the second.

The remaining two cardinal points are the *nodal points* (N′, N″), which correspond to the single optical centre of a simple lens.

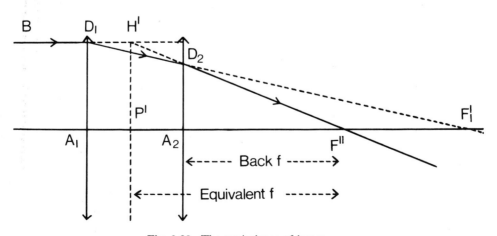

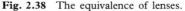

Fig. 2.38 The equivalence of lenses.

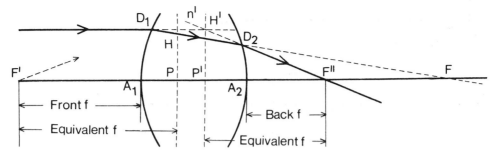

Fig. 2.39 The equivalence and vertex power of a thick lens in air. The first nodal point and the first principal points coincide; similarly the second.

Consequently (as will be seen from Fig. 2.18), an incident ray directed to the first nodal point (N') will emerge from the system in the same direction along a line which comes from the second nodal point (N'').

From the point of intersection of the rays passing through these points, the image (ab) of an object (AB) can be constructed (Fig. 2.37). The ray AQ, entering parallel to the axis, will run in the direction QF''. The ray AR, running through F', will emerge parallel to the axis. The ray AN' will leave the system as N''a. The intersection of any two of these three lines at a gives the position of the image of A.

Knowing any two of these cardinal points (the principal foci, the principal points and the nodal points) and their relationships, we can treat a complicated optical system theoretically as if it were composed of a single refracting medium subject to the comparatively simple laws with which we have dealt. We are now able to proceed to apply these principles to the optical system of the eye.

Reduced to its simplest terms, this construction can be readily adapted to determine the equivalence of a system of two lenses such as illustrated in Figure 2.35. If, for example, these two convex spherical lenses, represented by A_1 and A_2, are separated by 5 cm (Fig. 2.38) and each is of power 5.00 D, the incident parallel light would have a vergence of +5.00 D after passing through A_1 and would be brought to a focus at 20 cm (F'_1). When the light reaches A_2 it will be 5 cm nearer F'_1 so that its vergence will be 100/15 D. The second lens, A_2, provides another 5 D of convergence, making a total

convergence of 100/15 + 5 = +11.67 D. This is the *back vertex power* of the system and the emerging light will be brought to a focus at 8.57 cm at F'' (the second principal focus). If BD_1 and $F''D_2$ are produced to intersect at H', it can be seen that a single thin lens placed at this point, P'H', with a focal length P'F'' would have the same effect as the two lenses A_1 and A_2, i.e. the parallel rays would still be brought to a focus at F''. This lens at P' is called the *equivalent thin lens*, and the distance P'F'' is the *equivalent focal length* and its reciprocal is the *equivalent power* of the optical system formed by the two lenses.

Thick lenses

Up to the present we have been dealing with lenses which we have imagined to be so thin that their thickness has had no influence on the refraction of the rays of light passing through them. In practice, of course, this theoretical concept does not prevail. A thick lens, however, may be treated as two refracting surfaces separated by a medium of glass and not of air. The treatment of such a lens is evident from Figure 2.39. A ray entering the first surface at D_1 will be refracted so that it reaches the second surface at D_2 when it will be again refracted to cut the optic axis at F'', the second principal focus. With the general construction seen in Fig. 2.37, the initial and final paths of the ray are found to meet at H', the equivalent principal plane. The thick lens can therefore be treated as if it were a hypothetical thin lens situated at this point with an equivalent focal length P'F''. It is obvious that the equivalent power of the lens depends on the thickness of the glass, its refractive index and the refracting powers of the surfaces. In spectacle optics the only property of a lens that really matters is the vergence of the rays that leave the system, the *back vertex power*, a quantity determined by the dioptric value of the back vertex distance (A_2, F'').

The equivalent power of complex optical systems such as the eye, where the entrant and emergent media differ, is calculated in a manner similar to that we noted for a single refractive surface (p. 22) and is given by the product of the dioptric value of the second principal focal distance and the refractive index of the emergent medium.

3. The refraction of the eye — physiological optics

THE OPTICAL SYSTEM OF THE EYE

The roles of the cornea and lens

In order to understand the behaviour of rays of light on their way to the retina and the mechanism of the formation of an image there, it is necessary to study the various refractive elements in their path. The structures which are met with in their passage through the eye are seen in Figure 3.1. They are: the anterior surface of the cornea, the substance of the cornea, the posterior surface of the cornea, the aqueous humour, the anterior surface of the lens, the substance of the lens (which, as we shall see, is decidedly complicated), the posterior surface of the lens, and the vitreous humour.

This appears very involved, but as a matter of fact refraction takes place to any significant degree only at three out of the four surfaces, and we can ignore the refraction at the posterior

surface of the cornea. The reason for this is that the substance of the cornea has a refractive index which is practically the same as that of the aqueous humour. Furthermore, the refractive indices of aqueous and vitreous are similar. The light entering the eye is refracted markedly at the anterior corneal surface for two reasons: first because of its curvature, the central spherical part having a radius of curvature usually a little less than 8 mm, and secondly because of the big difference in refractive indices of air (1) and cornea (1.37). The light then undergoes little further refraction until it reaches the lens, at both surfaces of which it is again refracted. *Refraction by the eye therefore effectively takes place at two structures, the anterior corneal surface and the lens.* While the refractive index of the lens substance *is* significantly higher than that of aqueous and vitreous, the difference is not as marked as that between cornea and air. It follows that *the major part of the ocular refraction takes place at the anterior surface of the cornea*, the optical power of which (some 40–45 D) is over twice that of the lens (a little less than 20 D), in its place between the aqueous and vitreous.

Special features of the refraction caused by the lens

Both the corneal surface and the lens powerfully converge rays incident upon them, but while the cornea, as we have seen, acts largely as a single refracting surface the lens cannot simply be considered as two spherical surfaces enclosing a uniform substance and its refractive properties are complicated by the fact that it is not a homogeneous structure. On the contrary, it is made up of several layers, the central nuclear

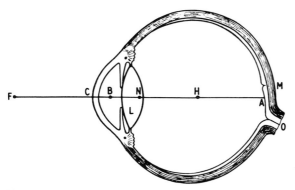

Fig. 3.1 The eye.
C, the cornea. B, in the anterior chamber, filled with aqueous. L, the lens. H, in the vitreous. M, the macula. O, the optic nerve. FA, the optic axis, meeting the retina at A. N, the nodal point. H, the centre of rotation.

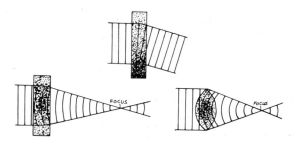

Fig. 3.2 Refraction of the lens.
The first illustration shows how a plate of glass, if of unequal optical density, will refract light. If the point of greatest density is in the centre, a plate with parallel sides will act as a converging lens, as is seen in the second figure. If, in addition, the sides are given a curvature, as in the third figure, the double influence of the refracting surfaces and the density will greatly augment the converging power.

Fig. 3.3 The structure of the lens.
The central nucleus is more nearly spherical, and the cortex may be considered as two encapsulating menisci. The greater curvature of the inner layers increases their refractive power.

having a higher index of refraction than the peripheral cortical layers. It will be readily seen from Figure 3.2 that this progressive increase in optical density will greatly augment its converging power, for even a plate with parallel sides, if constituted in this way, will act as a lens of considerable strength. In addition to this difference in refractivity, the converging effect is further augmented by the fact that the various layers are not strictly concentric. The curvature of the outer layers is less than that of the inner, so that the central nucleus compared with the outer part of the cortex is more nearly spherical (Fig. 3.3). Thus each successive layer, with its higher optical density and greater curvature, acts as an increasingly powerful lens.

The curvatures of the surfaces of the lens are unequal, the anterior being flatter than the posterior. The radius of curvature of the anterior surface is about 10 mm, while that of the

posterior is about 6 mm. The refractive index of the substance of the lens near the periphery is 1.386, while that of the nucleus is about 1.41, the mean value being approximately 1.39. Owing to the complexity of its architecture, however, the entire lens has a refractive power higher than these figures indicate, and would correspond to a uniform refractive index of 1.42 if the lens were homogeneous. Its total strength in situ is thus equal to that of a lens of from 16 to 20 D.

The comparatively greater refractive strength of the nucleus of the lens has a biological importance other than the ability to converge the rays of light effectively upon the retina. Its structure diminishes the optical errors of spherical and chromatic aberration, it reduces the amount of scattered light within the eyeball and, since the power of varying the refraction (that is the accommodation) depends upon the refractivity of the lens, the peculiar structure of this tissue enables it to exercise nearly double the range it could otherwise exert.

THE SCHEMATIC AND REDUCED EYES

The combination of the corneal and lenticular refraction

We have seen in the previous chapter that the refractive properties of a complex optical system can be reduced to the basis of a simple system by the application of the principles of the theorem of Gauss, provided the components of which it is formed are centred on the same optic axis. The eye forms, approximately, such a homocentric system.

We find its cardinal points to be as in Figure 3.4 and we refer to this analysis as the *schematic eye*. But the analysis can be made rather simpler when we notice that the two principal points and the two nodal points are very close together, so close, indeed, that no great inaccuracy will arise if we substitute for each pair an intermediate point and consider them as one. Without introducing any appreciable error, we can thus treat the optical system of the eye as if it were a single ideal refracting surface. This concept of a *reduced eye* was introduced by Donders, and it has the following properties:

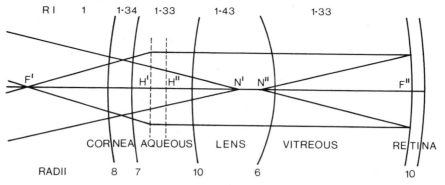

Fig. 3.4 The cardinal points of the eye.
F', the anterior principal focus, 15.7 mm in front of the cornea.
F", the posterior principal focus, 24.13 mm behind the cornea, that is, upon the retina.
H', H", the principal points in the anterior chamber.
N', N" the nodal points, in the posterior part of the lens. The refractive indices are approximate.

It is an ideal spherical surface, the radius of curvature of which is 5.73 mm, which separates two media of refractive indices 1 and 1.336. It lies about 1.35 mm behind the anterior surface of the cornea, that is in the anterior chamber. Its

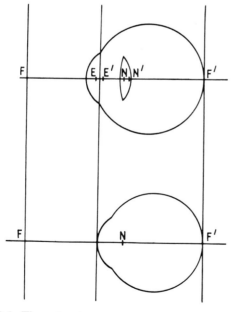

Fig. 3.5 The reduced eye.
The upper figure represents the normal eye, with the two focal points at F and F', the two principal points at E and E' and the two nodal points N and N'. The reduced eye, drawn in scale to correspond, is shown below, with the two principal foci at F and F', the single refracting surface corresponding to the mean of E and E', and the nodal point at N, corresponding to the mean of N and N'.

nodal point (optical centre) is therefore 7.08 mm behind the anterior corneal surface, that is in the posterior part of the lens. Its anterior focal distance is 17.05 mm (or 15.7 mm in front of the cornea), and its posterior focal distance is 22.78 mm (or 24.13 mm behind the anterior surface of the cornea), that is, in an average eye, upon the retina.

The formation of this reduced eye is shown in Figure 3.5. With it alone we will deal, and on its basis it is a simple matter to construct the nature of the images thrown upon the retina.

The formation of retinal images

The construction of a retinal image will be gathered from Figure 3.6. Since the nodal point (N) acts as the optical centre of the reduced

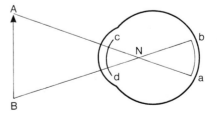

Fig. 3.6 The formation of retinal images.
The image *ab* of an object AB is formed by drawing lines from A and B through the nodal point N. *cd* is the position of the refracting surface of the reduced eye. ANB or *aNb* represents the visual angle.

optical system, rays which pass through it will not be appreciably refracted. If, therefore, an object (AB) is placed in front of the eye, its image (*ab*) may be constructed by drawing straight lines from the extremities of the object through the nodal point and producing them until they reach the retina. It is evident that the image thus obtained is inverted and diminished, just as are the images formed by a convex lens; it is reinverted psychologically in the cerebral cortex.

These two lines will enclose an angle at the nodal point; this, the angle ANB, is known as the *visual angle*, and is defined as the angle subtended by the object at the nodal point. It is, of course, equal to the angle *a*N*b*, subtended by the retinal image at the nodal point.

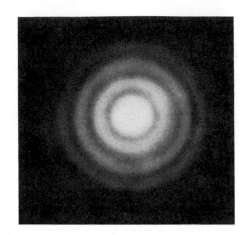

Fig. 3.7 The diffraction of light.
Light brought to a focus does not come to a point, but gives rise to a blurred disc of light surrounded by several dark and light bands (the 'Airy disc'). (W. H. A. Fincham.)

THE OPTICAL DEFECTS OF THE EYE

The accuracy with which any optical apparatus is able to form a clearly defined image is called its *resolving power*, which is thus an index of the efficiency of the system. Every lens system has inherent defects, in all of which the eye participates to some extent. However, the important thing to remember, is that, although the eye does possess these defects, it possesses them to so small a degree that, for functional purposes, their presence is immaterial; living organisms are never built to precisely applied mathematical laws, and any theoretical inaccuracies they may show in their configuration are more than counterbalanced by the adaptability and plasticity which their essentially flexible nature permits. The eye is by no means a perfect optical instrument, but its potentialities of accommodation, adaptation and retinal definition and differentiation render it unique. Some of these defects are inherent in the 'normal' eye, and are therefore physiological; others must be considered as abnormal.

PHYSIOLOGICAL OPTICAL DEFECTS

1. Diffraction of light

When a wave of light travels through space, the sides of the wave tend to deviate; expressed in popular language, having no support they tend to fall away from the main body of the wave. This effect is especially marked in a narrow wave, such as one which has passed through a pupillary aperture. The image, therefore, produced by a parallel bundle of rays, after passing through a converging lens, is not a mathematical point but a series of concentric rings of light with a bright spot at their centre; such an appearance is seen in Figure 3.7. In the eye with a pupil of 2 mm diameter, the diameter of this spot is 0.01 mm, and this inherent property of light thus sets a limit to the definition of the retinal image no matter how perfect the optical system itself may be. Diffraction has an effect which is the more serious the smaller the size of the pupil.

2. Chromatic aberration

White light is composed of rays of different wavelength, which, when taken separately, form the various colours of the spectrum. As we would expect, the short waves are retarded most in passing through a refractive medium, and hence on their way through a lens they are more acutely bent than the longer ones, so that they come to a focus in front of them. The short blue and violet rays therefore come to a focus in front of the long red rays. The effect of this phenomenon of the *dispersion of light* by a lens will be evident

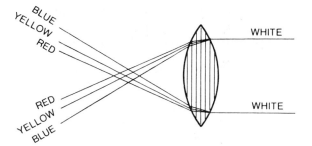

Fig. 3.8 Chromatic aberration.
The dioptric system of the eye is represented by a simple lens. The yellow light is focused on the retina, and the eye is myopic for blue, and hypermetropic for red.

from Figure 3.8. This to a certain extent reduces the definition of the retinal image, but the amount is small; it increases with the size of the pupil, and with a pupillary diameter of 2 mm approximately 70% of the light falls on an area of 0.005 mm diameter. Moreover, the effect is to a certain extent neutralised by the fact that the eye is normally focused so that the rays of greatest intensity (the yellow) form the most sharply defined image, while the colours of longer and shorter focus form circles of relatively low intensity compared with this and their images are therefore neglected. In this way the eye is hypermetropic for red rays and myopic for blue rays. Cobalt blue glass, for example, allows practically only red and blue rays to pass through it. If a white light be regarded through a piece of this glass, a position will be found when the red rays come to sharp focus and appear as a red spot while the blue form a blurred circle around them, while in another position the reverse will be evident — a blurred circle of red being obtained surrounding a sharply defined blue spot. As will be seen later, this forms the basis of a test for detecting refractive errors.

In optical instruments the effect of chromatic aberration can be abolished by combining glass of different refractive indices and different dispersions to form a compound lens. Thus flint glass gives a dispersion nearly double that of crown glass, and its index of refraction is 1.7, while that of crown glass is 1.5; hence, if we combine a convex lens of crown glass with a concave lens of half the strength composed of flint glass, the dispersion will be neutralised, while a considerable part of the

refractivity of the crown glass will still remain. Such a combination forms an *achromatic lens*.

The story of chromatic aberration is interesting, even among the many stories associated with the development of optical science, in showing how useful results may arise from wrong hypotheses. Newton concluded that dispersion was always proportional to refractivity and thus imagined that the realisation of an achromatic system was impossible; he therefore discarded his work on astronomical telescopes, in which the images are formed by refraction, and turned his attention to catoptric telescopes, which make use of reflected images. Euler, however, thinking that the eye was achromatic, stimulated an optician, Dolland, to construct achromatic lenses. Later, Wollaston, finding in controlled experimental conditions that the red end of the spectrum was sharply focused by the eye while the blue end was not, demonstrated that the eye was subject to chromatic aberration.

One consequence of chromatic aberration is to produce a *chromatic difference in magnification*.

Owing to the unequal refraction of light rays, not only are images formed at different distances from the cornea, but, when the object is a little to the side of the optic axis, the images produced by the short rays will be smaller than those formed by the long rays. We shall see that the fovea, which is the point of the retina with the greatest acuity of vision, is a little to the side of the optic axis, and consequently all images falling upon it must suffer from this error. This, however, has a beneficial rather than a disadvantageous effect, for it neutralises to a large extent the effects of chromatic aberration; indeed, it may be a teleological reason for the eccentric position of this important region.

3. Spherical aberration

The periphery of an optical lens has a higher refracting power than the central parts, and consequently the peripheral rays are brought to a focus more quickly than the central. Definition again suffers in this way, for the focus is not a point, as seen in Figure 3.9. The phenomenon, however, is little evident in the eye unless the pupil is widely dilated, for in ordinary circumstances the peripheral rays are cut off by the iris, a state of affairs opposite to that which holds in the case of diffraction. In any event the

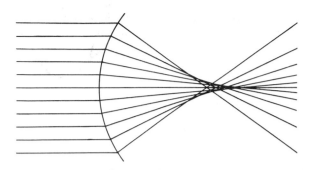

Fig. 3.9 Spherical aberration.

effects of spherical aberration are somewhat neutralised by the fact that, as we have already noted, the central portions of the lens of the eye have a greater density and are arranged in layers of greater curvature than the peripheral, thus tending to level up the general effect. Even when the pupil is dilated the error is to some extent remedied by the peculiar curvature of the cornea, which we have seen to be flatter at the periphery than at the centre. It may be taken, then, that the effects of spherical aberration are negligible.

The error is diminished by making the curvature of the anterior surface greater than that of the posterior; it is for this reason that the objectives of opera glasses bulge in front. The best forms are the so-called *periscopic* and *meniscus lenses*, where the radius of curvature of the posterior surface is greater than that of the anterior surface (see p. 206). This error can be eliminated by grinding lenses so that their curvature gradually decreases from the centre to the periphery. Such lenses are called *aplanatic*. In practice, by combining lenses of flint and crown glass of appropriate power in a suitable way, an achromatic and aplanatic combination can be made at the same time, thus eliminating both chromatic and spherical aberration.

4. Decentring

The formation of an ideal image would demand that the refractive surfaces in the optical system of the eye were accurately centred, that is that the centres of curvature of the corneal surface and the two surfaces of the lens were exactly on the optic axis. The centring of the eye is never exact, but the deviations are usually so small as to be functionally negligible. According to Tscherning, the usual defect is that the centre of

curvature of the cornea is situated (as much as 0.25 mm) below the axis of the lens. It is as if an optician in the making of an opera glass had placed one of the lenses a little below the axis of the instrument by a defect of workmanship.

We have noted that the fovea is not usually situated on the optic axis, but is placed about 1.25 mm downwards to its temporal side. Since this part of the retina is used for distinct vision, we do not look directly along the optic axis when we look at an object, but along a line joining the object (or the *fixation point*) with the fovea and passing through the nodal point (Fig. 3.10). This line (FNM) is called the *visual axis*. Sometimes the optic axis does cut the fovea, in which case it corresponds to the visual axis; usually it does not, but the visual axis cuts the cornea slightly up and to the nasal side of its centre, so that when the eye looks directly forward at an object, the optic axis is directed somewhat down and out. The angle formed at the nodal point between these two axes, that is the angle ONF, is called the *angle alpha* (α); its average size is 5°. It is as though, instead of looking directly along the central axis of an opera glass, we tilted it very slightly; the amount of tilt would then represent the angle α. We have seen that this deviation seems to have a teleological significance since it tends to correct chromatic aberration at the fovea.

When the visual axis cuts the cornea, as it usually does, on the nasal side of the optic axis, the angle α is designated *positive*; when the two axes coincide the angle is *nil*; sometimes the visual axis cuts the cornea on the temporal side of the optic axis, in which case the angle α is termed *negative*.

When movements of the eye-ball take place and the gaze is not directed straight forwards, a further complication occurs. These movements take place around a point situated in the middle of the eye on the optic axis called the *centre of rotation* (C, Fig. 3.10), and the line joining this to the point of

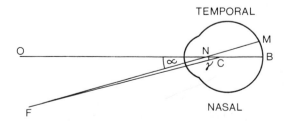

Fig. 3.10 The angles alpha and gamma. OB, the optic axis; FM, the visual axis, the two cutting at the nodal point, N. C, the centre of rotation, and FC, the fixation axis. The angle ONF is the angle α, the angle OCF is the angle γ.

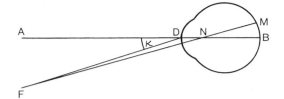

Fig. 3.11 The angle kappa.
ANB is the pupillary line cutting the cornea in D. FNM is the visual axis joining the object of fixation and the macula, and passing through the nodal point, N. If F and D are joined, the angle ADF is the angle κ.

fixation is called the *fixation axis* (FC). The angle between the optic axis and the fixation axis, that is the angle OCF is called the *angle gamma* (γ).

We shall see later that the measurement of these angles is of clinical importance in the question of squint. It is impossible in practice, however, to determine accurately the optic axis, for we cannot tell the exact centre of the cornea. It is much easier to estimate the centre of the pupil by an image (for example, of a light) on the cornea, and so we substitute for the optic axis a line, the *pupillary line* (AN, Fig. 3.11), perpendicular to the cornea and passing through this point. The angle formed between this line and the visual axis is called the *angle kappa* (κ). The centre of the pupil is somewhat to the nasal side of the centre of the cornea, but for clinical purposes the optic axis and the pupillary line may be taken as coincident, and the angle formed at the cornea (ADF) may be considered equal to that subtended at the nodal point (ANF).

5. Peripheral aberrations

Several optical considerations combine to make the images formed in the peripheral part of the retina less clearly defined than those in the central area. Some of the most important of these are the phenomena known as *coma, oblique astigmatism* and *distortion of the image*; but since most of them are to a large extent neutralised by the peculiar shape of the eye, they need not be discussed in detail. The curve of the retina has a very important effect on the efficiency of peripheral vision, and calculation shows that a very close approximation to the ideal optical conditions has been adopted. But although the ideal is not reached, the functional efficiency of the eye is greatly augmented by sacrificing the

definition of the marginal images to some extent in order to get the best possible condition for the central images.

CONSEQUENCES OF THE PHYSIOLOGICAL DEFECTS OF THE EYE

Circles of diffusion

While these aberrations may appear unimportant inasmuch as they occur normally and do not obtrude themselves into our consciousness in everyday life, we shall find that they require practical consideration when we are dealing with the correction of errors of refraction, especially the larger ones, by artificial lenses. In the normal eye their combined result is that no clear image is formed as a point focus on the retina, but only as a circle of light which involves a certain amount of blurring. Such a circle is called a *circle of diffusion*, and its nature will be gathered from Figure 3.12. It will be remembered that a line may be considered as a number of points, and therefore its image may be construed as a number of such circles superimposed the one upon the other so as to overlap to a large extent; a narrow line therefore becomes converted into a broad band (Fig. 3.13). The smaller these circles are, the greater will be the efficiency of vision, and thus to obtain the *circle of least diffusion* is our object in the correction of errors in the optical system of the eye.

Fig. 3.12 Circles of diffusion: the image of a point is a circle.

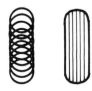

Fig. 3.13 Circles of diffusion: the image of a line is a broad band.

The size of the pupil: stenopaeic apertures

The beam of light within the eye takes the form of a cone, the base of which is formed by the pupillary aperture; the smaller this aperture is, the smaller will be the section of the cone. Since the periphery of the lens is largely responsible for the errors of spherical and chromatic aberration, the errors which these introduce will be correspondingly reduced. The beneficial effect of a small pupil will be more evident where the apex of the cone does not fall upon the retina, as when an error of refraction is present. Thus when an object O (Fig. 3.14) is regarded and the pupil contracts from the size aa to b, the diffusion circle formed by the image of O will be reduced from a_1a_1 to b_1, and will consequently have a less disturbing effect. If we suppose, for example, with the large pupil, aa, the converging pencil of rays covers an area in the macular region (a_1a_1) occupied by 100 cones, and if the pupil were contracted so that its radius were reduced to one-fifth of its original size, the area covered will be 1/25 in size (b_1), and only four cones will be involved. Theoretically, if the pupils were reduced to a point, one ray only would enter, one cone would be stimulated, and a clear image would be formed in all cases, no matter what the refractive error might be. The principle is the same as in the pin-hole camera (Fig. 3.15). This is taken advantage of in a clinical test (p. 145), wherein a *stenopaeic opening* ($\sigma\tau\acute{\epsilon}\nu o\sigma$, little; $\grave{o}\pi\acute{\eta}$, an opening) is put before the eye and the improvement of vision is noted. For this reason also, a hypermetrope prefers to read in brilliant illumination, so that the pupil is contracted down to a minimal size, and a myope gets into the habit

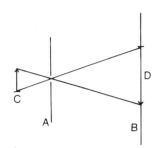

Fig. 3.15   The pin-hole camera.
To illustrate the principle of the stenopaeic opening. A candle flame, C, is held before a screen, B, separated by a diaphragm, A, in which is a minute hole. The diaphragm cuts off all the rays except those which can pass through the hole. Only a small pencil of rays from the top of the flame can reach the lower part of the screen, and so on throughout its extent. A clear inverted image, D, is therefore formed.

of looking at objects through the half-closed lids, gaining thereby the advantages of a stenopaeic slit.

Such a procedure, however, carries with it two disadvantages. When the pupil contracts not only does some degradation of the image occur because of diffraction, but also the amount of light entering the eye is correspondingly reduced and vision is rendered more difficult. There are thus two opposing tendencies, each making for visual efficiency up to a certain point, and the best results are obtained by taking a mean of both. The compromise which gives the best results varies with the illumination; where the illumination is high so as to produce a bright image, a small aperture can be used, but, where the illumination is poor, better results are obtained with a greater dilatation. In average conditions the best pupillary diameter is about 2 mm.

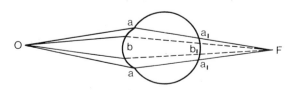

Fig. 3.14   The effect of the size of the pupil.
When the object O is looked at, the image is formed at F. At the level of the retina diffusion circles are formed. When the pupillary width is *aa*, the size of the circles of diffusion is a_1a_1; when the pupil contracts to *b*, the size of the circles of diffusion diminishes to b_1.

PATHOLOGICAL OPTICAL DEFECTS

The types of refractive error

We have seen that when parallel rays strike a physiologically normal eye they are refracted so as to converge upon the retina where they focus, forming a circle of least confusion; when these ideal optical conditions occur with the eye in a state of rest, i.e. without any accommodation, the condition is termed *emmetropia* ($\epsilon\nu$, within; $\mu\acute{\epsilon}\tau\rho\text{o}\nu$, measure; $\overset{\backprime}{\omega}\psi$, the eye).

It would be strange if this were a common state of affairs. It must be remembered that its attainment depends on an exactitude to within a fraction of a millimetre of such measurements as the length of the eye and the shape of the cornea and the lens; and such regularity and conformity to type as optical perfection would necessitate a mathematical accuracy which is nowhere realised in the constitution of living organisms. Emmetropia may be optically normal, but it is no more biologically normal than would be the universal attainment of a uniform height of 5 feet 6 inches. The opposite condition of *ametropia* ($\overset{\backprime}{\alpha}$, privative; $\mu\acute{\epsilon}\tau\rho\text{o}\nu$, measure; $\overset{\backprime}{\omega}\psi$, the eye), wherein parallel rays of light are not focused exactly upon the retina with the eye in a state of rest, is therefore much the more common; such an eye has a *refractive error*. When the refractive conditions of the two eyes are unequal, the condition is known as *anisometropia* ($\overset{\backprime}{\alpha}$, privative; $\overset{\prime}{\iota}\sigma\text{o}\varsigma$, equal).

Refractive errors may be of three main types: a principal focus may be formed by the optical system of the eye, but instead of being situated on the retina (as in emmetropia) it may be situated either behind it or in front of it. In the first case the eye is relatively too short, and the condition is then called *hypermetropia* (Fig. 3.16); in the second it is relatively too long, when the term *myopia* is used. Alternatively, the refractive system may be such that no single focus is formed, as in the case where *astigmatism* is present.

These refractive anomalies can obviously be caused by various conditions.

1. *The position of the elements of the system*
   a. The antero-posterior diameter of the eye is too short, and the retina is too near the optical system: *axial hypermetropia*.
   b. The antero-posterior diameter of the eye is too long and the retina is too far away from the optical system: *axial myopia*.
   c. *Lenticular displacement.* If the crystalline lens is dislocated forwards, *myopia* will exist; if backwards, *hypermetropia*.

2. *Anomalies of the refractive surfaces*
   a. The curvature of the cornea or of the lens may be too small, giving a *curvature hypermetropia*:
   b. or too great, giving a *curvature myopia*:
   c. or be irregular, varying in different meridians, giving *astigmatism*.

In *hypermetropic astigmatism*, the curvatures of both axes are unequal and too small; in *myopia astigmatism* they are both unequal and too great; when the two conditions are combined so that one axis is hypermetropic and the other *myopic*, the condition is termed *mixed astigmatism*.

   i. If the axes showing the greatest difference in curvature are at right angles, the condition is called *regular astigmatism*.
   ii. If they are not so related, the astigmatism may be called *bi-oblique*.
   iii. If there is no symmetry about the refraction and different groups of rays form foci at different positions, as occurs in the cornea after corneal ulceration or in the lens in developing cataract, the astigmatism is called *irregular*.

3. *Obliquity of the elements of the system*
   a. *Lenticular obliquity.* If the lens is placed obliquely or subluxated, astigmatism will result.
   b. *Retinal obliquity.* The posterior pole of the eye may be placed obliquely, as when it bulges backwards in a staphyloma in high myopia. If the summit of the staphyloma does not correspond to the fovea the rays will fall upon this region obliquely.

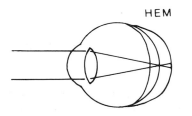

Fig. 3.16 Emmetropia, hypermetropia and myopia. In emmetropia (E), parallel rays of light are focused upon the retina. In hypermetropia (H), the eye is relatively too short; in myopia (M), it is too long.

4. *Anomalies of the refractive index*
   a. If the refractive index of the aqueous humour be too low, or that of the vitreous humour too high, there will be an *index hypermetropia*. If the refractive index of the aqueous is low, that is more nearly that of air, the refraction will be less. Similarly, when we consider the light travelling from the lens into the vitreous, if the refractive index of the vitreous be high, that is more nearly that of the lens, the refraction will again be less. Conversely, if the index of refraction of the aqueous be too high, or that of the vitreous too low, there will be an *index myopia*. Such changes are not clinically evident.
   b. If the refractive index of the lens as a whole be too low, there will be index hypermetropia, if too high there would be index myopia. If the index of the cortex increases relatively and approximates that of the nucleus, as it normally does in old age, the lens tends to act as a single refractive element, and consequently has less converging power than normal: the eye therefore becomes hypermetropic. Conversely, if the index of the nucleus increases, as frequently occurs in early cataract, myopia is produced. If the increase of the refractive index of the nucleus is very marked, a *false lenticonus* may be produced, wherein the central part of the pupil is myopic and the periphery hypermetropic. If the index of any part varies irregularly in different localities, as in developing cataract, an *index astigmatism* is produced.

5. *Absence of an element of the system*
Absence of the lens, a condition known as *aphakia*, produces hypermetropia.

The degree of refractive error

We denote the precise refractive error an eye demonstrates not only by its type but also by its degree. This last factor is easily derived from the strength of lens required to alter the vergence of

parallel rays so that the eye now focuses them on the retina. For example, in myopia a concave (or minus) lens is required which makes incident parallel light divergent to the appropriate degree (see Fig. 5.6) and conversely in hypermetropia a lens is needed which gives convergence to incident parallel rays.

It turns out that the strength required is that of the dioptric value of the far point distance. This is readily appreciated for the myopic condition but is a little more obscure in the case of hypermetropia where a theoretical 'far' point exists behind the eye. See Figure 4.1.

THE NATURE AND INCIDENCE OF REFRACTIVE ERRORS

The incidence of refractive errors is a subject of very considerable importance, for its study gives us an insight into their biological nature. Steiger, who first studied this subject scientifically by determining the incidence of the spherical refraction in large numbers of people, concluded that hypermetropia, emmetropia and myopia were not separate entities, but formed a single series around a common mean such as occurs in the case of many physiological variations in any large group of people with reference to any characteristic such as height and so on. Later research, however, has shown that this is not so.

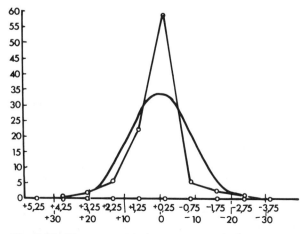

Fig. 3.17 The asymmetrical curve represents the incidence of refractive errors, and the symmetrical curve represents the theoretically derived binomial curve.

For example, the curve of Scheerer and Betsch, compiled from the examination of 12 000 eyes, is shown in Figure 3.17, where it is compared with a theoretically derived binomial curve. It is seen that the emmetropic cases are in excess of their theoretical value, and the myopic portion of the curve shows lengthening, that is there is a marked positive excess in the central values, a relative augmentation of the more extreme, and a definite 'skewness' towards the myopic side of the curve.

It is obvious, therefore, that we cannot consider the refraction as a whole, but must study the various component elements which combine to determine the optical system of the eye. The accurate measurement of the corneal curvature is easily accomplished, as we shall see, by the keratometer. The measurement of the optical constants of the lens can be similarly undertaken, but the technique is difficult and inaccurate. However, the fact that the dark-adapted retina responds to stimulation by X-rays was once utilised to devise methods of very considerable accuracy and wide clinical application whereby the axial length of the globe was measured and the total refraction estimated. In view of the fact that the depth of the anterior chamber is easily measured by several methods, the total refraction and all of its components can be determined so that the refractive power of the lens can be deduced. We are thus in a position to determine the influence of the various constituent elements upon the total refraction and to analyse the problem more fundamentally.

The measurement of the axial length

All modern techniques depend upon the use of ultrasonography, which has the value of being entirely objective (Fig. 3.18). When an ultrasonic beam is passed through the eye, peaks are seen in the echogram representing reflections from the various ocular interfaces; from the measurements thus obtained, the distances between these surfaces and the axial length of the eye can be calculated. The results given by these different techniques are remarkably consistent, average values for the axial length being between 23 and 24 mm for emmetropic eyes.

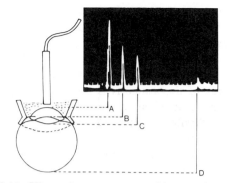

Fig. 3.18 Ultrasonic measurement of intra-ocular distances. The ultrasonic probe is inserted into a ring-shaped contact glass filled with water. The peaks in the echogram represent reflections at the anterior surface of the cornea (A), the anterior and posterior surfaces of the lens (B, C), and at the surface of the retina (D). AD is the axial length (see also Fig. 7.1).

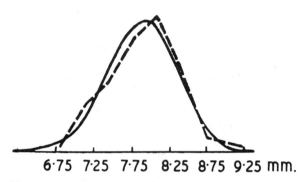

Fig. 3.19 The radius of the cornea.

It has been shown that all components in the optical system of the eye show a normal variation which does not differ greatly from the usual binomial curve with one exception — the axial length. Some of Tron's frequency curves illustrating this are seen in Figures 3.19 to 3.22. The variations that occur in these components must therefore be considered as normal. All these variants form components of the total refraction, so that different combinations of normal variations may result in emmetropia or a marked refractive error in the direction of either hypermetropia or myopia. Thus a myopic eye may have a shorter axial length than a hypermetropic. This again shows the impossibility of regarding hypermetropia and myopia as two distinct conditions. When we look at the axial length, however, the case is different,

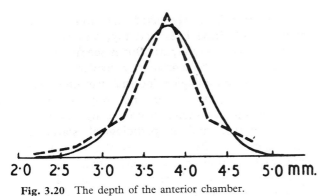

Fig. 3.20 The depth of the anterior chamber.

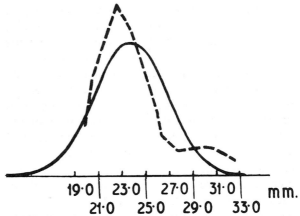

Fig. 3.23 The axial length in all cases of the series studied.

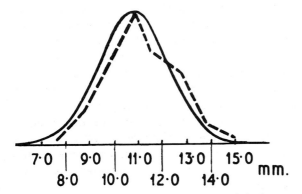

Fig. 3.21 The radius of the anterior surface of the lens.

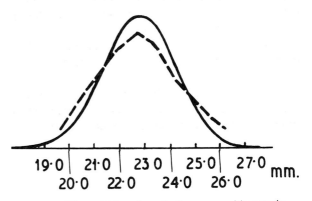

Fig. 3.24 The axial length excluding cases with myopia over −6 D.

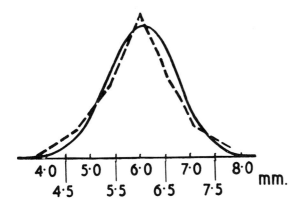

Fig. 3.22 The radius of the posterior surface of the lens.

for this curve of distribution differs from the binomial variation by showing both an excess above the mean and remarkable skewness (Fig. 3.23). There is a final point of interest. If myopes of above 6 D are eliminated from the calculation, Tron found that the error for the

axial length lost much of its peculiarities and the normal variation was again nearly attained (Fig. 3.24).

It seems obvious, therefore, that apart from high myopia the optical components of the eye show a normal chance variation, but the excess in the incidence of emmetropes (or near emmetropes) indicates that they do not vary independently from each other. As with other parts of the body, they are correlated and show a definite harmony in their construction so that there is a natural tendency for the total refraction to attain the ideal. Thus during the growth of the eye there is a high correlation between the corneal curvature and the axial length (the longer the latter, the flatter the cornea); while, again, the power of the lens bears a negative correlation with the axial length (the longer the axis, the flatter the lens). That this co-ordination is essentially genetically determined is seen in the high concordance not only in the total refraction but in the value of its separate components in uniovular twins and its discordance in binovular twins. The total refraction is thus not arrived at accidentally as the result of independent chance combinations, and the various optical components are not inherited independently of each other. It follows that biologically the emmetropic eye cannot be considered as normal, for it is not a separate group but merely an arbitrary limiting value between the two optical concepts of a hypermetropic and a myopic eye. All eyes with a refraction falling within wide limits around the mean refraction must equally be considered as fully normal, those in the extremes being the result of accidental but less favourable combinations of normal components.

The elongation of the curve in myopia requires a different explanation. It would seem that highly ametropic eyes differ biologically from the normal since the axial length falls outside the range of normal variation. We shall see that in the evolution of these eyes heredity, and to some extent disease, play a part. But it seems obvious that myopia can be legitimately divided into two types — a physiological normal variation in a large series differing in no way from its hypermetropic counterpart on the opposite side of the curve, and a pathological state, an aberration from the normal, as, of course, is the extreme hypermetropia of microphthalmos.

Simple refractive errors are thus largely hereditarily determined, owing to the co-ordinated combination of essentially normal elements of the optical system of the eye, are not progressive beyond the amount included within normal development, and are associated with good vision and require no treatment apart from their optical correction. *Pathological refractive errors*, on the other hand, are determined by abnormal developmental or acquired variations of the optical components of the eye, may progress beyond normal variational limits, may be associated with poor vision, and may require medical treatment to counteract a basic weakness.

Clinical anomalies

PART 1   Refractive errors

4. Hypermetropia

We have already defined hypermetropia as that form of refractive error in which parallel rays of light are brought to a focus some distance behind the sentient layer of the retina when the eye is at rest; the image formed here is therefore made up of circles of diffusion of considerable size, and is consequently blurred.

The possibility of such a condition was first suggested by a mathematician, Kästner (1755), and about a century later (1858) was put upon a sound basis by Donders, the ophthalmologist of Utrecht. He suggested the term *hypermetropia* ($\acute{\upsilon}\pi\grave{\epsilon}\rho$, in excess; $\mu\acute{\epsilon}\tau\rho o\nu$, measure; $\overset{\backprime}{\omega}\psi$, the eye). In the following year Helmholtz, writing on the subject, used the word *hyperopia*, although the shorter word is not etymologically so good as that introduced by Donders. Helmholtz in his later writings discarded it in favour of the original 'hypermetropia'.

The alternative name for hypermetropia, long-sightedness, is quite acceptable except in so far as it has given rise to confusion in the layman's mind. A patient will often describe himself as very long-sighted when what he intends to convey is that he sees well in the distance and presumes himself to be optically normal; it is, of course, true that early in life the hypermetrope sees as well in the distance as the emmetrope!

AETIOLOGY

It was at one time accepted that in the majority of cases hypermetropia was axial and the sentiment persists that in fact the hypermetropic eye has a shorter antero-posterior axis than normal. However, as we saw in the last chapter, it is quite possible for the hypermetropic eye to have a greater axial length than that of a myopic eye, and some uncertainty remains as to the relative importance of axial length and refractive power as influences in the cause of hypermetropia.

It is by far the commonest of all refractive anomalies, and indeed forms a stage in normal development. At birth practically all eyes are hypermetropic to the extent of 2.5 to 3.0 dioptres, and as the growth of the body proceeds the antero-posterior axis lengthens until, when adolescence is passed, the eye should theoretically be emmetropic. As a matter of fact, it is found that in over 50% of the population emmetropia is not reached, and some degree of hypermetropia persists; on the other hand, the mark may be overshot, and the eye may become myopic. Emmetropia should therefore be regarded as a stage in the development of the normal eye, and hypermetropia, while it is physiological in children, represents from the biological standpoint an imperfectly developed eye when it persists into adult life. Most primitive peoples and many of the lower animals are hypermetropic; Carnivora, for example, are almost constantly so.

As a rule, the degree of shortening is not great and rarely exceeds 2 mm. Each millimetre of shortening represents approximately 3 dioptres of refractive change, and thus a hypermetropia of over 6 dioptres is uncommon. Higher degrees, however, occur, cases up to 24 dioptres without any other pathological anomaly having been recorded; and, of course, in pathological aberrations of development such as microphthalmos, even this may be exceeded.

Shortening of the antero-posterior axis may also occur *pathologically*. An orbital tumour or inflammatory mass may indent the posterior pole of the eye and flatten it, or an intra-ocular neoplasm or oedema may displace the retina forwards at the macular region; a more pronounced condition may be caused by a detached retina, which may be displaced almost to touch the posterior surface of the lens. These, of course, form pathological instances wherein the refractive error occupies the background of the clinical picture.

Curvature hypermetropia occurs when the curvature of any of the refracting surfaces is unduly small. The cornea is the usual site of the anomaly, and it may be flattened congenitally (*cornea plana*), or as the result of trauma or disease. An increase of 1 mm in its radius of curvature produces a hypermetropia of 6 dioptres. In these cases, however, it is rare for the curvature to remain spherical and astigmatism is almost invariably produced. *Index hypermetropia* usually manifests itself as a decrease in the effective refractivity of the lens, and is responsible for the hypermetropia which occurs physiologically in old age, and for that which occurs pathologically in diabetics under treatment. Both of these will be noticed presently. A dislocation backwards of the lens also produces hypermetropia, whether it occurs as a congenital anomaly or as the result of trauma or disease; and a marked hypermetropia results from the absence of the lens, a condition which will be dealt with separately under the name of *aphakia*.

OPTICAL CONDITION

Whether the hypermetropia is due to a decrease in the length of the eye, a decrease of curvature, or to a change in refractive index, the optical effect is the same: parallel rays come to a focus behind the retina, and the diffusion circles which are formed here result in a blurred and indistinct image (Fig. 4.1). Moreover, since the axis of the eye is shorter and the retina is nearer the nodal point, it necessarily follows, as is obvious from Figure 4.2, that the image is smaller than in emmetropia. Conversely, rays coming from a point on the retina of the emmetropic eye will be parallel on leaving the eye, while in the hypermetropic eye they will be divergent. In the first case they will meet at infinity, in the second they will meet behind the eye (Fig. 4.3). It follows that with the emmetropic eye objects theoretically at infinity, or in practice at a

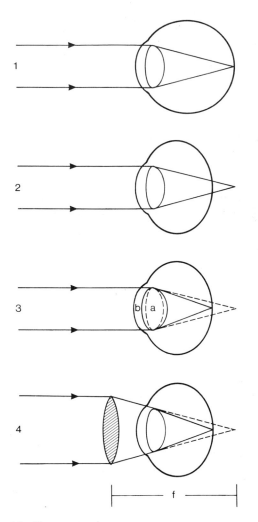

Fig. 4.1 Hypermetropia.
1. An emmetropic eye: parallel rays of light come to a focus upon the retina.
2. A hypermetropic eye: parallel rays of light come to a focus behind the retina.
3. A hypermetropic eye: parallel rays of light are brought to a focus upon the retina by increasing the refractivity by accommodation. The normal lens, *a*, becomes more convex, *b*.
4. A hypermetropic eye: parallel rays of light are brought to a focus upon the retina by increasing the refractivity by a convex spectacle lens. The degree of hypermetropia is given by the power of the lens, i.e. the reciprocal of *f* in metres.

distance of over 6 metres, are seen distinctly when the eye is at rest, while in hypermetropia the formation of a clear image of any kind is impossible unless the converging power of the optical system is increased. This may be done in

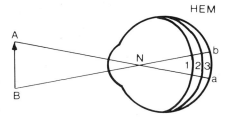

Fig. 4.2 The relative sizes of the image in hypermetropia, emmetropia and myopia.
AB is the object and N is the nodal point of the eye. The image *ab* is obtained by drawing straight lines from A and B through N to the retina. Since the retina in the hypermetropic eye (H) is nearer to N, and in the myopic eye (M) is further away than in the emmetropic eye (E), it follows that the image of the first (1) is smaller and that of the second (3) is larger than the image in the emmetropic eye (2).

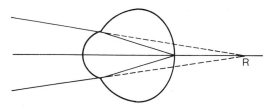

Fig. 4.3 The emergent rays in hypermetropia.
Rays coming from a point on the retina are divergent and appear to come from a point (R) behind the eye.

two ways — by the eye itself, or by artificial means. The curvature of the crystalline lens, and therefore its converging power, may be increased in the effort of accommodation [Fig. 4.1 (3)]. Alternatively, a convex lens may be placed in front of the eye in the form of spectacles [Fig. 4.1 (4)].

The accommodation in hypermetropia

It will be noted that the contraction of the ciliary muscle in the act of accommodation increases the refractive power of the lens so that it can correct a certain amount of hypermetropia. Normally there is an appreciable amount corrected by the contraction involved in the physiological tone of this muscle, and consequently the full degree of hypermetropia is revealed only when this muscle is paralysed by the use of a drug such as atropine. The moiety which this ciliary tone normally corrects is called *latent hypermetropia* (*Hl*). In

contradistinction, the remaining portion, which in normal circumstances is uncorrected, is termed *manifest hypermetropia* (*Hm*); and the two added together equal the *total hypermetropia* (*Ht*).

As a rule the latent hypermetropia amounts to only 1 dioptre, and so, in order to try to get a clear image, an individual with an error greater than this will usually supplement the tone of the ciliary muscle by an effort of contraction. He may correct part of his error in this way, or he may be able to correct the entire error and thus be able to see distinctly. In either case the amount corrected is spoken of as *facultative hypermetropia* (*Hf*). If the error is large and by no effort of accommodation can he see objects clearly, the amount of hypermetropia still remaining uncorrected and which cannot be overcome by accommodation is called *absolute hypermetropia* (*Ha*).

Total hypermetropia may therefore be divided into:

1. Latent hypermetropia, overcome physiologically by the tone of the ciliary muscle.
2. Manifest hypermetropia:
   a. Facultative hypermetropia, overcome by an effort of accommodation.
   b. Absolute hypermetropia, which cannot be overcome by accommodation.

The relationship between these may probably be best understood from the method employed to determine them clinically. Let us suppose a hypermetrope cannot see a distant object clearly. We then place convex lenses of gradually increasing strength in front of his eyes until he can just see clearly; at this moment the lens and his accommodation are both acting so that with the combination of them both a distinct image is seen. The amount of hypermetropia corrected by the lens, that is the amount which his efforts of accommodation cannot correct, is the absolute hypermetropia; and it is measured by the weakest convex lens with which maximum visual acuity can be obtained.

We now add stronger lenses until we reach the strongest with which clear vision is still maintained. During this process we have been substituting the converging power of the effort of his accommodation by the lenses and measuring the amount of hypermetropia he can correct in this way by his own efforts. This is the facultative hypermetropia; and it is determined by the difference between the strongest and the weakest convex lens with which maximum visual acuity is obtained. The limit we have reached, that is the strongest lens, is the measure of the manifest hypermetropia. We now instil atropine, and when the ciliary muscle has been paralysed and its tone thus abolished, we again find the strongest lens with which maximum visual acuity can be obtained. This is the total hypermetropia; it will be found to be a little more than before by an amount which represents the latent hypermetropia.

It thus appears that a high hypermetrope, or a low hypermetrope with no accommodative power, can see nothing distinctly, but if the accommodation is active and the error low and within his facultative limits, he can see clearly. To a certain extent this may be an advantage, and the variability of focusing of which he is capable has been aptly compared to the position of an observer looking down a microscope with his finger on the fine adjustment. On the other hand, the constant accommodative effort which is made automatically in the instinctive attempt to obtain distinct vision may lead to fatigue and distress, to a disorientation between accommodation and convergence, and to other troubles which we will consider later.

The normal age variation

We have seen that in the normal individual at birth 2 to 3 dioptres of hypermetropia are present; this may increase slightly in the first years of life but thereafter gradually diminishes as growth proceeds, until after puberty the refraction tends to become emmetropic. Thus in general terms it may be said that 90% of children at the age of 5, and only 50% at the age of 16, are hypermetropic. After the period of growth has passed the refraction tends to remain stationary, until in old age a further tendency to hypermetropia is evident. This is due to two causes, both associated with the lens. In the first place, in the continuous growth of the lens which occurs throughout life the outer cortical layers have a smaller curvature than the inner, a circumstance which decreases the converging power of this tissue. A second important influence is a change in the refractivity of the different layers. In youth the index of refraction of the cortex is considerably less than that of the nucleus, and this inequality, resulting in the formation of the combination of a central lens surrounded by two converging menisci (see Fig. 3.3), increases the refracting power of the whole. In old age the index of the cortex increases, so that the lens becomes more homogeneous; acting thus as a single lens, it has less converging power than it had before, and the eye becomes hypermetropic. Thus an eye which was emmetropic at 30 years of age may show 0.25 dioptre of hypermetropia at 55, an addition of 0.75 dioptre may be evident at 60, of 1 dioptre at 70, and at 80 years this may increase to about 2.5 dioptres. Hypermetropia of this origin is frequently designated *acquired hypermetropia*. It is to be noted that, if the nucleus also increases in optical density, the original relative difference will remain or may even be increased, an effect which is seen to a marked degree in the excessive nuclear sclerosis which sometimes occurs in early cataract when the opposite change of myopia is frequently produced.

This increase of hypermetropia with age is real; an *apparent increase* due to the progressive failure of accommodation also occurs with advancing years. As the tone of the ciliary muscle decreases, some of the latent hypermetropia becomes manifest; and as the range of accommodation gets smaller and the possibility of correction less, more of the facultative hypermetropia becomes absolute. In early life, unless the error is unusually large, the accommodative power can correct it all and none of the hypermetropia is absolute; after 65 practically all of it becomes absolute, and therefore apparent.

CLINICAL PATHOLOGY

The hypermetropic eye is typically small, not only in its antero-posterior diameter but also in all directions. The cornea is small, and since the lens varies little this structure is relatively large, thus making the anterior chamber shallow. The eye is therefore of the type which is predisposed to closed-angle glaucoma, a point which should be remembered in the administration of drugs which dilate the pupil. In the extreme degrees of the condition developmental aberrations, such as colobomata, microphthalmos, may be present.

Ophthalmoscopically the fundus may have a characteristic appearance which, although by no means confined to the hypermetropic eye, occurs much more commonly in the higher degrees of this refractive condition than in any other. The retina appears to have a peculiar sheen — a reflex effect — the so-called *shot-silk retina*. The optic disc sometimes has a characteristic appearance which may resemble an optic neuritis (*pseudo-papillitis*). It assumes a dark greyish red colour with indistinct and sometimes irregular margins, the haziness of which may be accentuated by a grey areola around it or by grey radial striations emanating from it, while an inferior crescent is occasionally present. The condition is congenital, its ophthalmoscopic appearance is largely accentuated by reflex disturbances, and it involves no appreciable diminution of vision. The vascular reflexes may be accentuated and the vessels may show undue tortuosity and abnormal branchings; such an eye should be watched lest the diagnosis has been mistaken.

It sometimes happens that the face is asymmetrical, in which case the most markedly hypermetropic eye is usually found on the side which shows the least perfect development. This asymmetry is often seen in the eye itself, for the condition of hypermetropia is more often than not associated with astigmatism.

The macula is generally situated further from the disc than is usual in the emmetropic eye, and the cornea is more decidedly decentred; the visual axis consequently cuts the cornea considerably to the inside of the optic axis, thus making a large positive angle alpha (Fig. 4.4). This in its most marked degrees frequently gives rise to an apparent divergent squint, a condition the opposite of that found in myopia.

CLINICAL FEATURES

Symptoms

As we might expect, because accommodation occupies a crucial position in the ability to

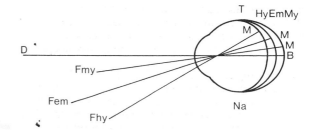

Fig. 4.4 The size of the angle alpha.
T, temporal side; Na, nasal side; DB, the optical axis; FM, the visual axis, cutting at the nodal point, N. The varying positions of the macula in hypermetropia (Hy), emmetropia (Em) and myopia (My) determine the fact that the angle α in the hypermetropic eye (DNFhy) is greater than that in the emmetropic eye (DNFem), while in the myopic eye it is smaller (DNFmy).

overcome the effects of hypermetropia, the principal symptom of the condition is blurring of vision for close work. However, this statement needs qualifying. First, if so much accommodation is available in relation to the degree of hypermetropia, as for example in a young subject with a low degree of error, there may be no symptoms; indeed, the condition may be unsuspected. Secondly, symptoms may not be present in the early years but may appear pari passu with the decline of accommodation later in life. Again, they may come on at times of physical debility or emotional stress. If the accommodation available is quite inadequate to cope with the degree of hypermetropia then blurring of vision may occur not only for close work but also for distance. This last condition can occur in the young with marked degrees of hypermetropia but it also affects all hypermetropes once they reach an age when they have little accommodation left.

In any event, if symptoms do occur, the greatest difficulty occurs in looking at near objects, for here an additional amount of accommodation is required, and starting with a certain amount of deficit the hypermetrope is put in a disadvantageous position. Thus an emmetrope requires 3 dioptres of accommodation in order to read at 33 cm but a hypermetrope of 2 dioptres will have to exercise 5 dioptres to get the same optical effect.

Obviously the trouble will be aggravated by

long-continued application to close work; for example, after reading for some time the vision becomes blurred and indistinct, and only recovers when the patient ceases temporarily and rests his ciliary muscle.

Symptoms of eye-strain are therefore frequent in these conditions. The headaches and the general disturbances to which this may give rise have been already described, and it has been explained that the syndrome is due to the excessive accommodation and to the forced dissociation between it and convergence. The condition is one of *accommodative asthenopia*. In the case of a seamstress or a compositor who works over a long day, or a student who reads closely for many hours on end, the strain thrown on the ciliary muscle is similar to that imposed upon the leg muscles in a correspondingly long and forced march; and it is not surprising in those whose physical or nervous condition is not of the best, or whose surroundings, from bad ventilation or other causes, are not conducive to rapid recovery from muscular fatigue, that the symptoms of distress thus produced may be considerable.

If this state of affairs persists, more definite results may ensue. Temporary *failure of the ciliary muscle* to maintain contraction may result in obscurations of vision, or the opposite condition of *excessive accommodation* or even *spasm of the ciliary muscle* may produce a condition of artificial myopia. The desire for accommodation in excess of convergence leads to a dissociation of muscle balance, and the struggle to maintain binocular vision in these circumstances leads to further strain. Sometimes, particularly in the young, if the fusion faculty is defective or ill-developed, the advantages of binocular vision are abandoned in favour of the more obvious advantages of clear vision; one eye only — usually the better eye — is used to the neglect of the other, and an accommodative *convergent squint* is produced.

Finally it should be mentioned that occasionally hypermetropes of moderate or high degree may present because of a history of holding a book too close to the eyes, a habit more suggestive of the opposite refraction, myopia. By doing so the hypermetrope gets enlargement of the retinal image which compensates for its indistinctness.

Treatment

It may be taken as a general rule that, if the error is small, the visual acuity is normal, and the patient is in good health and complaining of no symptoms of accommodative asthenopia and showing no anomalies of muscle balance, treatment of hypermetropia is unnecessary; but if any of these conditions are violated, spectacles should be prescribed.

In young children below the age of 6 or 7, some degree of hypermetropia is physiological, and a correction need be given only if the error is high or if strabismus is present. In those between 6 and 16, especially when they are working strenuously at school, smaller errors may require correction. If an accommodative squint is present, or definite symptoms of subnormal visual acuity or ocular fatigue appear, any error should receive attention. If a suspicion of strain is suggested by more indefinite signs — a complaint of headache or unaccountable lassitude, a dislike of work and an early tiring after it is begun, rubbing the eyes and complaints of their itching, or a combination of these — an examination should be made. If the error is greater than 3 dioptres, it is probably wise to advise that correcting lenses be worn constantly; if below, it may suffice that they be used for near work alone.

In all these cases the examination should be conducted under a cycloplegic. As a general rule, in ordering the spectacles, 1 dioptre is deducted from the objective findings to allow for the tone of the ciliary muscle. This rule may not always be adhered to in cases of strabismus, when slightly less may be deducted; but in younger

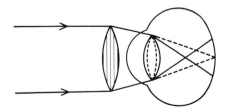

Fig. 4.5 Artificial myopia produced by too full a hypermetropic correction. The dotted lens and rays indicate the optical state measured with accommodation more relaxed. When accommodation is more active, myopia is produced.

children below the age of 6, especially if the error is high, more should be deducted. At this age subjective tests are not available or are of little value, and 1.5 or 2 dioptres can well be deducted.

In older children, as close an approximation to this generalisation as possible should be attempted, and far and away the wisest routine is to base the correction on a subjective test carried out after cycloplegia has worn off. This is, of course, time-consuming, but it is much better to do so than to order a child a lens by rule of thumb which then turns out to be too strong, blurring the distance vision because of the artificial myopia produced (see Fig. 4.5). It is usually safest to prescribe the fullest correction consistent with good vision which he will accept. If the symptoms indicate that a determined attempt should be made to reduce his refraction as nearly as possible to emmetropia, as for example in cases of squint, weak atropine may be given every second day for a week or two until the ciliary muscle becomes accustomed to its new conditions of work.

It is important to remember that in all these children hypermetropia tends normally to diminish with growth, and consequently the refraction usually approaches emmetropia gradually until adolescence is passed. Children should thus be examined once a year and their spectacles changed if necessary, lest a lens which is overcorrecting their error may induce an artificial myopia. For this reason it is the rule that spectacles of progressively diminishing strength are required, until finally, in many cases, they may safely be discarded altogether.

In older people the advisability of wearing spectacles depends upon the degree of vision and the symptoms. Young adults with an error less than 3 dioptres who have normal vision and *are without symptoms* should rarely be corrected. Conversely, as is the case with children, the decline of accommodative power in middle and later life makes lenses of gradually increasing strength necessary. An adult with 3 dioptres of hypermetropia may be comfortable at 25 but at 35 the additional accommodation required for near work will begin to tax his declining power and he may require correcting lenses for reading; in such a case, if the spectacles do not improve

distant vision and there are no symptoms of asthenopia, they need not be worn constantly but only for close work. But in later life, when his accommodation has gone and all the hypermetropia has become absolute, distance spectacles also will be required if he desires to see well; if he does not, of course, they are not necessary.

If complaint is made only of visual symptoms and the refraction is not done under a cycloplegic, it is usually sufficient to order the strongest lenses with which maximal visual acuity can be obtained with both eyes: this will be found to be slightly higher (about 0.25 D) than the correction which each eye will tolerate separately. If circumstances indicate that a cycloplegic should be used, there is some difference of opinion as to the amount of the total hypermetropia which should be corrected. It might be thought that it would be advisable to correct the whole of the hypermetropia and thus place the patient in the position of the emmetrope; but it must be remembered that such a course frequently results in the patient being unable to see at all efficiently whenever he removes or is deprived of his spectacles. It would seem advisable, therefore, to undercorrect the total hypermetropia. On the other hand, it frequently happens that the headaches, the asthenopia, and the referred symptoms return if a part of the hypermetropia remains uncorrected; we are thus faced with a dilemma, the solution of which frequently calls for no little judgment.

In such cases it is quite inadequate to be guided by hard and fast rules, such, for example, as the deduction from the total hypermetropia of 1 dioptre if it is estimated under atropine, or 0.50 if cyclopentolate is employed. Donders advised that the lens ordered should correspond to the manifest hypermetropia plus one-quarter of the latent, a suggestion which has received very general acceptance. The most practical method is to consider each case individually on its own merits, to determine the manifest hypermetropia and order lenses on this basis, correcting the patient as nearly to his total hypermetropia as possible, while remaining within the limits consistent with comfort and good vision, at the same time paying regard to his age, to the state of his accommodation, his symptoms, his muscle balance, his general physical and nervous state and his vocation.

The younger a patient is, the more active is his accommodation, and the more we may undercorrect. The greater the latent hypermetropia, that is the greater the residual accommodation, the more we undercorrect. On the other hand, if his symptoms of eye-strain are marked, especially if indicated by mental or general physical state, we correct as much of the total hypermetropia as possible, trying as far as we can to relieve the accommodation. When there is spasm of the accommodation we correct the whole of the error, as also when there is a tendency to a latent convergent squint, with a view in the first case to forcing rest upon the ciliary muscle and in the second to relieving convergence indirectly by relieving accommodation. In both cases we insist that the spectacles are worn constantly. Conversely, if there is a latent divergent squint we undercorrect in the hope that, by stimulating accommodation, we may stimulate convergence. On the whole, if the patient leads a sedentary and studious life, we tend to correct more of the hypermetropia than we would if he had little to do with the study or the desk and lived mainly out-of-doors.

Generally, the more fully the error is corrected, the better the result, always provided that the lenses are compatible with good vision; but if the amount which we would like to give is refused on this account, it is usually well to temporise. As a compromise in a difficult case, it may be well to undercorrect considerably at first, and to strengthen the lenses at intervals of a few months until the full correction is comfortably borne; or it may help to advise weaker lenses than are correct for distance and the full correction for close work.

Finally, it is to be remembered that the symptoms of accommodative asthenopia frequently have a significance deeper than their superficial consideration would indicate. The delicate adjustment of the eye serves as an index of the general constitutional state, and the onset of fatigue here should suggest its imminence elsewhere: the eye-strain is a symptom of general strain. Treatment, if it is to be adequate, should not be confined to the correction of the optical apparatus alone, but should include an inquiry into the general physical and nervous state and, if necessary, should involve a reorganisation of the habits and activities of the individual so that he lives within the limits of his capabilities. Thus typical symptoms come on in the child starting school, in the youth studying for an examination, in the girl leaving the comparative ease of home life and setting out in business, in the adult in periods of overwork and anxiety, and in them all in states of physical debility and mental depression. Interpreted in this light, the development of failure to compensate for hypermetropia may be the means of calling attention to the existence of a more deeply seated trouble before it would have otherwise enforced recognition — it is an 'early symptom'; and if its true significance is neglected and treatment is confined to the ocular condition alone, sufficient relief and encouragement may be given to the patient to make it possible for him to carry on until a breakdown of a more serious nature may be unavoidable.

Surgery for high hypermetropia is in its infancy. Thermokeratoplasty, in which corneal curvature is increased by appropriately sited burns, produces such variable effects as to vitiate its widespread acceptability at present. The use of the Excimer and Holmium lasers is under investigation.

5. Myopia

Myopia ($\mu\acute{v}\omega$), I close; $\overset{\backprime}{\omega}\psi$, the eye), or short sight, is that form of refractive error wherein parallel rays of light come to a focus in front of the sentient layer of the retina when the eye is at rest; the eye is thus relatively too large, and the condition is the opposite to that of hypermetropia.

The term myopia was introduced from the habit which short-sighted people frequently have of half-closing the lids when looking at distant objects so that they may gain the advantages of a stenopaeic opening (see p. 145). Occasionally a term in conformity with other refractive designations — *hypometropia* — has appeared in American writings. The first satisfactory definition of the condition was stated by Kepler in 1611, and Plempius (1632) first examined the myopic eye anatomically and attributed the condition to a lengthening of its posterior part. Donders (1866) established its pathological basis, and detailed its clinical manifestations.

AETIOLOGY

In the great majority of cases, certainly in the higher degrees, myopia is *axial*, that is it is due to an increase in the antero-posterior diameter of the eye.

Curvature myopia may be associated with an increase in the curvature of the cornea or one or both surfaces of the lens. An increased curvature of the cornea not infrequently occurs, but it is usually evident as an astigmatic rather than a spherical error. Small deviations from the normal are common, since the radius of the normal cornea has been found to vary within the limits of 7 to 8.5 mm, and these may be of considerable importance since a variation of 1 mm results in a refractive change of 6 D. This factor has no influence on the occurrence of the usual axial type of myopia, for in this condition the cornea is usually flatter than normal. Pronounced cases of a true increase of corneal curvature only occur in diseased conditions, such as ectasias or conical cornea.

Increase of lenticular curvature is also rare; in fact, corresponding to the state of the cornea, the lens is usually flat in typical axial myopia tending, as it were, to correct the error. Conditions of anterior and posterior lenticonus occur, which may involve a marked degree of myopia. The curvature of the surfaces is also increased whenever the suspensory ligament is relaxed, as occurs in spasm of the accommodation or in the most extreme degrees when the ligament is ruptured and the lens dislocated.

As far as *index myopia* is concerned, a change of refractive index of the aqueous or vitreous can never be so great as to exercise any appreciable effect. On the other hand, changes in the lens can certainly induce myopia. It is possible that a decrease of the refractive index of the cortex plays a part in diabetic myopia. An increased refractivity of the lens nucleus is responsible for the myopia found with incipient cataract; indeed, the lens may not go opaque but its nucleus may simply become more and more hyper-refringent pari passu with which there develops a progressive myopia.

In *buphthalmos*, a condition of congenital or infantile glaucoma due to defective development, the whole eye is enlarged, and the antero-posterior diameter greatly increased. The axial myopia which is produced in this way, however, is much less than might be expected, for it is counteracted to a large extent by the flatness of the cornea and lens and the displacement backwards of the latter.

We have seen that in the newborn the normal eye is hypermetropic and that, as age progresses and growth proceeds, this tends to diminish. In some cases the hypermetropia remains, in others emmetropia is reached and development becomes stabilised at this point, while in some the tendency progresses and a greater or less degree of myopia results. The period of growth is therefore the crucial one from the standpoint of myopia.

The *aetiology of axial myopia* has given rise to a very large amount of speculation and controversy, and numberless theories have been put forward at various times to explain its incidence.

The classical view is that two types of the condition exist. First there is the group of cases which are physiological variants of the normal such as are found in any large biological series (see Fig. 3.17); this we refer to as *simple myopia*. Secondly, so far as the higher degrees are concerned, the condition is clearly of a more serious nature determined by heredity or post-natal factors; this is *pathological (or progressive) myopia*. Simple myopia is a condition of limited progression, whereas pathological myopia may increase apace, to such a degree that it merits consideration as a medical entity on its own.

There is some support for a subdivision of the condition known as simple myopia, into *physiological* and *intermediate*. The precise defining criteria are not universally applicable but generally speaking in physiological myopia the ocular components are all within the normal distribution range and there are no typical fundus changes. The development of early signals of globe enlargement such as a temporal, not inferior, crescent and perhaps supertraction of the disc is quoted as justifying a more severe category–intermediate myopia.

The aetiology of pathological myopia is obscure; it used to be generally considered that the main factor in the determination of this type of myopia was weakness of the sclera and its consequent inability to withstand the intra-ocular pressure without giving way and stretching. It was generally held that the changes in the fundus were due to this stretching; but it seems more likely that they are usually due to a genetic developmental defect which affects the whole of the posterior segment of the eye. The changes do not vary in degree with the myopia, they may be extensive in eyes which have a shorter axial length than the normal emmetropic eye, and they do not usually appear in marked degree, at any rate until the third, fourth, or even fifth decade, long after the period of active elongation has passed.

Whatever the cause it is probable that the primary fault is an aberration of development. This is seen in the fact that the condition, while rarely congenital, may come on very early in life, is typically hereditary and to some extent racial. Myopia may be said to develop only during the period of active growth, for elongation of an eye which has remained of normal dimensions up to the age of 25 is rare. The eye shares with the brain the peculiarity of having a precocious growth, for at the age of 4 the brain is 84% of its full size, the eye 78%, and the rest of the body only 21%. After this both eye and brain increase slowly in size until at about 20 years the adult dimensions have been reached. It has been suggested that myopia results from a continuation of this precocity, owing to a failure of the arresting influence to act. The nature of this influence is not definitely known, and which tissue is primarily at fault is also obscure. Many of the older writers considered that in the sclera lies the key to the problem and, since one of the controlling factors which regulate the activities of fibroblastic cells (for of such the sclera is composed) is the endocrine system, more especially the pituitary body, myopia has been compared with such a condition as acromegaly. The frequent onset or, alternatively, the rapid progress of myopia at puberty has been considered to be significant in that at this period the endocrine system is unusually active and unstable.

On the other hand, more cogent arguments can be adduced that the primary fault lies in the retina. Experimental embryology has shown the very great influence this tissue has upon the surrounding structures. When one remembers that it has been shown that a transplanted optic vesicle may convert the ectodermal structures of the abdominal wall into a lens, it can be easily conceded that the retina can exert a profound influence on the tissues in contact with it. The retina develops very considerably in post-natal life, almost doubling its area, and it is quite conceivable that, as Vogt contended, the axial length of the eye accommodates itself to this tissue; when the retina grows more rapidly and extensively than normally, the sclera becomes stretched and myopia results. On the same basis it may be argued that the myopic changes in the fundus are essentially hereditarily determined developmental aberrations — an early breakdown after a precocious growth — showing a considerable similarity to abiotic degenerations at the macula.

However this may be, it seems beyond question that, in addition to the primarily developmental fault which must be postulated in the aetiology of myopia in its higher degrees, *adjuvant factors* may have some influence in its progress, the most important of which is physical debility; even an emmetropic young adult may develop several dioptres of myopia after a long exhausting illness.

It is difficult to assess the importance of near work in the aetiology. Statistics show that the proportion of myopes increases rapidly and steadily during the years of school and university life, and is common in those occupations in which the eyes are assiduously used for study or the close inspection of minute objects. These statistics, however, are in many ways open to question, for the school age happens to be the age at which myopia normally develops and, just as the short-sighted child will rather sit and read at home than join his fellows at play outside, a myope will choose preferentially an occupation which involves close work. In addition, it is to be remembered that the condition does occur in the illiterate and in those who do little or no close work, while the highest degrees are as common among them as among the better educated, among some primitive as among cultured peoples. Moreover, large numbers of those who are exposed to close work in the most adverse conditions never develop myopia. On the whole it would seem reasonably certain that the influence of close work is secondary and incidental in the aetiology of a condition which is essentially predetermined and constitutional

and not environmental, effective — if at all — only insofar as it is associated with bad ocular and general hygiene and lack of adequate facilities for normal and healthy development.

A very large number of further theories has been suggested. Excess of accommodation has been indicted, in that it raises the intra-ocular pressure — which is untrue — or that the ciliary muscle pulls upon the choroid. Convergence has been blamed, acting either by the muscles pressing directly against the globe, or by their obstructing the outflow of the vortex veins; some have regarded the recti as the offending muscles, others the superior oblique. Congestion has been said to be conditioned by manual labour, especially when stooping, while the shape of the orbits has been called into question, since it is said to influence the shape of the eyes or, by increasing the inter-pupillary distance, to increase the effort necessary for convergence and thus influence the degree of muscular pressure upon the eye. These, and many more: most of them more remarkable for their ingenuity than their value.

For an up-to-date discussion of theories of the aetiology of myopia consult *The Myopias* by B. J. Curtin (Harper & Row 1985).

The progress of myopia

We have seen that myopia is very uncommon at birth, although in certain cases it is congenital and in many of these cases the condition is static. Some are associated with prematurity.

As has been noted, a change in refraction in the form of decreasing hypermetropia is the usual condition in childhood, and in most of the cases destined to end up in the category we have called simple myopia the change does not lead to symptoms until the early teens, although it may pre-date this in some subjects. Thereafter such cases generally progress to the level of 5 or 6 dioptres over the succeeding few years, finally stabilising at about the age of 21 or slightly younger in women.

It is very uncommon but far from unknown for myopia to commence after adolescence is over. Here one must be careful to eliminate other causes for the myopic condition such as early diabetes and, of course, the presentation of the myopic state at this period of life may not absolutely indicate its origin at that time — it may have commenced earlier but was simply ignored until then. If the error progresses rapidly in early youth, it is less likely to become stationary, and may finally amount to 20, 25, or even 30 dioptres; in these cases the period of most rapid progression is usually from 15 to 20 years. After this the process usually tends to slow down, but in the later decades of life in the higher degrees of the defect, degenerative changes tend to occur so that vision may steadily deteriorate until at about 60 virtual blindness may ensue. In the less degrees, the tendency to hypermetropia owing to the changes in the lens which occur in old age may appreciably diminish the myopia.

Clinical types

It is clinically impossible to draw a distinct line of demarcation between the types of myopia in the early stages. In general, however, it may be said that no pathological changes are evident in physiological myopia while characteristic changes appear in the other types. In both physiological and intermediate varieties, the great majority of eyes remain healthy and visual acuity can be corrected to the accepted standard with the appropriate lenses. In pathological myopia the earliest signs of deterioration may be an unaccountable loss of visual acuity, an accentuated foveal reflex and slight degenerative changes in the vitreous, to be eventually followed by the characteristic severe changes in the retina. Nevertheless it is to be remembered that these are not necessarily comparable with the degree of myopia for they may be marked when the myopia is relatively slight and absent when it is gross.

CLINICAL PATHOLOGY

The elongation of the eye which results in pathological myopia is almost entirely confined to the posterior pole, for the anterior half of the globe is relatively normal (Fig. 5.1). The entire eye, however, is obviously large and prominent, and when it is turned strongly inward so that the equatorial region appears in the outer part of the palpebral fissure the flatness of its curvature is obvious. The anterior chamber is deep, and the pupil usually large and somewhat sluggish. The absence of any stimulus to accommodate may

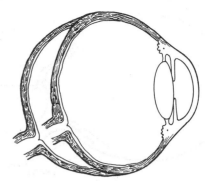

Fig. 5.1 The deformation of the eye in myopia. An emmetropic and a myopic eye compared. It is seen that the deformation affects the posterior part of the globe only, while the anterior part is normal. (After Heine.)

allow the ciliary muscle, especially its circular part, to become atrophied. The posterior segment of the sclera is thinned, and in extreme degrees may be reduced to a quarter or less of its normal thickness.

Ophthalmoscopically, the main changes observed are the generalised atrophy of the retina and choroid, the myopic crescent at the disc, the disturbances at the macula, the occurrence of a posterior staphyloma, the almost invariable appearance of cystoid degeneration at the ora serrata, and the presence of Weiss's reflex streak.

The changes in the choroid and retina are marked (Plate 1). The pigmented layer of the retina loses much of its pigment, so that the fundus is tigroid and the choroidal vessels are well seen. Patches of choroidal atrophy may appear in the fundus, especially in the posterior region, leaving white areas often surrounded by pigment, and the process may result in haemorrhages; finally, an accumulation of large white patches associated with splotches of pigment may be scattered widely over the posterior part of the fundus. At the macula such an atrophic patch is common, and this is accompanied by the abolition of central vision. A similarly disastrous result is produced by the appearance of a dark pigmented area in this region (the Förster–Fuchs fleck, Plate 2). This is relatively rare and may occur suddenly, when it is probably caused by proliferation of the pigmentary epithelium associated with an intra-choroidal haemorrhage or thrombosis.

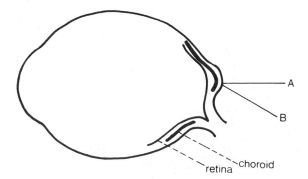

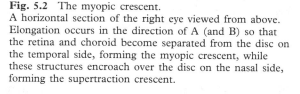

Fig. 5.2 The myopic crescent.
A horizontal section of the right eye viewed from above.
Elongation occurs in the direction of A (and B) so that
the retina and choroid become separated from the disc on
the temporal side, forming the myopic crescent, while
these structures encroach over the disc on the nasal side,
forming the supertraction crescent.

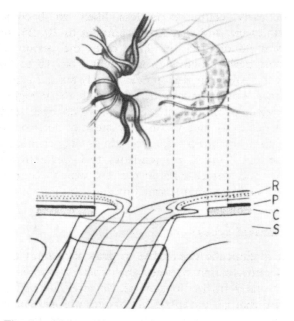

Fig. 5.3 The myopic crescent and supertraction. The
clinical appearances are seen above and the corresponding
structural changes below. On the left is the phenomenon
of supertraction; on the right a myopic crescent consisting
of an area of bare sclera surrounded by a crescent in
which the choroidal structure is visible. R, retina; P,
pigmentary epithelium; C, choroid; S, sclera.

Small dark spots resembling haemorrhages are
relatively common near the macula, but since
they sometimes undergo no change for an
indefinite time these are probably bunches of
dilated choroidal capillaries or aneurysmal
dilatations.

At the disc the elongation tends to produce the
characteristic crescent. The bulging backwards of
the posterior pole (A, Fig. 5.2) results in a
separation of the retina and choroid from the
temporal margin of the disc, leaving an atrophied
part through which the sclera is seen as a white
area (the *myopic crescent*), while on the nasal 'side
the retina extends over the edge of the disc, thus
blurring its margin and conditioning the so-called
supertraction crescent (Fig. 5.3). The myopic
crescent is usually temporal, but it may run as
an annular ring all the way round the disc (see
Plate 2). In the higher degrees the whole of the
posterior pole of the eye may herniate backwards
as a *posterior staphyloma*. This is a rare
phenomenon recognised ophthalmoscopically by
the sudden kinking of the retinal vessels as they
dip over its edges in the same way as they dip
into a glaucomatous cup. Pathologically, such a
state results in gross atrophic changes, and
optically, of course, its effect is disastrous.
Around the periphery of the retina, cystoid and
other degenerative changes are so common as to
be regarded as almost universal.

These changes by no means always run pari
passu with the degree of myopia, and very high
errors may exist with few gross lesions in the
fundus. In all cases the condition of the choroid
is one of atrophy with no evidence of
inflammation, while the retinal changes are
similarly degenerative. Similar mechanical and
degenerative changes occur in the vitreous.
Detachment of the vitreous may occur at the
posterior pole, and the reflex streak described by
Weiss may be seen ophthalmoscopically on its
posterior face in front of the retina; the vitreous
itself frequently liquefies, obvious muscae
volitantes are almost invariable, and large floaters
are common.

Complications usually take the form of tears and
haemorrhages in the retina, and its more or less
extensive detachment: this may be associated
with trauma but, on the other hand, may occur
spontaneously, probably most frequently
associated with the degenerative areas in the
periphery giving way on traction by the

framework of the vitreous, which tends to adhere to it most closely in this region. Some loss of vision may also be determined by the degenerative changes in the vitreous, while similar processes in the lens may lead to the formation of opacities, the most typical of which is posterior cortical in site.

OPTICAL CONDITION

In the myopic eye parallel rays of light come to a focus in front of the retina; the image on the retina is therefore made up of the circles of diffusion formed by the diverging beam [Fig. 5.4 (2)]. It follows that distant objects cannot be seen clearly; only divergent rays will meet at the retina, and thus, in order to be seen clearly, an object must be brought close to the eye, so that the rays coming from it are rendered sufficiently divergent [Fig. 5.4 (3)]. This point, the furthest at which objects can be seen distinctly, is called the *far point* (*punctum remotum*). In the emmetropic eye it is at infinity; in the myopic eye it is a finite distance away, and the higher the myopia, the shorter the distance. This distance is thus a measure of the degree of myopia; if the far point is 1 metre from the eye, there is 1 dioptre of myopia; if it is 2 metres away, there is 0.5 dioptres, and so on.

If they are to be brought to a focus at all, parallel rays coming from distant objects must be rendered more divergent, and this we can do by placing a diverging lens in front of the eye [Fig. 5.4 (4)]. If the far point is 1 metre away, a lens of the strength −1 D will render parallel rays as divergent as if they came from this point, and therefore the weakest concave lens with which normal distant vision is attained is a measure of the degree of myopia. To some small extent the myope compensates for his poor visual acuity, for, since the nodal point is further away from the retina, the image here, as is seen in Figure 4.2, will be appreciably larger than it would be in the emmetropic eye.

There may be an apparent convergent squint due to the presence of a negative angle alpha.

CLINICAL FEATURES

Symptoms

Blurred distance vision is the most prominent symptom of myopia. Where good visual acuity at a distance is required, even the smaller errors are

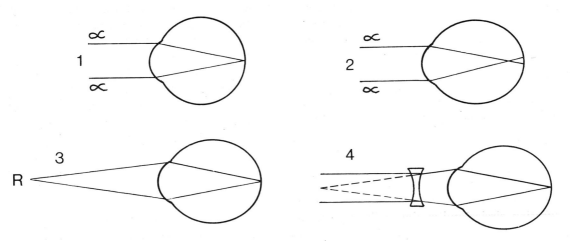

Fig. 5.4 Myopia.
(1) An emmetropic eye, parallel rays being focused upon the retina.
(2) A myopic eye, parallel rays being focused in front of the retina.
(3) When looking at a near object (R), the divergent rays are focused upon the retina. R is the far point.
(4) A similar divergence may be given to parallel rays by a concave lens so that a focus is again formed upon the retina. The degree of myopia is given by the reciprocal of the far point distance in metres, i.e. the power of the appropriate lens.

incapacitating, and if the myopia is present in any marked degree the visual disability is always serious.

Apart from the physical disability and the economic disadvantages which this necessarily entails, such a condition usually reacts upon the psychological outlook of the individual. This is most strikingly seen in children, especially in short-sighted children who are allowed to grow up with the error uncorrected. They develop in a limited world wherein they are at a considerable disadvantage in comparison with others, a handicap which may entail a seeming limitation of intelligence and a curtailment of interests which are frequently put down to stupidity and backwardness or to naughtiness, while they are really due to the physical defect. When the error is adequately corrected, these considerations do not necessarily apply; and even when it is not, in many instances interests suitable to their case and other compensatory factors more than make up for their disability. But as a general rule in these cases, much that is going on in the world — especially the more subtle things — escapes them; avoiding outdoor sports and prone to introspection, and finding free intercourse with their fellows difficult, they frequently tend to grow up with distinct mental habits and peculiarities.

Curiously, in its slighter degrees short sight may often appear to be an advantage. Accustomed to defective vision from the time when he began to look upon the world intelligently, the myope frequently fails to recognise his limitation. Especially when his close attention is required largely for near work, as so often happens in the conditions of civilised life, he accepts as normal and neglects the blurring of distant objects. In middle life, when his accommodation fails, he has the added advantage that he does not require spectacles for reading; and in old age, as his contracting pupil cuts down the diffusion circles and as the senile changes in his lens bring on a relative hypermetropia, he is in the happy position of finding his vision gradually improving. And so it happens that at 80 he is the envy of his hypermetropic contemporaries and the pride of his bespectacled presbyopic children. In the smaller degrees of error especially, symptoms of *eye-strain* are evident, although generally not so obviously as in the case of the hypermetrope. The excess of convergence for close work disorientates the accommodation which is not required. The physiological impulse for the two related functions to work together may have one of two opposite results. The accommodation may attempt to equal the convergence, thus inducing ciliary spasm and artificially increasing the amount of myopia. Alternatively and more frequently, the attempt at convergence is given up, its latent insufficiency gives rise to the troubles of muscular imbalance, until finally the advantages of binocular vision are abandoned, one eye alone is relied upon and the other deviates outwards, the usual apparent convergent strabismus giving place to a true divergent squint.

Complications

The situation may not be nearly so happy for the high myope in later life. If atrophic retinal patches appear, actual scotomata result, a complication which is seen in its most incapacitating form when the macular region is affected and central vision is lost. The degenerated and liquefied vitreous abounds in muscae volitantes and floating opacities, and these, throwing abnormally large images upon the retina, although their actual significance is small, cause a great deal of annoyance and anxiety to the patient. Matters may tend to progress slowly and relentlessly, the patient all the while never using his eyes with comfort until finally no useful vision may remain, or until the occurrence of a sudden calamity, such as a gross macular lesion or a retinal detachment, brings about a more dramatic crisis.

Prognosis

The prognosis of myopia depends very largely upon the age of the patient. Any degree occurring in a child under the age of 4 should be regarded as potentially serious requiring observation. Above this age, and certainly above the age of 8 or 10, low degrees up to −6 D may be looked upon with less alarm; care should be exercised especially about the time of puberty, and if the age of 21 is passed without serious progression the condition may be expected to remain stationary and the prognosis may be taken as good. In the higher degrees the prognosis should always be guarded; it must be based on the appearance of the fundus and the acuity of the vision after correction. In all cases the possibility of a sudden haemorrhage or a retinal detachment should be borne in mind.

Prophylaxis

In view of the hereditary nature of both myopia and the degenerative conditions asssociated with it, the evidence is sufficient to warrant the adoption of prophylactic eugenic measures. There need be no restraint on marriage and procreation among simple myopes; but a parent with degenerative myopia should be warned that any offspring will be liable to the same disability according to the laws of recessive Mendelian inheritance. Two highly myopic adults with degenerated fundi should never — from the medical point of view — have children. The children of such parents should be closely supervised from their earliest years, and if an increase in refractivity appears to evolve more rapidly than would be normally expected they should be treated as if they were 'pathological' myopes, particularly if the early clinical signs suggestive of degenerative myopia appear.

Treatment

The optical correction

Although there seems little scientific justification for the claim commonly advanced that the constant wearing of meticulously correct spectacles prevents the progress of the myopia or preserves vision, nothing but good can accrue from the elimination of visual strain and the proper training of visual habits, particularly in children. Their value is also obvious in assisting mental and educational development by opening out the world to their observation. After the growing period has passed and visual habits have

been established, if for any reason, aesthetic or otherwise, the spectacles are not worn continuously, and if a blurred world is accepted without the exercise of constant visual strain to overcome the disability, it is probable that no medical harm results.

In cases of *low degrees* of myopia (up to −6 D) in young subjects, while the defect should never be overcorrected, a full correction should be ordered and advised for constant use. By giving him his full correction, we place the patient in the position of the emmetrope, and accommodation and convergence resume their natural balance. It should be impressed upon him that, in the matter of near work, his glasses are not intended to improve his vision but to make him read at the proper distance and bring his eyes into their normal relationships. In adults above that age receiving spectacles for the first time, it will frequently be found that the ciliary muscle is not equal to the unaccustomed task of accommodating efficiently so that a lens of slightly lower power (1 or 2 D) may be prescribed for reading, especially if engaged in to any great extent. Above the age of 40, of course, when accommodation fails physiologically, a weaker glass for near work is essential.

At various times public attention is drawn to night myopia — a refractive change occurring in reduced illumination which is very variable in degree between different subjects but rarely amounts to more than 0.5 D. Its cause is probably multiple, cone rod shift in the retina, pupillary dilatation, ciliary muscle activity, etc. In those few cases where it is felt there is a serious impairment of night vision an appropriately increased myopic correction should be given.

The devotees of muscle, internal or extrinsic, aetiologies of myopia have recommended optical corrections in accord with their theories. The excessive accommodation school advises bifocals, or perhaps spectacles for distance only. The overconvergence proponents favour the incorporation of base-in prisms. None of these has the universal support of properly controlled studies.

In the case of *high myopes*, the full correction can rarely be tolerated. A compromise must therefore be adopted, and, while we attempt to reduce the correction as little as is compatible with comfort for binocular vision, we prescribe the lens with which the greatest visual acuity is obtained without distress. The amount which has to be deducted usually varies from 1 to 3 D, but in the highest grades lenses even weaker than these will be found necessary. The correction needed, as indeed with any high refractive error, will in any case be heavy, and special dispensing techniques may be advisable (high-index glass or plastic lenses, lenticular forms, etc., see p. 200). In those high myopes who are over 20 years of age, weaker lenses for near work are found even more necessary than in the lower degrees of error. In the most pronounced cases, especially where much pathological change is present in the fundus, little benefit may accrue from the use of any spectacle lens. So far as reading is concerned, some of these patients are helped by compound telescopic spectacles, which reduce the field of vision but magnify considerably (see p. 279), while others appear to get about more comfortably unaided. In attempting to look at near objects, they see most efficiently by bringing the object close up to the eye in order that they may obtain the benefit of an enlarged image.

Contact lenses have their most important role in the optical correction of myopia. They have undoubted cosmetic advantage for simple myopes, and in the much higher degrees considerably superior optical benefits accrue. As they move with the eye, contact lenses are free of the aberrations which are the unavoidable optical defects of thick spectacle lenses.

There are many assertions in the literature as to the beneficial effect of contact lens wear on the progression of myopia. It was certainly observed in hard lens wearers that their prescriptive power seemed to require less or less frequent change than in spectacle wearers. This was attributed to corneal flattening or perhaps overpowerful initial prescribing. Less has been heard of this phenomenon recently, and it seems not to apply to soft lens wearers in any case.

A myope wearing a full contact lens correction has a higher requirement for accommodation as compared with a spectacle wearer, a fact which seems to contradict the 'excess accommodation' theory of myopia, if contact lens wear does actually slow down myopic deterioration.

The *general hygienic treatment* is no less important than the provision of spectacles. Particularly is this the case with children. The general health should be maintained with an abundance of fresh air, exercise and wholesome food, especially protein.

Visual hygiene is also of importance. During close work the illumination should be good and adequately arranged, the posture should be easy and natural, the clarity of print should be carefully supervised and undue ocular fatigue should be avoided. Especially is this so in children in whom progressive myopia should call for unusual care. It would seem reasonable to suggest that, so long as the corrected visual acuity is adequate, proper care of visual hygiene is maintained and the general health is good, education will not be seriously curtailed. The amount of work should be adjusted to the general physical and mental development of the child rather than to the degree of the myopia. It is certainly the case that the regime of many modern schools imposes too much application to books upon young children at an age when they require all their available vitality for physical growth and development, a generalisation which applies particularly to girls at the age of puberty. In the exigencies of our artificial civilisation, early application to work with neglect of open-air pursuits may be an advantage in some respects, but it is an advantage sometimes gained at the cost of the retention of good vision in the middle years of life in the high myope.

In the choice of a career, if it seems possible that progressive myopic changes will involve visual deterioration in later life, it is obviously economically unwise to choose work requiring constant study of books or figures and better that interest should be diverted to a vocation of a less visually exacting nature, preferably one which can to some extent be continued if the central vision eventually fails.

In advanced and progressive cases, only when the corrected visual acuity is inadequate for ordinary reading need the child be sent to a school where special non-visual educational methods are employed. In such institutions an attempt should be made as far as possible to provide individual tuition whereby the cultivation of associative memory is made the first consideration, the sense of touch is relied upon as well as sight, and oral tuition takes the place of reading out of books, while the eyes are required only for looking at bold blackboard drawings and for large-typed and well-spaced printing.

Pharmacological therapy for myopia, apart from the speculative description of vitamins, includes the use of cycloplegic drugs, for example cyclopentolate 1% drops at night time, on the grounds that excessive accommodation in the myopic subject may be followed by inadequate relaxation of the ciliary muscle or incomplete return of the lens to its unaccommodated state. The value of such therapy in slowing or arresting the progression of myopia is as unconfirmed as its theoretical basis.

The manifest enlargement of eyes with congenital glaucoma has prompted the idea that ocular pressure reduction might help to prevent the ocular enlargement of the progressive myope; again this claim has not been substantiated nor have treatments, pharmacological or surgical, based on the theory, been proven to have any effect in arresting the progression of the condition.

Surgery for myopia

Listed here for the sake of completeness are some of the surgical procedures which are or have been suggested as helpful in the condition of myopia.

Alterations of corneal shape — flattening the corneal apex. This is the basis of the present popular surgical procedures. It is important for the refractionist to know something about it because myopes will often ask about what non-optical treatment is offered. The force with which to advise to proceed to surgery is given depends to some extent on the temperament of both examiner and the subject, and of course on the climate of expectation prevailing in the part of the world concerned.

A consensus view is that surgery should be considered only when there is real difficulty in or objection to wearing spectacles or contact lenses. This may consist of the distortion and minification of high minus spectacle corrections, physical intolerance of contact lenses or a working condition that proscribes both glasses and contact lenses. Ideally the subject has stable myopia, which usually means an age over 20 years, by which time the natural progression of myopia is likely to have ceased.

Whatever the indication, the procedures themselves fall into several categories related to the degree of myopia. For the lower degrees, up to −5 D (some put the limits much higher), radial keratotomy is the popular surgery. Several radial incisions (initially 16, now down to four) are made in the cornea between the periphery and its optical zone. The incisions are made almost down to the level of Descemet's membrane, and their length is gauged so as not to encroach on the pupil in average light circumstances, but glare may nevertheless be a problem post-operatively. Vision may also show fluctuations according to the period of day. There is in addition some evidence that the initial effect may very slowly increase, possibly because there is subtotal healing of the incisions, and this may proceed even over a period of years, converting what was originally a satisfactory reduction or abolition of myopia to an overcorrection.

However that may be, a 75% success rate is standard, with the remaining 25% showing a variety of complaints relating to vision and fluctuation, glare, over- or undercorrection, etc. Operative complications such as inadvertent perforation of the cornea, infection or cataract are very uncommon.

Intentional perforation of the cornea employed in the original operation by Sato, 60 or more years ago, led inevitably to corneal decompensation, and the procedure was abandoned until reintroduced as partial thickness incisions.

Once one is dealing with higher degrees of myopia, over −6 D and certainly over −8 D, more complex procedures are usually required if surgery is indicated.

Keratomileusis is the operation of corneal reshaping. In autoplastic myopic keratomileusis, useful up to about −15 degrees of error, the patient's own cornea is reshaped, a segment being removed frozen and then lathed to the appropriate shape before being reattached. It can produce excellent results but is not easy to perform.

In homoplastic surgery a keratectomy is followed by replacement with a pre-shaped lenticule supplied from a laboratory, or with a lenticule fashioned by the surgeon from a donor eye. Preserved donor lenticule is simply corneal stroma plus Bowman's membrane; there are no living cells in it, but when in position it becomes epithelialised and populated with host keratocytes. The use of donor tissue means that recovery is not as rapid as with the autoplastic technique, but higher degrees of myopia can be corrected up to 25 D.

Epikeratophakia is also useful for such high degrees, certainly up to 20 D. In this operation the epithelium is removed, a pocket is fashioned under the edge of the remaining epithelium and into this is inserted a cryolathed donor homograft. Preserved material may also be used.

Other techniques for changing corneal curvature involve the insertion of specifically shaped *inlays* into the stroma. Such inlays can correct up to −9 D of error. They are made of polysulphone, which is impervious, or of hydrogels. Results are only fair, often on account of the variability of the refractive change induced. The most recent innovative refractive alteration technique is the use of the Excimer laser operating at UV light of 193 nm. This effects ablation of concentric areas of the superficial stroma of the central cornea and in consequence the corneal surface flattens. Various keratoscopic devices are used to ensure accurate centration, and the laser energy power is computed according to the degree of error; the procedure may be painful as the epithelium is taken off. After prolonged animal experimentation human trials are now proceeding with so far very promising results.

Although doubts remain about the clarity of the cornea, which often appears hazy after treatment, and about the permanence of the refractive change usually induced, *photo-refractive keratectomy* (PRK) is certain to become widely practised, once the possibility of long-term complications has been excluded.

The stromal haze and the epithelial disturbance may initially give rise to glare and haloes round lights, as well as some impairment of contrast sensitivity.

Corrections to within ±1 D can be anticipated in myopes up to −6.00 D and, although more complex versions of the technology may be available for higher degrees (up to −20 D), predictability is erratic over −6.00 D. The fall off of effect is anticipated by aiming for an initial over-correction and it may be 3–6 months before the final refraction is reached. In any case accurate retinoscopy is often difficult in the early weeks after the procedure.

Several ingenious masking techniques are in use to vary the intensity of the treatment in different axes of the cornea so as to correct associated astigmatism. The introduction of wider laser beams masked axially, to treat hypermetropia, is under way.

Non-corneal interventions

Removal of the clear lens. An operative treatment for myopia suggested by Boerhaave in 1708 was popularised by Fukala in 1889. We have seen that the aphakic eye is normally strongly hypermetropic. If an eye with an axial myopia of about −24 degrees is deprived of its lens it will become emmetropic without any correcting lens, inasmuch as parallel rays of light will be focused upon the retina. Retinal images moreover will be larger than in emmetropia, but at the same time it must be remembered that all accommodation will be abolished; nevertheless the immediate result is frequently a dramatic improvement in visual efficiency. It has to be borne in mind, however, that the highly myopic eye is often a diseased eye and is by no means an ideal one to withstand surgical procedures. The two main dangers from which complications may arise are loss of vitreous, which is peculiarly fluid in the high myope, and the predisposition to retinal detachment. Both of these factors are much less likely to occur during modern extra-capsular as compared to classical intracapsular cataract extraction, and in some quarters this approach, which had previously been largely abandoned, has now been revived.

Lens implantation. Increasing confidence in the safety of modern lens implantation procedures during and after cataract surgery has prompted a trial of anterior chamber lenses for high myopia. A negative power lens is implanted and the eye's own lens is not interfered with. Optical results are said to be very acceptable, but a question mark must remain over the long-term results in view of possible later corneal decompensation.

Surgery to prevent posterior retinal changes. There is no evidence whatever that alteration of the refractive state of a highly myopic eye in any of the means we have discussed influences the development or progression of the posterior segment pathology of such cases. Pressure-reducing surgery has been abandoned as totally ineffective if not dangerous. One promising technique is that of scleral reinforcement, in which the posterior part of the globe is strengthened by strips of fascia lata.

It goes without saying that laser and cryotherapy techniques are widely employed in the prophylaxis of high myopia's most serious surgical complication — retinal detachment.

6. Astigmatism

Astigmatism ($\overset{\circ}{\alpha}$, privative: $\sigma\tau\acute{\iota}\gamma\mu\alpha$, a point) is that condition of refraction wherein a point focus of light cannot be formed upon the retina. Theoretically, no eye is 'stigmatic', and in practice we include under this form of ametropia those anomalies in the optical mechanism wherein an appreciable error is caused by the unequal refraction of light in different meridians.

Sir Isaac Newton, who himself appears to have been astigmatic, first considered the question of astigmatism in 1727. This optical error received its first detailed investigation from that many-sided scientist, Thomas Young, in 1801; he had 1.7 D of astigmatism, and since it remained on his immersing his head in water and thus eliminating the influence of the corneal refraction, he attributed his defect to the lens. The Cambridge astronomer, Airy (1827), was the first to correct the defect by a cylindrical lens; but it was largely the work of Donders (1864) which impressed the ophthalmological world with the prevalence and importance of this anomaly.

AETIOLOGY

Astigmatism may be an error either of curvature, of centring, or of refractive index.

Curvature astigmatism, if of any high degree, has its seat most frequently in the *cornea*. The anomaly is usually congenital, and ophthalmometric measurements show that its occurrence in small degrees is almost invariable. The most common error is one wherein the vertical curve is greater than the horizontal (about 0.25 D). This is known as *direct astigmatism* and is accepted as physiological; it is presumably due to the constant pressure of the upper lid upon the eye. It has been found by Marin Amat that, whereas at birth the cornea is normally almost

spherical, this type of astigmatism is present in 68% of children at the age of 4 years and in 95% at the age of 7. There is evidence that it tends to increase to a very slight extent with advancing years, but in age it tends to disappear or even reverse itself to an *inverse astigmatism* with the vertical curvature less than the horizontal.

An acquired astigmatism is not infrequently seen. Disease of the cornea results in its deformity; an extreme example of this is seen in conical cornea, while inflammations and ulcerations produce the same effect. Traumatic interference with the cornea may bring about the same result; in this category we should include surgical trauma, particularly operations for cataract, now of such clinical importance (see Ch. 7) as to spawn a new buzz word, *astigmia*.

Furthermore, corneal astigmatism can be induced by the pressure of swellings of the lids, whether the humble chalazion or a true neoplasm. A transient deviation from normal can be produced by finger pressure on the eye, by contraction of the lids, or by the action of the extra-ocular muscles.

Curvature astigmatism of the *lens* also occurs with great frequency. In the great majority of cases such anomalies are small; but on occasion, as in lenticonus, they may be marked. Not uncommonly the lens is placed slightly obliquely or out of line in the optical system (see p. 34), and this, causing a certain amount of *decentring*, produces a corresponding astigmatism; a traumatic subluxation of the lens has similar results. Finally, a small amount of *index astigmatism* occurs physiologically in the lens. This is usually slight, and is due to small inequalities in the refractive index of the different sectors, but it may be accentuated to produce considerable distortion or even polyopia in the grosser changes of cataract.

OPTICAL CONDITION

The manner of the refraction of parallel rays of light by an astigmatic system has already been described (p. 21). Instead of a single focal point, there are two focal lines (B and F, Fig. 2.31), separated from each other by a *focal interval*. The length of this focal interval is a measure of the degree of astigmatism, and the correction of the error can only be accomplished by reducing these two foci into one. It will be remembered that a cylindrical lens refracts rays of light in one plane and leaves unaltered the rays in the plane perpendicular to this (that is, in the plane of its axis). If the two principal meridians of the astigmatic system are at right angles to each other, the error can be corrected by the use of a suitable cylindrical lens which, acting in the plane of one meridian, so changes the refraction of the rays that they are brought to a focus at the same distance as those of the other meridian, when the whole image (theoretically) becomes a point.

Types of astigmatism

This type of astigmatism where the two principal meridians are at right angles, and which is therefore susceptible of correction, is called *regular astigmatism*. In the great majority of these cases the meridians of greatest and least curvature are close to or actually vertical and horizontal, or vice versa. Should this not be so and provided the greatest and least meridians are at right angles, we speak of this type of regular astigmatism as *oblique astigmatism*. When the axes are not at right angles but are crossed obliquely, the optical system, as will be seen later, is still resolvable into a sphero-cylindrical combination, and the condition may be called *bi-oblique astigmatism*; it is not of very common occurrence.

Where there are irregularities in the curvature of the meridians so that no geometrical figure is adhered to, the condition is called *irregular astigmatism*; it does not lend itself to adequate correction by spectacles.

REGULAR ASTIGMATISM

Regular astigmatism may be classified thus (Fig. 6.1):

1. *Simple astigmatism*, where one of the foci falls upon the retina. The other focus may fall in front of or behind the retina, so that while one meridian is emmetropic the other is either hypermetropic or myopic. These are respectively designated *simple hypermetropic* and *simple myopic astigmatism*.

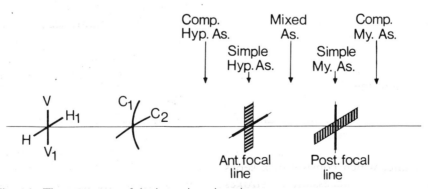

Fig. 6.1 The appearance of the image in astigmatism.
A cross with a vertical (VV_1) and horizontal (HH_1) limb is the object. Corneal astigmatism of the direct type is present wherein the vertical diameter (C_1) is more curved than the horizontal (C_2). The arrows indicate the site at which the image is formed in different types of astigmatism, and the appearances of the image at the anterior focal line (in simple hypermetropic astigmatism) and the posterior focal line (in simple myopic astigmatism) are shown.

2. *Compound astigmatism*, where neither of the two foci lies upon the retina but both are placed in front of or behind it. The state of the refraction is then entirely hypermetropic or entirely myopic. The former is known as *compound hypermetropic*, the latter as *compound myopic astigmatism*.

3. *Mixed astigmatism*, where one focus is in front of and the other behind the retina, so that the refraction is hypermetropic in one direction and myopic in the other.

The usual physiological type of astigmatism, wherein the vertical curve is greater than the horizontal, ' is termed *direct astigmatism* or astigmatism 'with the rule', in contradistinction to the opposite condition of *indirect astigmatism* or astigmatism 'against the rule'.

CLINICAL FEATURES

Symptoms

When the degree of astigmatism is of appreciable size, since in no circumstances can the eye form a sharply defined image upon the retina, the diminution of visual acuity may be very considerable. In his endeavour to see clearly the patient attempts to focus not the central circle of least diffusion, but one or other of the focal lines. Other things being equal, the meridian which approaches most nearly the emmetropic condition is chosen, and if the two are approximately equally in error the vertical focal line is as a rule preferentially chosen. This is a natural adaptation, for most objects and certainly printed matter are least indecipherable when they are distorted vertically. Since a focal line is made the object of attention, the vision of the astigmat shows peculiarities other than indistinctness on account of the elongated form of the diffusion circles which he has to interpret. Circles become elongated into ovals; a point of light appears tailed off; and a line, which consists of a series of points, appears as a succession of strokes fused into a blurred image. Let us imagine an astigmatic person focusing on the vertical focal line and looking at two straight lines standing the one perpendicular to the other (Fig. 6.1). We may imagine the lines made up of an infinite

number of points, each of which appears on his retina as a short vertical stroke (or, more correctly, an ellipse). The horizontal line therefore appears as a series of such vertical strokes, which coalesce into a broad blurred band, while in the case of the vertical line the vertical strokes are superimposed and cover each other, so that the whole line appears sharply defined, with only the uppermost and lowermost of the constituent strokes extending beyond it, giving it a tailed-off appearance and making it seem longer than it really is. Conversely, if the horizontal focal line is focused, the vertical lines become blurred. Thus in every case of regular astigmatism there is one direction in which lines appear most distinct, and one in which they appear most confused. This is taken advantage of in the detection of astigmatism by a fan-shaped figure (see p. 182). If the axis of the cylinder is oblique, the head is frequently held to one side so as to reduce the distortion, a habit which may in children lead to the development of scoliosis; and in all cases there is a tendency to half-close the lids in order to make a stenopaeic slit, so that by cutting out the rays in one meridian, the object may appear more distinct.

The continuous strain thrown upon accommodation in the attempt to see clearly is a prolific cause of the symptoms of *asthenopia* and *eye-strain*. Particularly is this so in the case of small astigmatic errors, for here the measure of success which the accommodative effort achieves stimulates it to greater endeavour. Thus, as we have seen in an earlier chapter, the most marked symptoms are associated with the greatest retention of visual acuity, and when the error is so gross as to make any correcting effort useless, none is made and visual symptoms only are evident. Considered as a whole, of course, in the great majority of cases these small errors give rise to no discomfort; they may be accepted as physiological and do not require treatment. In other cases, however, all the symptoms already considered in the chapter on eye-strain may be present — headaches varying from a mild frontal ache to violent explosions of pain, and a whole gamut of reflex nervous disturbances such as dizziness, neurasthenia, irritability and fatigue. The most severe symptoms are usually seen in cases of hypermetropic astigmatism, in which the accommodation makes further efforts to overcome the hypermetropia.

Treatment

Optical treatment

Provided they produce no deterioration of the visual acuity, and provided they are giving rise to no symptoms of asthenopia and eye-strain, the smaller astigmatic errors (0.5 D or less) generally do not require correction; but if either of these two conditions is present, the error should receive attention. It is obvious that in their correction the utmost care is to be exercised, for any difference that remains is left for the patient to correct by his own efforts, and if he is forced to do this the symptoms of eye-strain may continue or even be exaggerated.

As a rule, every attempt should be made to correct the cylindrical defect fully, and this applies with more force when a complaint of eye-strain is made. It sometimes happens, however, that, in adults with high errors who have never worn glasses, the unaccustomed effect of cylinders of considerable power makes objects appear distorted and causes distress, and in these it may be well to undercorrect the error until they have become used to them, when, at a later date, the full correction may be worn comfortably. The spherical correction should be treated on the lines already indicated.

Contact lenses can play an important role (p. 259).

Surgery for astigmatism

This is usually reserved for iatrogenic astigmatism, i.e., that arising after cataract or corneal transplant surgery. However such are the advances in this field that the technique may well become widely applied to those developed astigmats for whom cylindrical spectacle corrections and contact lenses are unsatisfactory. The surgical intervention is to decrease the curvature by relaxing incisions (T-cuts) in the axis of the more plus cylinder or alternatively to increase the curvature by placing extra sutures in the axis at right angles to this. Similar effects are promised by the use of the Excimer laser. The problem of post-cataract surgery astigmatism is dealt with elsewhere.

IRREGULAR ASTIGMATISM

In irregular astigmatism the refraction in different meridians is quite irregular. A small degree of this defect occurs physiologically owing to minute differences in the refractive index of the lens; but its effect is so small as to be inappreciable. It is only when the difference in the refractivity is accentuated, as in incipient cataract, that symptoms are caused; indeed, in this condition the distortion may be so great as to lead to polyopia.

A marked degree of irregular astigmatism is commonly found only in pathological conditions of the cornea, when it is usually the result of irregular healing after traumata or inflammations, particularly ulceration. Here the visual defect caused by the optical error is accentuated by the presence of opacities, and the combination of the two makes any attempt to improve vision by lenses frequently difficult or impossible.

Another, not uncommon condition is *conical cornea (keratoconus)* (Fig. 6.2) wherein the cornea is bulged forwards into the shape of a cone, the

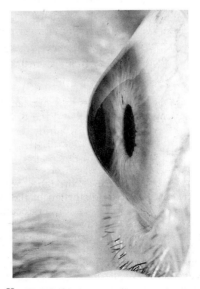

Fig. 6.2 Keratoconus.

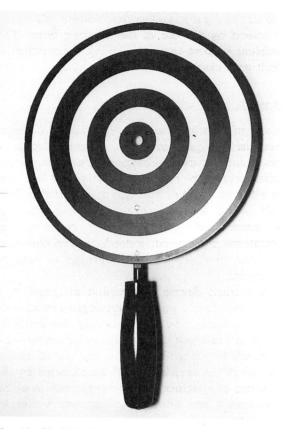

Fig. 6.3 Placido's disc.

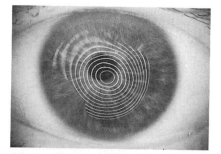

Fig. 6.4 The appearance seen by keratoscopy in irregular astigmatism (T. A. Casey).

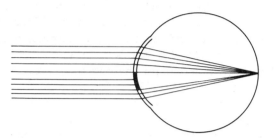

Fig. 6.5 The effect of a dense corneal opacity. The effect of such an opacity is to cut off completely all the rays incident upon it. The area of the retina behind the opacity is reached by rays coming in through the more peripheral parts of the cornea.

apex being slightly below the centre. The eye becomes myopic, but owing to the hyperbolic nature of the corneal curvature the refraction is irregular. The difficulties of adequate correction are increased by the progressive nature of the disease so that the optical conditions tend constantly to change.

The condition of irregular corneal astigmatism is most easily recognised by observing the distortion of the corneal reflex. This is best done by holding up a large flat disc painted with concentric black-and-white circles (Placido's disc or keratoscope, Fig. 6.3) in front of the eye; the reflex is observed (or photographed) through a hole in the centre of the disc, and the distortion of the circles is readily appreciated (Fig. 6.4). In keratoconus when the eye is examined with the ophthalmoscopic mirror at 1 metre distance, a ring shadow is seen in the red reflex of the fundus, which alters its position on moving the mirror. This ring appears dark because none of the rays from the fundus passing through it enter the observer's eye, the rays

on the central side being convergent, and those on the peripheral side being divergent.

A condition of somewhat similar nature is seen in *lenticonus*. This is due to a similar deformation of the curvature of the anterior or posterior surface of the lens or of the configuration of its nucleus. It is a rare congenital anomaly the precise origin of which is in doubt. The centre of the pupillary aperture has a myopic refraction while the periphery is relatively hypermetropic, and the difference may be so great as to make two images of the fundus appear. Ophthalmoscopically, a dark disc is seen situated in the centre of the pupillary aperture; its appearance is due to the same optical phenomena as the similar zone in conical cornea.

Treatment

The optical treatment of all these varieties of irregular astigmatism is often unsatisfactory. Conforming to no geometrical system, their refraction must be estimated by a time-consuming method of trial and error, which is frequently unrewarding. Improvement with spectacle lenses will in many cases be disappointingly small, but determined attempts to improve the vision by this means should be made as the results may occasionally be surprisingly satisfactory.

Typically in conical cornea but even in other cases with actual opacities present, an immense visual improvement may be obtained by employing contact lenses (p. 261).

In other cases operative measures may be indicated, and where the condition is serious keratoplasty in the central area of a conical cornea or excision of a scar and its replacement by a graft is the most effective method of treatment. Of recent years attempts are being made to reshape the cornea, keratomileusis, but this is usually reserved for regular astigmatism.

Minor, surgical procedures are now only of historic interest. These included, for example, an optical iridectomy, which may improve vision where there is an opaque central cornea and clear periphery, although the aberration associated with the peripheral refraction lessens the optical value of the result. Cauterisation of the tip of the cone may stay the progress of a conical cornea. A thin translucent nebula situated in the centre of the pupillary area may be benefited by being made quite opaque by tattooing with platinum chloride. In this condition, if light is allowed to pass through the nebula, it is refracted irregularly and renders the whole retinal image blurred; but a complete opacity allows the passage of no rays, and since the rays from the periphery can reach the part of the retina directly behind the blocked-out area in the cornea a more clearly defined, although fainter image may be formed   (Fig. 6.5).

Removal of the lens may place a patient with gross lenticonus in a more comfortable condition by rendering him aphakic.

7. Aphakia and pseudophakia

Aphakia ($\overset{\text{'}}{\alpha}$, privative; $\phi\alpha\kappa\grave{o}\zeta$, lens), although the term suggests an absence of the lens from the eye, is usually taken to embrace those conditions wherein the lens is absent from the pupillary area. In the vast majority of cases the lens has been removed by operation, sometimes it has been lost through a perforating wound, it may be absent as a congenital defect, or it may be displaced from the pupil by dislocation. We use the opposite term phakic to describe an eye with its lens in place.

The vision in aphakia

An aphakic eye is usually strongly hypermetropic; in the absence of the lens, other things being normal, parallel rays of light are brought to a focus 31 mm behind the cornea, while the average antero-posterior diameter of the eye is only 23 to 24 mm. The dioptric system must therefore be supplemented by a strong converging spectacle lens, usually, if the eye were originally emmetropic, of about +10 D.

The optical conditions are completely changed, for the dioptric apparatus has been reduced to a single refracting surface (the cornea) bounding a medium of uniform refractive index (the aqueous and vitreous humours). The nodal point of the eye is thus moved forwards. The anterior principal focus, for example, is 23.22 mm in front of the cornea instead of 17.05 mm.

The disadvantages of aphakia

Enlargement of the image

Since the size of the image varies with this distance, the size of the image of the (corrected) aphakic eye (if the correcting lens were placed at this point) will therefore be in the ratio of 23.22 to 17.05 or 1.36 to 1. The nearer the correcting lens is to the eye, the smaller will be this difference (p. 209); nevertheless the result is that the image in an aphakic eye, corrected by spectacles in their usual position, is about 25% larger than when the eye is phakic. The visual acuity is therefore theoretically worse than is indicated by the usual clinical tests; when vision is interpreted in visual angles, a vision of 6/9 in a corrected aphakic eye corresponds to an acuity of only 6/12 in an eye with its optical system unaltered.

The relative magnification just noted introduces a false spatial orientation of familiar objects, which, being of unusual size, are judged to be nearer than they actually are. The patient is thus visually unco-ordinated, knocking over china and pouring water onto the table instead of into a glass, with disastrous and humiliating results until eventually, usually after some months of trial and error, he learns a new visual co-ordination of eye and hand.

The difference of retinal image sizes, aniseikonia, between the phakic and aphakic optical state presents special problems to binocular vision in a patient where one eye has its lens in situ and the opposite eye is aphakic. This matter will be considered elsewhere.

All accommodation is abolished

Consequently the patient should theoretically be provided with a pair of spectacles for every distance at which he desires to see clearly. In practice it is usually sufficient to provide a lens for distant vision, one for reading distance, with in addition, in many cases, one for an intermediate position. A convex lens becomes stronger if it is moved away from the cornea (see p. 209), so that a certain amount of artificial accommodation may be attained by the patient if he moves the spectacles up and down his nose, whereby his point of distinct vision is removed or brought nearer. A further considerable disadvantage is the *limitation of the visual field,* for the spectacles do not move with the eyes, and the prismatic effects produced by their periphery are great. The patient has to learn to move his head rather than his eyes, especially on looking downwards, so that he always uses the central portion of his lenses. Until the patient gets accustomed to the condition and has learned to make allowances for it, the lack of accommodation and limitation of the field may cause a considerable amount of inconvenience, and at the beginning great patience is often necessary before he can tolerate the new optical conditions (see further p. 219).

In addition, two optical defects inseparable from the use of strong lenses exist — the distortion of peripheral objects due to spherical aberration (p. 218) and the existence of a blind area due to prismatic deviation at the periphery of the lens which gives rise to a ring scotoma (p. 219), both of which phenomena are much more accentuated on moving the eyes. These defects will be discussed at a subsequent stage.

It should be remembered that operative interference for cataract may leave the eye highly astigmatic as well as aphakic, and this may add to the difficulties of proper optical correction with distortion of the image so that floors or tables seem to slope.

Treatment

The traditional management of the aphakic is to order a spectacle correction which is based on accurate refraction, due attention being paid to the back vertex distance of the trial frame lenses (see p. 209 and Table 5, Appendix I).

Although many of the difficulties of aphakia have been progressively eliminated in clinical practice by contact lens correction instead of spectacles (p. 263) and within the last 15 years the almost universal practice, at least in developed countries, of intra-ocular lens implantation, there remain cases, however, where for economic, social or clinical reasons neither of these approaches is available.

The ophthalmologist should explain the optical difficulties which may arise from aphakic spectacles before surgery is undertaken to avoid post-operative disappointment, and during the initial post-operative period he must take trouble to assist sympathetically in the visual reorientation of his patient. It is true that some patients accept their new visual world rapidly and almost without complaint, but it is equally true that others of a less adaptable character are never able to reconcile themselves to their aphakic spectacles, remaining completely disorientated and distressed and preferring to grope about the world with uncorrected misty vision using their spectacles only when sedentary and usually for reading. Nevertheless the dramatic improvement in vision following surgery encourages most aphakics to persist in their efforts of visual rehabilitation, and some of the problems can be mitigated by the provision of modern designs of aphakic spectacles. Desirable features of an aphakic spectacle correction include aspherical or lenticular lens forms with relatively flat base curves, lightweight high-refractive lens material (p. 200) and substantial but light spectacle frames which sit properly on the nose bridge. Pantascopic tilt should not be more then 7 degrees, so as to avoid an unwanted cylindrical effect.

And finally, if it seems that the patient is quite intolerant of either aphakic spectacles or of contact lenses, then consideration should doubtless be given in appropriate cases of secondary intra-ocular lens implantation.

PSEUDOPHAKIA

The proximity of an aphakic contact lens to the eye leads to considerable reduction of retinal image size to perhaps within 5% of the phakic level, but an intra-ocular lenticulus (referred to as IOL) offers an almost normal optical situation, and lens implantation is standard practice, so much so that a whole section of ophthalmic optics is now exclusively concerned with the clinical condition of *pseudophakia*. Suffice it to say here that the problems of retinal image size are largely eliminated. There is of course no peripheral distortion of images, and surprisingly many patients combine with good unaided distance vision some degree of useful near vision even without any particular spectacle reading supplement — a condition referred to as pseudo-accommodation. Of course the discomforts of heavy spectacle wear or of contact lenses are absent.

Pseudophakic calculation

Any modern account of the refraction of the eye must refer to the calculation of the power required of a lens to be implanted during the course of or subsequent to cataract surgery, as this has become such a routine part of ophthalmology, at least in developed countries. The subject is complex and constantly evolving, embracing the sciences of optics, physics, mathematics, computing and electronics as well as surgical technique.

Initially it was believed adequate to make an intelligent guess at the required power of an intra-ocular implant based on the patient's optical state and history. In its simplest form such an approach led to the use of a standard lens power employed where there was reason to suppose that the patient had always been emmetropic, with a fairly normal distribution of ocular parameters. Going by the rules of effectivity, powers of standard lenses increased according to their position. An anterior chamber lens might be of +17 D, a pupil-supported lens +19 D and a posterior chamber lens +20 or +21 D.* Variations from this 'standard lens' approach were made according to the patient's actual refraction, as estimated when stripped of any ocular effect of the cataractous process itself.

The standard lens method may still have a place in circumstances which preclude more

sophisticated estimations where perhaps a very limited range of implant powers is available. However its widespread use rapidly revealed that there were occasional unexpected and unsatisfactory results deviating very widely from the targeted final refraction, whether this was for emmetropia or a particular degree of ametropia.

Biometry

From this dissatisfaction the mini-science of *biometry* has arisen and, though still not quite perfect, it is now established as a routine prior to modern cataract surgery.

Basically this consists of a keratometry reading together with an ultrasonic measurement of the axial length of the eye, perhaps with a measurement of anterior chamber depth. This information is fed into a variety of formulae (six at least), which appear to be of two kinds.

In one group, typically the Binkhorst formula, the power of the intra-ocular lens is predicted on the basis of the optical situation as it is presumed will be obtained, without reference to the individual characteristics of the surgeon or of the lens implanted.

Calculations from this type of what is known as 'theoretical formula' have to make assumptions about the post-operative anterior chamber depth.

Another type of formula is based on, perhaps bulk, experience of surgeons looking retrospectively at their results, thenceforth characterising a particular style of intra-ocular lens. The most popular of these 'regression formulae' is that of Sanders, Retzlaff and Kraff. As noted below this involves a constant, the A constant, which is supposed to be peculiar to the form of lens being implanted. However the individual surgeon will use his 'personalised' A constant, modified from the given one by the results of his own cases.

The two groups of implant power calculation formulae have been progressively modified for a variety of reasons. In general, since their initial exposition, surgical technique and lens styles have been continually altering. Thus, for example, the assumed values for post-operative anterior chamber depth used in theoretical formulae now have correction factors applied to them before

---

*Note that these are the powers of the lenses in situ, in ocular 'medium', not their power in air, which may be four or more times as much.

introduction into the more up-to-date versions of each of these.

As an example of one of the original *theoretical* formulae, here is the Binkhorst formula originally for an anterior chamber implant modified for posterior chamber implant.

$$P = \frac{1336\ (4r - a)}{(a - d)\ (4r - d)}$$

where P is the required dioptric power of the implant, in aqueous, r is the corneal radius in mm (average), a is the axial length in mm and d is the assumed post-operative anterior chamber depth plus corneal thickness (values for d of 3.19 mm or later 4.2 mm for posterior chamber lenses were used). The problem of the assumed post-operative anterior chamber depth is not resolved (d in the above formula). Correction factors have been applied relating mainly to the measured axial length of the eye.

The Colenbrander–Hoffer formula is

$$P = \left(\frac{1336}{a - d - 0.05}\right) - \left(\frac{1336}{\dfrac{1336}{K} - d - 0.05}\right)$$

where K is the average keratometry reading in dioptres.

The most widely used *regression* formula is that based on the original suggestion of Sanders, Retzlaff and Kraff (SRK I),

$$P = A - 2.5\,L - 0.9\,K$$

where P is the required dioptric power of implant, L is the axial length in mm and K is the average K reading in dioptres. The A constant was something to be ascribed to each style of IOL as noted above. In the early usage of this formula the lenses employed were either pupil supported or anterior chamber implants. With the increasing use of posterior chamber lenses it was recognised that this formula works well for eyes with axial lengths of 22–24.5 mm, which make up about three out of four cases, but that for shorter or longer eyes modifications are required to improve predictability.

The SRK II formula recognises this as follows:

Short eye:
axial length 21–22 mm, add 1 to usual A constant
axial length 20–21 mm, add 2 to usual A constant
axial length less than 20 mm, add 3 to usual A constant

Long eye:
over 24.5 mm subtract 0.5 mm from usual A constant

To produce an intentional ametropia the calculated power for emmetropia is modified as follows:

$$P_{AM} = P_{EM} - \left(\frac{P_{SP}}{R_F}\right)$$

where P_{AM} is the required IOL power to produce a final spectacle power of P_{SP}, P_{EM} is the IOL power calculated to produce emmetropia, $R_F = 0.8$ for $P_{EM} > 14$ D and $R_F = 1$ for $P_{EM} \leqslant 14$ D.

With most modern formulae a result within 1 D of the predicted refraction obtains in two-thirds to three-quarters of cases, but the search for even greater accuracy continues, and the latest modification 'theoretical' formulae have had 'regression' formulae information introduced. The collective term for these modifications is the 'fudge factor', which relates to the individual surgeon's results. Conversely, the SRK formulation has been updated to include theoretical elements, the SRK (T), which is said to give even greater predictability for very long eyes. What this appears to amount to is a Binkhorst type formula where the estimate of post-operative anterior chamber depth derives ultimately not only from pre-operative axial length and corneal curvature measurements but also from the surgeon's individual A constant.

The limits of predictability of intra-ocular lens power

Perfect predictability of IOL power is probably unattainable for many reasons. There are inherent limitations of the accuracy of biometric measurements. These are either in the instruments or in their operation. Ultrasonic axial length measurements, however electronically controlled or computerised, have to make assumptions about the speed of sound in normal and pathological ocular tissues; an estimate may need to be made of the retinal thickness of perhaps 0.5 mm; the true axiality of the measurement is subject to observer error, and experience with a particular machine is very valuable. The method of coupling the ultrasonic probe to the eye is also important, whether by the immersion method, the patient being supine, or the applanation technique, the probe replacing the tonometer prism of the Goldmann applanation tonometer (Fig. 7.1). Keratometry is also a technique liable to observer error, but the increasing use of auto-keratometry eliminates this.

The form of the implanted lens has some bearing on the power required. The common forms are plano-convex with the plano surface posterior, and biconvex; to some extent these variations may be taken care of by varying the A constant of the SRK formula. The degree to which the loops of the lens are backwardly angled may influence the precise lens position, which is also of course dependent on their site, either in the ciliary sulcus, i.e. immediately behind the iris root, or further back in the capsular bag. Sulcus as distinct from bag fixation requires a lens of relatively lower power by perhaps 0.5–1.5 D. This is only one of a number of features of surgical technique which influences the final refraction. The matter will be discussed further below.

Factors other than biometry in IOL power selection

Whichever of the formulae is used for computing IOL power, it is mandatory to look at the actual results obtained by the surgeon, and it is of course recommended by their proponents that this should be done. The A constant of the SRK formula can be personalised for a particular style of lens used by one particular surgeon.

The state of the fellow eye must always be considered. There are several situations that may obtain, and it must be admitted that in many cases there is no absolute consensus about the objectives to be sought, particularly where the fellow eye or indeed both are or have been known to be grossly ametropic. Underlying the difficulty is the possibility of post-operative anisometropia leading to aniseikonic problems, perhaps compromising binocularity. The pre-operative state of the latter is itself a factor in lens power selection.

Having said this, where such problems are not in prospect, the aim will be for emmetropia or nearly so, although many surgeons tend deliberately to go for a correction on the side of a low degree of myopia (see below for discussion of reading vision). However if the fellow eye is markedly ametropic and either free from cataract or with little prospect of surgery for it, a decision to aim for near emmetropia may be unwise. To aim for example at about 3 D less myopia than a highly myopic but cataract-free

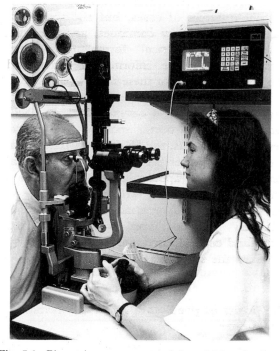

Fig. 7.1 Biometric measurement of the axial length of the eye.

contralateral eye may be best, but it must be admitted that very much wider differences in post-operative refraction are often surprisingly well tolerated. It seems that at least in some cases the aniseikonia resulting from pseudophakic anisometropia is either non-existent or within clinically tolerated limits.

Again the nature of the ametropia needs consideration. Bilateral nuclear cataract producing high myopia may indicate an objective of emmetropia, any resulting co-ordination problems indicating early surgery for the fellow eye even with relatively reasonable vision on that side.

If the other eye is already pseudophakic, this will be of direct influence on the lens power now to be selected. A further consideration is the reading vision. The opportunity obviously exists to aim for -2 or -2.5 D myopia even with a pre-operatively emmetropic eye, leaving the subject in a position where the sacrifice of true binocularity may be rewarded by a spectacle-free existence. This as with all decisions on IOL power obviously requires particular discussion pre-operatively with the patient. A similar situation exists in the contact lens field, and in both supplementary spectacles for distance may be advisable for driving, to bring up the distance vision of the eye habitually used unaided for near.

Finally, however, it should be pointed out that where, pre-operatively, each eye is of a similar type of ametropia, to end up with one eye significantly myopic and the other hypermetropic is a situation best avoided.

The reading vision in pseudophakia

Another matter relating to reading vision is the question of so-called pseudophakic accommodation, a rather inflated expression for the ability of pseudophakic subjects wearing the best distance correction (which may be nil) also at the same time to have a very useful degree of near vision.

The influences responsible for this are probably multiple: the miosis of near viewing, the possibility that the capsular bag may carry the pseudophakos forward in 'accommodation' and the value of residual post-operative myopic astigmatism, accidental or intended (see below).

A more recent development is the bifocal or multifocal intra-ocular lens. Long-term evaluation of these is still in progress, but their advantages when successful are obvious. As with contact lenses there are segment and concentric types of lens style. Surprisingly, some eccentricity of the implant may not be very serious. Nevertheless, good centration of the implant, already hotly debated by surgeons, has clear advantages for the bifocal type; and proponents of the current wave of enthusiasm for the continuous tear small anterior capsulotomy technique, associated with phacoemulsification, point to the advantage this offers for an intact capsular bag remnant and consequent excellent centration.

With bifocal IOLs some degree of simultaneous distance reading vision requires the patient to ignore the unwanted image, and inevitably some loss of quality for both far and near, and sometimes results in ghost imaging. An unfortunate feature of one of the diffractive types of multifocal implants is that the best near vision, although usually adequate, is not perfect and may not be improved by spectacles. Furthermore, there appears to be a loss of contrast sensitivity to higher frequencies, as well as a susceptibility to glare and to chromatism.

The management of pseudophakic optical problems

These may arise in several ways. First, there may be a large spherical element disparity between what was planned and what has resulted. Secondly, significant astigmatism may be present, although this is only exceptionally due to the implant itself and is much more likely to be corneal in origin (see below). Thirdly, aniseikonic problems may lead to problems with binocular co-ordination. Grossly eccentric lenses may give annoying multiple or flared images if the lens edge or a dialling hole is opposite the pupil. The management of these will depend on their severity, and only as a last resort should lens replacement be considered. Special spectacle correction of appropriately advantageous modified forms and perhaps compromising in power on the visual acuities of the two eyes may help binocular problems. Contact lens wear should also be addressed, although it will seem a pity to end up with mandatory contact lens use when the whole object of the exercise is to avoid it.

As mentioned above, binocular problems following pseudophakic implantation in one eye may prompt more rapid surgery on the fellow eye in order to balance things up.

SURGICAL TECHNIQUE AND POST-OPERATIVE OPTICS

Astigmatism

Cataract surgery without implantation necessitates the wearing of a powerful convex glass, and to have to incorporate in this a correction for astigmatism might be considered merely a marginal extra disability to those already conferred by aphakic spectacles. Nevertheless, the distortion given by a powerful cylinder is very real and may add to the problems of enlargement of the image, etc.

Even with modern microsurgical methods of wound suture the problem of astigmatism has not been eliminated. Because of this the visual result of pseudophakic surgery intended to produce emmetropia may be compromised. Significant astigmatism in these circumstances may not only necessitate a distance correction but lead to difficulty in binocular co-operation when this is worn although again, perhaps surprisingly, not inevitably so.

The factors concerned in the genesis of this astigmatism are multiple and not completely understood. It is widely accepted that these include large incisions, corneal rather than limbal or scleral, and closely placed long tight sutures. In recognition of this there is a strong advocacy of small-incision single-suture or sutureless cataract surgery, usually involving phacoemulsification for nucleus removal and a small foldable intra-ocular lens implant. The ins and outs of such surgery are beyond the scope of this work, but it is certainly claimed that these

techniques lead to more rapid stability of the pseudophakic refraction, though the degree of astigmatism may be only marginally better than finally obtained after larger, conventional cataract incisions.

Some control of astigmatism is of course possible prophylactically by recognising and avoiding accepted factors producing it; intraoperative keratometry (the Terry keratometer for example) is helpful in some cases. If it is excessive post-operatively then it may be dealt with by selectively removing sutures, this being an argument in support of those surgeons who advocate interrupted rather than continuous sutures. The rule is to remove the suture in the axis of the plus cylinder. In many cases but not invariably that is at the 12 o'clock meridian, the induced astigmatism present being of the 'with the rule' variety.

As we noted above some advantage may actually accrue from a moderate degree of myopic astigmatism. It has always been recognised that the (phakic) myopic astigmat previously uncorrected develops presbyopic symptoms later than the 40–45 age of onset of the emmetrope. Such a pseudophakic result therefore often confers useful unaided near vision as well as reasonable distance acuity.

Perhaps because the difference of refractive index between implant material (say 1.49) and that of the medium on either side (1.336) is so small, eccentricity and tilt, unless extreme, of the pseudophakos have a remarkably small effect on the total astigmatism of the eye. Even though these may cause some difficulty in interpreting the retinoscopy reflex, subjective testing often gives very good acuities and, curiously, in many instances the power of the cylinder required in subjective testing is often much less than retinoscopy might indicate.

Some of the other visual problems that arise following implantation are not strictly in the optical field, such as distorted images due to the edge of dialling hole of a poorly centred lens. In severe cases of astigmatism specialised corneal surgery may be indicated if routine optical devices and spectacles or contact lenses do not give a satisfactory clinical result.

The stability of the refraction in cataract operated patients

After either simple or pseudophakic cataract surgery refraction takes time to settle down and, in the initial period, the rapidity with which this occurs is inversely related to the size of the incision. Refractive stability is soonest obtained with the modern small-incision single-suture technique; in classical large-section methods the refraction may alter until 6 weeks post-operatively on average, and ordering spectacles is usually delayed until that date, the patient being tided over with temporary corrections such as plastic +10 D spheres (with or without a bifocal element), for cases where a pseudophakos has not been used.

All this of course depends on straightforward wound healing. Should this not occur because of inadequate closure technique or inadvertent inclusion of extraneous material such as lens capsule or vitreous strands, the refraction may take a great deal longer to reach an unchanging state, and in many of these cases there may be a persisting unpleasantly high astigmatic element.

Late changes in refraction may occur not only in power but also in cylinder orientation. A slightly tight suture may fray, a cystoid wound may go on altering, a lens implant may undergo some intra-ocular movement if capsular bag shrinkage occurs, although posterior capsular thickening, whatever its effect on vision, in itself does not necessarily alter the refraction.

In any event the best test of the optical stability is of course to confirm it by repeating the refraction at whatever interval is appropriate to the period after surgery, that is to say frequently in the immediate post-operative period and at longer and longer gaps between routine revisits.

Further interventions for optical anomalies following cataract surgery

Marked astigmatism may call for one of several techniques if a contact lens cannot give a satisfactory result, either because of poor vision or poor tolerance of the lens. Tactically-placed extra sutures or T-cuts performed surgically, or more recently by the Excimer laser, have all been employed to reshape the cornea.

In children where difficulties with contact lens wear are experienced or anticipated epikeratophakia (p. 63) has been successfully tried.

8. Changes in refraction

Although, as a general rule, the refraction of a particular eye is a relatively stable and constant quantity, there is always a tendency towards slow and gradual changes. These vary from time to time and from individual to individual; usually the changes are not great in degree, but their occurrence renders it necessary that the eyes should be examined and the lenses changed, if necessary at periodic intervals.

Physiological changes

To a large extent these changes may be erratic, but there are certain well-defined tendencies of general occurrence which may be considered physiological. Most of these have already been alluded to in the previous chapters and it will be sufficient here merely to recapitulate them: the change from hypermetropia at birth to emmetropia as growth proceeds, a change which may progress to the development of myopia; the *apparent increase of hypermetropia* which accompanies advancing years and which indicates a decrease in the power of accommodation; and an *absolute increase in the hypermetropia* with age, as a result of changes in the size and refractivity of the lens. In astigmatism also there is frequently a tendency to gradual change. As we remarked elsewhere, the curvature of the cornea is usually slightly greater in the vertical meridian than in the horizontal in the early years and this tends to change to the opposite condition later in life. Thus in hypermetropic astigmatism the axis of the correcting plus cylinder swings from vertical towards the horizontal; in myopic astigmatism the correcting minus cylinder moves from axis horizontal towards axis vertical. This is by no

means constant or invariable, and when it does occur it usually involves a very slow transition of only one or two degrees a year.

Pathological changes

The first of these are *changes in the dynamic refraction* due to conditions of spasm or paralysis of the ciliary muscle. The effect is typically seen in the 1 dioptre of hypermetropia which is revealed by the ciliary paralysis following the instillation of atropine. The same effect is seen in those *neurological disorders* which similarly affect the ciliary muscle. *Trauma* to the eyeball may act in the same way, and many cases of transient refractive changes have been reported as a result of an accident involving a blow. A *displacement of the lens* backwards or forwards will have the same optical effect, while a subluxation and tilting of the lens will produce a marked degree of astigmatism. The myopia which accompanies spasm of the ciliary muscle is sometimes met with in *iritis*, the spasm being due to the irritant effects of inflammatory products.

A transient myopia occurring in various *toxic states* such as jaundice and influenza and after the administration of drugs such as the *arsenicals* and *sulphonamides* is now well annotated in the literature. More recent chemical relatives of the sulphonamides such as the carbonic anhydrase inhibitors (Diamox) and the thiazides (hydrochlorothiazide) have been held responsible. As a rule the myopia does not occur when the drug is taken initially but during a subsequent period of dosage suggesting that a sensitivity develops. The mechanism is by no means clear, nor is it by any means certain that the cause in every case is the same. Most writers ascribe the phenomenon to an irritative, toxic ciliary spasm which may be due to a central toxic irritation of the parasympathetic nerves or centres. In other cases the myopia has been found to be unchanged by atropine and in these, whatever the mechanism, lenticular changes seem the basis for the optical change. It is interesting that as a rule the myopia, varying from 1 to about 4 D in degree and from a few days to a few weeks in duration, is frequently the only toxic symptom.

Slight refractive changes may occur in *glaucoma*. A small degree of myopia, due to an antero-posterior stretching, may occur in the course of this disease, but it is neither common in incidence nor great in amount because an increase of tension rarely stretches the dense adult sclera. On the other hand, in the congenital condition of buphthalmos, when the pressure makes itself evident before the tissues are fully consolidated, such an effect becomes apparent to a marked degree; here, incidentally, the optical effect is largely neutralised by the depth of the anterior chamber and the relative displacement backwards of the lens.

After operation any shallowness of the anterior chamber invariably produces a marked myopia, and in the period following the operation the re-establishment of the chamber and the recession of the lens are accompanied by the gradual development of hypermetropia.

A much more significant happening in glaucoma is a loss of accommodation because of pressure on the ciliary muscle, and its occurrence is a sign of some diagnostic importance. The accommodative loss may vary rapidly in states of temporarily raised tension in closed-angle glaucoma so that the print in reading suddenly becomes blurred; while in simple glaucoma a permanent loss of accommodation may develop more rapidly than would normally be explained by the physiological development of presbyopic changes (p. 91).

When the coats of the eye are diseased refractive changes are produced more readily. This is most obvious in *corneal disease*, such as ulceration or stromal keratitis, when an irregular astigmatism usually results, a deformity largely cicatricial in nature. A softening of the cornea may result in a progressive keratoconus; severe *scleritis* has been recorded as producing a considerable degree of myopia; while a similar occurrence has been noted as a sequel of *choroiditis*. Myopia may also result from *constitutional disturbances* which may undermine the strength of the sclera. It has been noted accompanying dyscrasias of the pituitary gland, goitre, and obesity; and it appears to form an occasional complication of such diseases as malaria, tuberculosis and acutely debilitating illnesses such as the exanthemata.

Refractive changes of considerable importance are associated with alterations in the refractivity of the lens. The most common of these is the gradual myopic change which accompanies the early stages of *cataract*. It is the result of the increase in the optical density of the lens which occurs in this disease and is most evident when the nuclear portions are particularly involved. The most interesting and dramatic changes of this class, however, are those which occur very frequently in *diabetes*.

In this disease the essential features are that the changes of refraction come on suddenly and bilaterally, that a myopic trend is associated with a rise, and a hypermetropic with a fall, in the sugar concentration of the blood, and that the hypermetropic trend seems not to occur as an initial phenomenon but to follow a myopic change. If the blood sugar concentration varies clinically, the refractive state of the eye may follow, altering from hypermetropic to myopic and vice versa. The cause of these refractive changes has excited much speculation. It is evident that they arise from events in the lens. It may be that the myopia associated with a rising sugar concentration is due to hydration of the cortical layers of the lens relative to the nucleus. As the blood sugar rises, provided the available water reserve is maintained, the osmotic pressure of the aqueous tends to decrease, largely owing to the great elimination of osmotically active substances from the blood in the increased flow of relatively concentrated urine. In order to establish osmotic equilibrium, fluid tends to flow into the lens from the chambers of the eye. This tissue therefore swells and is deformed, its curvature being increased; further, the optical density of its peripheral layers becomes diminished while the nucleus remains unaltered. On both counts its refractive power is increased, and the eye becomes myopic. On the other hand, it has been suggested that with a fall of sugar concentration a reverse osmotic flow is inaugurated and a condition of hypermetropia is produced, hydration of the nucleus of the lens being responsible for the hypermetropic change. In hyperglycaemia there may be a retention of salt in the tissues which on diminution of the sugar is followed by hydration. The lens may share in these changes, the phenomenon being more marked in the nucleus since the cortex finds rapid equilibrium with the aqueous.

Whatever the causes of the changes a sudden and seemingly inexplicable myopia should always suggest the possibility of diabetes and direct attention to the urine; occurring in a known diabetic it should suggest an inadequate control of the disease. On the other hand, a sudden hypermetropic change, indicating, as it does, a general disturbance in the water balance of the body, points to treatment being too suddenly undertaken or too rigorously applied. In either case the treatment should be directed not to the eye but rather to the constitutional disease, for the refractive change is transitory and invariably returns to normal provided metabolic equilibrium can be re-established. If spectacles are to be prescribed, they need be considered only as an emergency and temporary measure.

Finally, pressure on the globe from outside may produce slight changes of refraction mechanically. Thus, depending on its point of pressure, an orbital tumour may bring about hypermetropia or hypermetropic astigmatism from axial pressure. An orbital inflammation has been noted to induce a similar transitory myopia. Pressure by the finger or a tumour or swelling in the lids may also involve a transient astigmatic change. A similar change may follow a tenotomy or advancement operation on the extra-ocular muscles or a buckling procedure for a retinal detachment.

Changes in refraction following cataract surgery are dealt with in Chapter 7.

Clinical anomalies

PART 2   Accommodation and its disturbances

9. Accommodation

Hitherto we have concerned ourselves mainly with the mechanism by means of which parallel rays of light are brought to a focus upon the sentient layer of the retina. We have seen that this is accomplished by the refractive system of the emmetropic eye without effort and that, in consequence, objects which are a considerable distance off are seen distinctly. It is obvious that if the eye is to function adequately it must be able to vary its focus so that it can adapt its refractive mechanism to allow objects which are near at hand to be seen clearly. Thus in Figure 9.1 parallel rays coming from an object (theoretically) infinitely far away are focused upon the retina; if the object is brought nearer (to A), the image will be formed at the conjugate focus (A′) behind the retina, and the large diffusion circles at the level of the retina will allow only a blurred image to be seen. If it were possible to increase the converging power of the eye so that the focus would be brought nearer to lie upon the retina (from A′ to R), a distinct image could still be retained; this power of changing the focus is called *accommodation*.

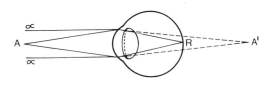

Fig. 9.1 Accommodation.
In the emmetropic eye rays from infinity are brought to a focus upon the retina at R. When a near object, A, is looked at, a focus is formed behind the retina at A′ (the conjugate focus). In order to bring this focus forwards to R, the lens increases its convexity as illustrated.

There are four obvious ways in which accommodation could be brought about. In the first place, the eye could be made to elongate so that the retina was moved out to A′; this is the method adopted to alter the focus of a camera when the photographic plate is moved, and a somewhat similar arrangement is seen in the eye of the mollusc *Pecten*. Thomas Young, however, showed that it did not occur in man. Having particularly prominent eyes, he found that by rotating his eye strongly inwards, he could affix two clamped iron rings, one in front of the cornea and the other immediately behind the macula; then on strong accommodation he found that the phosphene caused by the pressure of the posterior ring did not alter, and so concluded that his eye did not elongate.

In the second place, an increase of converging power might be attained by increasing the curvature of the cornea; this, indeed, is the mechanism seen in some birds. Again the ingenuity of Thomas Young disposed of this possibility in the case of man. He immersed his eye in water, thus eliminating the effect of the cornea, replaced the corneal refraction by a suitable convex lens, and then found that his power of accommodation was unaffected.

A third method by which this end could be attained would be by altering the position of the lens and making it advance forwards. This occurs in fish, but in the human eye Tscherning showed that an advance of about 10 mm would be necessary to give full range which occurs normally, and this, of course, is outside the bounds of possibility, since the depth of the anterior chamber is only 2.6 mm. This leaves us with a fourth suggestion which attributes the mechanism of accommodation to an increase in the refractivity of the lens.

THE MECHANISM OF ACCOMMODATION

There is still a considerable amount of controversy as to the precise nature of the mechanism of accommodation. Everyone is agreed that the essential feature is an increase of the curvature of the lens which affects mainly the anterior surface. It can be shown that in the state of rest the radius of the curvature of this surface is 10 mm, while during accommodation it decreases to 6 mm; this alteration in shape increases the converging power of the eye so that the focus can be altered as is required. Helmholtz considered that the lens was elastic, and that in the normal state it was kept stretched and flattened by the tension of the suspensory ligament. In the act of accommodation the contraction of the ciliary muscle lessened the circle formed by the ciliary processes, and thus relaxed the suspensory ligament; relieved of the strain to which it had been subjected, the lens then assumed a more spherical form, increasing in thickness and decreasing in diameter, showing at the same time a protrusion forwards at the centre and a relative flattening at the periphery.

Although this view has been disputed, most modern views of the mechanism of accommodation are based upon the central idea of Helmholtz's theory which is that the suspensory ligament is in tension in the unaccommodated state of the eye and that it relaxes during accommodation, allowing the lens to change its shape.

The general concepts which were developed by Hess, Gullstrand, Fincham and others from the Helmholtz theory have been considerably amplified and amended in recent years by the view of Weale (Fig. 9.2) and the considerable experimental and theoretical contributions of Fisher.

There have always been two central problems to which the Helmholtz concept gave rise. First, exactly how does the lens alter its shape when the tension in the suspensory ligament is relaxed?

Secondly, what is responsible for the decline in the power of accommodation with increasing age?

As far as the former is concerned, much of the recent work has concentrated on the interplay of force between the capsule and the substance of the lens. It had previously been assumed that the latter was a passive plastic substance. It was known to Fincham that if the capsule of the

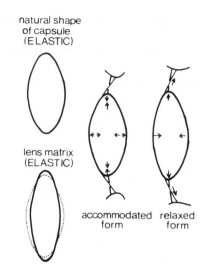

Fig. 9.2 The lens in accommodation.
To show the deformation of the lens in the normal and accommodated state owing to the opposing factors of the elasticity of the lens matrix and the capsule (R. Weale).

isolated human lens was removed the lens substance assumed a more unaccommodated, flatter shape. Fisher has now shown that for centrifugal radial forces the lens substance is truly elastic and that the interplay of the elasticity of the capsule and the lens substance is what determines the shape of the whole lens. Related to these findings, Fisher has been able to make measurements of the physical properties of the lens substance and of the capsule at various ages so as to indicate what takes place in presbyopia, the natural decline of accommodation with age. Here it is seen that there is progressive weakness of the capsule's ability to deform the lens substance from the unaccommodated shape it naturally tends to assume. In particular the three ageing factors Fisher incriminates are a decrease in the elastic modulus of the capsule, an increase in that of the lens substance and a flattening of the lens as a whole.

The precise way in which the capsule alters the shape of the lens has led to some speculation about the role of its various regions. It was at one time held that when the zonule was relaxed the capsule became relieved of strain and, having been previously compressed, the lens substance now bulged preferentially at its poles, especially the anterior, the posterior being resisted by the vitreous. On this view the capsule was thought to be thicker at the zonular attachment. It now seems that this is not so and that the capsule is thicker at this site only in old subjects in whom accommodation has ceased. It is thickest at the equator in younger subjects.

The modern version of the Helmholtz theory is that during accommodation the ciliary muscle contracts, the suspensory ligament relaxes and the elastic capsule of the lens then acts unrestrainedly to deform the lens substance into the more spherical, perhaps conoidal, accommodated shape that its own natural elasticity resists. With increasing age in spite of unimpaired power of the ciliary muscle, changes in the lens capsule leave it with less ability to alter the mass of increasingly resistant lens substance.

It has long been generally accepted that the contraction of the ciliary muscle was induced by the third (parasympathetic) nerve and the adjustment of the dioptric mechanism for distant vision was considered to be determined by a relaxation of the accommodative act for near vision. It is now known that the parasympathetic system is not alone concerned with this mechanism, but that, while accommodation for near vision is effected, as in the classical view, by a contraction of the circular fibres of the ciliary muscle (Müller's muscle) brought about by the parasympathetic nerve, an active accommodation for distant vision is effected by a contraction of the meridional fibres of the ciliary muscle (Brücke's muscle) which have an action antagonistic to the circular fibres and are mediated by the sympathetic. It has been found experimentally that stimulation of the sympathetic brings about a flattening of the lens, and that removal of the superior cervical ganglion (in the cat) involves a permanent decrease in hypermetropia. It would seem, therefore, that there is a mutually antagonistic activity in accommodation — a sympathetic mechanism focusing for distant vision and a parasympathetic mechanism focusing for near vision. Such a theory brings accommodation into line with pupillary activity which shows a reciprocating contraction and dilatation, both of which are active but in which the parasympathetic component of miosis greatly preponderates over the sympathetic component of mydriasis.

Physical and physiological accommodation

It is obvious that two factors enter into the efficiency of the act of accommodation: the ability of the lens to alter its shape and the power of the ciliary muscle. If the substance of the lens becomes inelastic, as it does with advancing age so that it can no longer change its shape, accommodation cannot be effected even if the ciliary muscle contracts violently. On the other hand, a weak or paralysed ciliary muscle will not be able to induce changes even in a lens of normal elasticity. There are thus two distinct considerations entering into the mechanism of accommodation, and these Fuchs has differentiated as *physical* and *physiological accommodation*. Physical accommodation is an expression of the actual physical deformation of the lens, and it is measured in dioptres. Thus if the converging power of the eye is increased by 1 D, we speak of the expenditure of 1 D of accommodation. The physiological component has as a unit the *myodioptre*, which is taken as the contractile power of the ciliary muscle required to raise the refractive power of the lens by 1 D.

These two elements are fundamentally distinct, and although they normally correspond during the first half of life they may become dissociated, and when they do so they entail different pathological effects. Physical accommodation fails in later life when the lens becomes hard in the condition known as *presbyopia*. From Fisher's work we may take it that changes in the physical properties of the lens alone can account for this; accommodation is therefore difficult, while at the same time the available ciliary power is unimpaired. Conversely, a failure of the physiological power of the muscle may appear in states of debility at any age, diminishing or abolishing accommodation although the lens is eminently deformable. Since an attempt is made to overcome the muscular deficiency by a sustained and exaggerated ciliary effort, such a weakness may be responsible for the distressing symptoms of asthenopia and eye-strain.

The range and amplitude of accommodation

The furthest distance away at which an object can be seen clearly is called the *far point* (*punctum remotum*). In order to see such an object the parasympathetic component of the ciliary muscle is relaxed, and the refractivity is at a minimum. When the maximum accommodation is in force, the nearest point which the eye can see clearly is called the *near point (punctum proximum)*. At this point the refractivity of the eye is at a maximum. The distance between the far point and the near point, that is the distance over which accommodation is effective, is called the *range of accommodation*. The difference between the refractivity of the eye in the two conditions — when at rest with a minimal refraction and when fully accommodated with a maximal refraction — is called the *amplitude of accommodation*.

In the first case, where no conscious effort is involved, we call the refraction *static*; when the refraction is altered by the exercise of accommodation, it is spoken of as *dynamic*.

The distance of the far point in metres is traditionally referred to as r, and R denotes the refractive power of the eye when accommodated for r; p refers to the distance of the near point and P to the refractive power of the eye in accommodation for p; a refers to the range of accommodation, and A to the amplitude. It follows that $a = r - p$ and $A = P - R$.

The accommodation is usually measured in dioptres, but since 1 dioptre represents a focal distance of 1 metre, the two are easily interchangeable, the refractive power, as we have seen (p. 22), being the reciprocal of the focal distance in metres. Thus if r is 1 metre, R is 1/1 D, i.e. 1 D. If p is 10 cm, then P is 100/10, or 10 D. Thus, in order to focus an object at 10 cm (10/100 metre), we require 10 times as much accommodation as is required to focus it at 1 metre.

In an *emmetrope* r is at infinity and $R = 1/\infty = 0$. For distant vision, therefore, the eye is at rest. If the near point is 10 cm away, $p = 10$ and $P = 100/10$ D. This latter figure gives the amplitude of accommodation (10 − 0), and the range of the accommodation is infinite ($\infty - 10$).

The *hypermetrope* on the other hand, in order to see clearly at a distance, has to exert an amount of accommodation equivalent to the amount of his hypermetropia, and to see an object at 10 cm he must add to this an amount of 10 D to put him on an equality with the emmetrope. Thus, although his range of accommodation is the same ($\infty - 10$), the amplitude is necessarily greater.

This can be readily calculated from the same formulae, always remembering that distances behind the eye are negative. If he has a hypermetropia of 5 D, so that his far point is 1/5 metre behind the eye, and if his near point is 10 cm away, the amplitude of accommodation is represented by $P - R$, i.e. 100/10 − (− 5) or 10 + 5, i.e. 15 dioptres. If we were to replace his accommodation by lenses, we would need to place a + 5 D lens before his eye when he was looking at distant objects, and when he wished to see an object distinctly at 10 cm a lens of +15 D would be required. While, therefore, a hypermetrope has the advantage that he can compensate for his refractive error by accommodative effort, this faculty brings with it the disadvantage that if he is to see distinctly he must make continual use of it, and when he does near work the demands made upon the ciliary muscle must be still greater.

A *myope* has a far point at a finite distance in front of his eye. Suppose he can only see objects distinctly at a distance of 20 cm away, his refractive error will be corrected by a lens of this focal distance (1/5 metre), and thus he will have a myopia of −5 D. Let us imagine that his near point is 10 cm away from his eye. His range of accommodation is therefore 20 − 10 cm, i.e. 10 cm. At this point the refractive power of his eye will be +10 D, and the amplitude of accommodation will therefore be $P - R$, i.e. 10 − 5, or 5 dioptres. A myope, then, although he cannot see distant objects clearly by any effort of accommodation, has the advantage that he can see near work with considerably less effort than the emmetrope or the hypermetrope, being, in a sense, partially accommodated in his normal state.

There is no evidence of the accommodative effort acting unequally in order to counteract an astigmatic error, and so it follows that a distinct image is never obtained in *astigmatism*. Similarly, since the accommodative effort of the two eyes cannot be dissociated, the error of an *anisometrope* cannot be corrected by his accommodation, so that when correcting lenses are not worn the image of one eye is always blurred. Especially where the error is small, however, the slight difference may act as an incentive for its correction, and since the end is never achieved and the stimulus is always there, just as occurs in astigmatism, a considerable amount of accommodative strain may result.

The availability of accommodation

We have seen that the range of accommodation is not by any means proportional to the amplitude. In the emmetrope, an infinitely large alteration from infinity to 6 metres can be accomplished practically without effort, and the nearer we get to the eye a progressively shorter distance will require an ever-increasing power to cover it. Again, a hypermetrope will need to employ a greater amount of accommodation to see distinctly at a distance of 10 cm than an emmetrope, and a myope may be able to see at this distance without effort. The range cannot therefore be taken to express the work done in accommodation; this can only be appreciated by a consideration of the amplitude. On the other hand, the range is an indication of the *availability of accommodation* in that it gives us an idea of the distance at which clear vision is possible. Thus an emmetrope or a low hypermetrope with active accommodation is able to see distinctly over all ranges which may be considered to exist in practical life; a high hypermetrope may be incapacitated from all near work without the artificial aid of spectacles; while a myope may have his far point so close to his eye that without spectacles his vision is extremely limited and his range so small as to render his accommodation practically useless.

Phenomena associated with accommodation

There are two phenomena which are associated with accommodation, in that, although not necessarily accompanying it on all occasions or to the same degree, they usually act in concert with it. Such an associated action has been called a synkinesis (σύν, with; κίνησιζ, movement).

When looking at a distant object, the eyes are directed straight forwards, or approximately so, in order that the rays of light, which may be considered parallel, can fall upon both maculae; but if a near object is to be studied close up to the eyes, they must be turned inwards so that their visual axes are both directed upon it. The nearer the object the greater will need to be the convergence and, at the same time, the greater the accommodation.

Further, in looking at such a near object the pupil contracts. To some extent this action increases the acuity of vision by cutting off the outer parts of the lens and thus diminishing optical aberrations, but it also helps to cut off the relative increase of light which enters the eye from near objects. Convergence is accomplished by the medial recti and the pupillary contraction by the sphincter pupillae, while the ciliary muscle governs accommodation; the close physiological association of these three synkinetic movements is seen in the supply of all these muscles by the same nerve — the third cranial.

Fatigue of accommodation

The fatiguability of accommodation is most easily measured by a technique initiated by Lucien Howe of Buffalo and amplified by Berens. It is a modification of Mosso's classical method of studying fatigue in skeletal muscle. In brief, it consists of repeatedly approximating to the eye a target carrying as object a dot or minute type until it becomes blurred, the excursion of the target being recorded automatically on a drum. There should be no evidence of diminution of the excursion in 15 minutes, whereafter the factor of general fatigue may make itself obvious. It is to be noted that the response of the two eyes may be different and that of either may differ from binocular records. On the whole, in the normal eye it is difficult to fatigue accommodation, and in a considerable proportion of cases its excessive use leads to the development of a greater amplitude. If, however, visual tasks are continued at a range near the punctum proximum over any length of time, fatigue appears even in the normal emmetropic and orthophoric individual.

10. Presbyopia

When discussing the mechanism of accommodation we saw that the increased refractivity of the eye was probably brought about by a change in the balance between the elasticity of the matrix of the lens and that of its capsule, allowing it to assume a more globular shape. As age advances, however, several factors combine to diminish the accommodative power. The lens becomes harder and less easily moulded so that the elastic force of the capsule is no longer greater than the resistance of the lens substance. The lens tends therefore to set in an unaccommodated form. Moreover, the progressive increase in the size of the lens together with similar changes in the ciliary body reduce the circumlental space so that the zonule becomes slackened and works at a disadvantage, making the amplitude of accommodation less. Although there is evidence that some weakening of the ciliary muscle occurs as age advances, especially in the later years of life, it is now clear from the work of Fisher that presbyopia can be explained solely by the physical changes in the lens itself.

As a result it becomes more and more difficult to see near objects distinctly; that is, the near point gradually recedes. This loss of accommodation is not to be considered as abnormal, and it proceeds gradually throughout the whole of life without any sudden alterations. At first no inconvenience is experienced, but eventually a time comes when the near point has receded beyond the distance at which the individual is accustomed to read or to work or beyond the distance at which his arms allow him to hold the printed page, and then, being unable to see clearly, he becomes seriously inconvenienced.

Such a condition is called *presbyopia* ($\pi\rho\acute{\epsilon}\sigma\beta\upsilon\zeta$, old; $\grave{\omega}\psi$, the eye).

The variation of accommodation with age

The variation of the power of accommodation with age can be gathered from Figure 10.1, which was compiled by Fisher from various sources. The diagram is a representation of the average of the results, on many subjects.

It is seen that in the early years of life the amplitude of accommodation is about 14 D, and that the near point is situated at 7 cm distance.

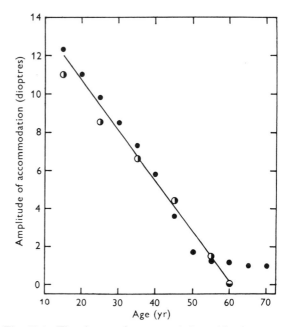

Fig. 10.1 The change of accommodation with age.

91

Thereafter it gradually and uninterruptedly recedes; at the age of 36 it has reached 14 cm, when the amplitude of accommodation has become halved and is now 7 D instead of the original 14 D. At the age of 45 it has reached 25 cm, and the amplitude of accommodation is only 4 D; at the age of 60 only about 1 D of accommodation remains.

In the majority of cases near work is done at an average distance of 28 to 30 cm away from the eyes, and therefore in the emmetrope the actual limit of clear vision is reached at 45 years when an amplitude of 3.5 to 4 dioptres of accommodation remains. This, however, would entail working at the near point continuously and thus exercising the whole of the accommodation to obtain useful vision, a condition of strain that can rarely be tolerated over any length of time. Comfort demands that about one-third of the accommodation be kept in reserve, so that when this limit has been reached and the near point is at a distance of 22 cm presbyopia may be said to have set in. In the emmetrope this occurs between 40 and 45 years of age, although there is some geographical, perhaps racial variation: an earlier age of onset may occur in those living in the tropics. Thereafter the accommodation must be supplemented by a convex lens if near work is to be done without strain.

A hypermetrope starts life with this near point considerably further away than that of an emmetrope so that the symptoms of presbyopia will come on earlier. Thus a hypermetrope with an error of +3 D will require to exercise 7 D of accommodation to give himself an amplitude of 4 D; he may therefore show presbyopic symptoms at about 25 years of age. In a myope, on the other hand, the opposite conditions hold, and if he has an error of −4 D presbyopia will never occur.

Presbyopia is thus a relative term, depending not only on the age but also on the refraction. It also varies with the individual and with his habits. A person who has the habit of reading with his book on his knees complains of discomfort later than one who is used to reading more closely; and the carpenter or the book-keeper or the musician will be comfortable at his work at 30 or 35 cm or over, while the seamstress or the compositor or the engraver of the same age and with the same refractive state will have been forced to use spectacles in order to see at his working distance of 20 cm. Or again, the ciliary muscle may fail in states of debility or disease and the physiological accommodation be at fault. There is thus no fixed presbyopic point, and there can be no rational rule-of-thumb treatment.

Symptoms

The failure of accommodation becomes evident gradually, and as a rule becomes apparent first in reading. Small print becomes indistinct, and in order to get within the limits of his receding near point the patient tends to hold his head back and his book well forward until a distance is reached when clear vision in any circumstances is difficult. Trouble is experienced at first in the evening when the light is dim and the pupils are dilated, permitting large diffusion circles; at this time, too, after the work of the day, fatigue comes on easily. The presbyope consequently likes to read by brilliant illumination, and he tries if possible to get the light between the book and his eyes or to read in the sunlight so that his pupils may be forced to contract down and diminish the aperture. For this reason, in more advanced years when the pupils become smaller in senility, an old person with no accommodation may see near objects with a fair degree of detail.

Paradoxically, early presbyopia may be marked by ciliary spasm which produces temporarily blurred distance vision on changing from near to far.

Complaint is usually made of visual failure rather than visual fatigue. Sooner or later, however, symptoms of eye-strain appear. The ciliary muscle working near its limit becomes fatigued, and the accommodative effort, strained in excess of the convergence, gives rise to distress. Headaches may occur, and the eyes feel tired and ache and sometimes tend to assume a chronically suffused appearance.

Treatment

The treatment of presbyopia is to provide the patient with convex lenses so that his accommodation is reinforced and his near point brought within a useful working distance. To do this adequately we must first know the working point of the individual, estimate his refraction and, in theory, determine the amplitude of his accommodation, and then supplement this by the appropriate strength of lens allowing him a sufficient reserve accommodation.

Thus, if the patient is emmetropic and wishes to work at 25 cm, he will require an amplitude of accommodation of 4 D. Let us suppose that his near point has receded to 50 cm: he has, in this case, 2 D of accommodation of his own. But he must, if he is to work comfortably, be able to keep one-third of this in reserve, so that he has an amplitude of 1.3 D, i.e. $\frac{2}{3}$ of 2 D. The lens he requires theoretically is therefore one of 2.7 D. If he were ametropic, his refraction must be determined, and his near point estimated whilst wearing the correcting lenses which render him emmetropic.

The techniques for determination of the accommodation and the other tests of near vision will be discussed later and should certainly be applied in appropriate circumstances. However, in practice a knowledge of the patient's static refraction and of the distance at which close work is carried out is usually sufficient to allow the refractionist to proceed to a subjective test of near vision with the addition of appropriate convex lenses and to prescribe on the basis of the results.

The appropriate strength of these additions raises important questions. It is certainly true that presbyopic spectacles should never be prescribed mechanically by ordering an appropriate addition based on the age of the patient. Each patient should be tested individually and those lenses should be ordered in each case which give the most serviceable and comfortable, not necessarily the clearest, vision for the particular work for which the spectacles are intended. Nevertheless, there is not a great variation between individuals in the way that their accommodation declines. While it is wrong to give a dogmatic rule such as the addition of 1 dioptre for every 5 years above 40, most refractionists formulate their own loose relationship between the age and the presbyopic correction needed by the average patient. It is customary to start with an addition of +0.75 D to the distance correction in the first reading spectacles prescribed for a presbyope

showing the typical early symptoms of difficulty with newsprint in the evenings or in poor illumination, and it is a safe rule to be wary of increasing a reading addition by more than this amount (0.75 D) for the presbyope whose near correction is no longer adequate.

In all cases *it is better to undercorrect than to overcorrect* since, if the lenses tend to be too strong, difficulties will be experienced with the association of accommodation and convergence and the range of vision will be inconveniently limited. Short of a formal determination of the positive and negative relative accommodation (p. 133), a good practical hint is to make sure that with the reading correction it is intended to prescribe the patient is able to read the near-vision chart satisfactorily not only at his reading distance but also some 12 to 15 cm further away. This will guard against overcorrection.

The average subject's accommodation declines so that in the late 50s an addition of about +2.50 D becomes necessary and thereafter little further change is required. In any case, a lens which brings the near point closer than 28 cm is rarely tolerated (that is, a total power of 3.5 D), and if for any reason the demands of fine work require a higher correction, the convergence should be aided with prisms as well as the accommodation with spheres. Unequal or very powerful additions for near work are often indicated in the presence of medical lesions causing poor visual acuity in one or both eyes. Thus patients with early cataract will often be enabled to read more comfortably with a +3.5 D or +4 D addition. Even higher additions may be considered as visual aids.

In the normal subject however, it cannot be too strongly emphasised that the usual cause of strain and discomfort following the prescription of spectacles for presbyopia is overcorrection. If the lenses can be reduced in strength without causing a serious deterioration in visual acuity for work at the required range, they should be so reduced; but if this is impossible, the discomfort is usually relieved by adding to the lenses a prism with the base inwards or, alternatively, by decentring the lenses by a corresponding amount. Thus, while the sphere relieves the accommodation, the prism relieves the convergence.

This author does not totally disapprove of over-the-counter purchase of reading spectacles (ready made up convex spheres of various powers, equal for the two eyes). In choosing them, a self-performed subjective test is being carried out and, as long as the wearer realises that ability to read with them is no guarantee of absolute ocular health, no harm is done, even if the correction is not exactly what would be prescribed following a formal refraction. Obviously such corrections may be much less helpful if significant astigmatism or anisometropia is present.

11. Anomalies of accommodation

Accommodation has a fairly wide range which may be looked upon as normal (see Fig. 10.1), but variations in either direction, above or below that range, are by no means uncommon.

INCREASED ACCOMMODATION

Excessive accommodation

We have seen that a certain degree of sustained accommodation is not infrequently found in young hypermetropes, but this is to be considered as a physiological adaptation in the interests of clear vision. A similar condition, however, is also found in myopes, especially in young subjects who are doing much near work, and it also on occasion accompanies astigmatic errors. It usually occurs in association with excessive convergence, and in many cases appears to be part of an attempt to obtain clarity of vision in spite of the presence of an optical anomaly. It is seen most frequently in young people, but it is not unknown in middle life when presbyopia is beginning to become apparent and the accommodation is being strained by an amount of work which it can accomplish only with difficulty.

A large amount of near work is an important factor in the aetiology of this condition, especially when the work is habitually undertaken in deficient or excessive illumination; a refractive error is usually but not invariably present or, alternatively, the wearing of improper or ill-fitting spectacles may cause it; and its occurrence may be associated with general debility and ill-health, physical or mental.

The condition involves the production of an artificial myopia which varies from time to time, sometimes in the most bewildering fashion: a hypermetrope appears myopic, and a myope more so. Both the far point and the near point are brought nearer to the eye, and distant vision becomes blurred. Vision is therefore improved by concave lenses, and these may perhaps be prescribed unwittingly, in which case, by thus catering for the spurious myopia, the condition becomes aggravated. In the more marked degrees near vision also suffers, and after reading for some time the printed page becomes confused, an effect which clears up only after a temporary rest. Meantime, typical symptoms of accommodative asthenopia are usually present, with headaches and a feeling of fatigue and discomfort in the eyes themselves.

Normally, after the exhibition of atropine and the abolition of the tone of the ciliary muscle, the refraction becomes hypermetropic by about 1 dioptre; the diagnosis of these cases of excessive accommodation is clinched by the discovery of a greater difference than this after the instillation of a cycloplegic. The dynamic refraction is incomparable with the static refraction.

The prognosis of such a condition is good, and the treatment usually effective. The refraction should be done under full cycloplegia, and the correction as found when the ciliary muscle is paralysed in this way should be ordered, deducting therefrom only about 1 dioptre. In the worst cases the eyes may well be kept mildly under the influence of atropine for a week or two in order to ensure absolute rest and allow the overexcited ciliary muscle to recover from its condition of irritability. The general treatment is usually more important than the optical correction. Near work should be forbidden for a period, and thereafter its amount should be curtailed and the conditions in which it is undertaken supervised. The general condition of the patient's health should receive attention, for most of these subjects are ailing or overworked or neurotic; a holiday with a change of air usually has a greater beneficial effect than anything else.

An occasional association of excessive accommodation is difficulty in refocusing from near to far. Having stimulated the accommodation for close work, it takes the subject some time to relax it for clear distance vision.

Spasm of accommodation

Something approaching spasm may be experienced by young glaucoma subjects using pilocarpine drops, especially if myopic. In many cases the spasm becomes less pronounced with continued use of the drops, but in some it is severe enough for this form of medication to be discontinued. Indeed the advocates of the beta-blockers argue their superiority over the parasympathomimetics precisely because of this spasm. The slow-release pledgets of pilocarpine — 'Ocuserts' — may avoid or mitigate this problem.

True spasm of the ciliary muscle, a condition similar to that brought about by miotics such as eserine is rare, and very few authentic cases have been reported. The spasm is usually out of the control of the patient, and its amount may reach 10 dioptres or more, a high degree of myopia being produced. The patients are very frequently neurotically inclined. With this may be associated some precipitating factor: a marked degree of muscular imbalance, trigeminal neuralgia, a dental lesion, or a general intoxication. Cases of iridocyclitis or those exhibiting a toxic reaction to some drugs may show similar symptoms (p. 79).

The most effective method of treatment is the production of complete ciliary paralysis with atropine, and the cycloplegia must be kept up for a long time — 4 weeks or more. Even then the spasm not infrequently returns whenever the influence of the drug has passed off, when a

further period of atropinisation must be prescribed. Correcting spectacles should be worn immediately the eyes are used again, and the general health and habits of the patient should be supervised as already indicated.

A well-developed condition of ciliary spasm is associated with the phenomenon of *macropsia* ($\mu\alpha\kappa\rho\delta\zeta$, large; $\dot{\omega}\psi$, the eye). Here, objects appear larger than they really are as a result of a delusion of distance induced by the disturbance of the accommodation. An object close at hand appears larger than one normally a considerable distance away, and thus the size tends to convey an impression of distance. When the accommodation is in spasm, the amount of additional voluntary effort to see a near object distinctly is small, and consequently, making little or no accommodative effort to see it, we judge it some considerable distance off, and are therefore led into the delusion that it is larger than it actually is.

DIMINISHED ACCOMMODATION

Insufficiency of accommodation

In the condition of insufficiency of accommodation the accommodative power is constantly below the lower limit of what may be accepted as the normal variation for the patient's age. It is a relatively common condition and may be caused by one of two factors.

The failure may be *lenticular* in origin, arising from an undue sclerosis of the lens. It is thus in essence a premature presbyopia and affects the physical accommodation only. This is a stable condition and gives rise to no symptoms except those of presbyopia which sets in at an earlier age than usual.

On the other hand, the failure may be due to *weakness of the ciliary muscle* and thus involve the physiological accommodation. Such a condition is usually labile, and varies within wide limits from time to time. Its aetiology embraces all the causes of muscular fatigue, and it is often associated with general debility, anaemia and malnutrition, accompanied by an excessive use of the eyes, especially for close work undertaken in unfavourable surroundings. Failure of accommodation may also occur in the prodromal stages of simple glaucoma.

The symptoms may be productive of much

discomfort. All the features of asthenopia and eye-strain may be present, with headaches, fatigue, and irritability of the eyes. Near work is blurred and becomes difficult or impossible, and the accommodative failure is frequently accompanied by a disturbance of convergence. Sometimes the attempt to accommodate brings on an excessive amount of convergence, but more often this associated function also fails. The duration of the condition is dependent upon the cause; with an improvement of the exciting factors a betterment in the general health, or a relaxation from overwork or worry, the ocular condition may considerably improve, only to relapse at a later date if the same conditions again prevail.

When tests of the amplitude of the accommodation reveal the presence of such an accommodative insufficiency, and when it is giving rise to symptoms, treatment may be prescribed which usually brings a great deal of comfort. In the first place any refractive error should be corrected, and if vision for near work is seriously blurred and reading is therefore difficult, distance spectacles correcting the refractive error should be supplemented by an additional pair for reading, the procedure adopted being the same as that described for presbyopia. If there is an associated convergence excess, such glasses should be prescribed unhesitatingly, for by relieving the effort to accommodate much of the stimulus to converge is removed. On the other hand, if there is convergence insufficiency, the addition of prisms, bases in, may add considerably to the patient's comfort. The prismatic correction added should as a rule be such as brings the near point of convergence to the same distance as the near point of accommodation, and it generally corresponds to the spherical addition required. In all these cases only the weakest convex lenses which will allow adequate vision should be ordered so that the accommodation may be exercised and stimulated rather than relieved. For the same reason, as soon as recovery takes place the additional correction for reading should be made progressively weaker from time to time.

Meantime, the accommodation may be considerably improved by the practice of *exercises* provided the patient is intelligent enough to undertake them properly. The most simple of these involves the use of the accommodation test-card (a black vertical line drawn on a white card is sufficient), and he is instructed to practise with this at short periods throughout the day. The card is held a considerable distance away and then brought closer to the eye until the line appears blurred and indistinct; by repeating this he should be encouraged to attempt to bring his near point as close as possible, and to maintain his accommodative effort as long as he can with comfort. Such exercises will defeat their own ends unless they stop short of producing fatigue and distress, and if they are to be undertaken successfully the patient should be one who can appreciate the physiological limits of his powers. The exercises should be undertaken only in those cases which are the result of ciliary underactivity, and in patients who are not in a state of general debility, in whom the condition of the ciliary muscles is merely the local expression of generalised muscular weakness. In cases of early cataract wherein the condition is stable and visual symptoms characteristic of presbyopia only are evident, such exercises are worse than useless in that they merely force the ciliary muscle to attempt the impossible. During the exercises the patient should wear his distance correction. Where there is an excess of convergence, one eye only should be used at a time and the other should be covered; where convergence also is deficient, both eyes should be exercised simultaneously and other measures should be undertaken for the stimulation of this function (see p. 138).

At the same time, treatment should be directed to the cause of the weakness, if that is discoverable. Work and the conditions of work should be regulated, the general health should be improved in every way, and any suggestive toxic state should be dealt with on its merits.

Ill-sustained accommodation

Ill-sustained accommodation is essentially the same condition as insufficiency but less accentuated. The range of accommodation is normal, but on any attempt to use the eyes for near work over a prolonged interval the accommodative power weakens, the near point gradually recedes, and the near vision becomes blurred. Frequently it is the initial stage of a true insufficiency. The causes of the condition are the same as those just reviewed and it is common in convalescence from debilitating illnesses. The treatment is essentially the same, and is to be directed mainly to the reduction of work within the limits of the patient's capabilities and general tonic measures.

Such a condition in a mild form is relatively common in those who read in the evening when they are tired, or in bed when they are physically relaxed. This, of course, is by no means surprising. The ocular muscles share in any general state of fatigue, and when the other muscles are tired and have demanded and have obtained relaxation it would be strange if the former should be prepared to carry on without complaint. In these circumstances and in convalescence from illness, it is too often forgotten that reading or sewing entails muscular work in as true a sense as any other exercise, and these should be regulated on this understanding.

Inertia of accommodation

Accommodative inertia is a somewhat rare condition wherein the patient experiences some difficulty in altering the range of his accommodation. It takes some time and involves some effort for him to focus a near object after looking into the distance. It rarely assumes serious proportions, but on occasion may give rise to some trouble and annoyance. For its relief, any refractive error should be corrected and accommodative exercises should be undertaken.

Paralysis of accommodation

This may occur from local or general causes; the most important local cause is the exposure of the eye to parasympatholytic (i.e. cycloplegic) medication, atropine drops for example. Occasionally trauma to the eye may be responsible.

More general causes act either on the midbrain or on the parasympathetic nerve supply in the oculo-motor nerve or on the ciliary muscle itself. Central neurological causes are uncommon but include vascular disorders, cerebral syphilis, and, historically, encephalitis lethargica.

Other infectious causes act either centrally or by peripheral neurotoxic action. Cases have been recorded in those suffering from mumps, infectious mononucleosis, tonsillitis, herpes zoster and pneumonia. Rarer causes include diphtheria, botulism, and typhoid.

Non-infective toxic states may also be responsible, such as chronic alcoholism, belladonna intoxication and also in certain cases of diabetes.

Failure of accommodation and convergence occasionally results from head injury even of mild degree. Near paralysis or at least weakness of accommodation is often a feature of an eye demonstrating Adie's myotonic pupil.

In paralysis of the accommodation the near point recedes and approximates the far point so that objects close at hand appear blurred. Vision in the distance, however, is not necessarily impaired, although the enlarged pupil which usually accompanies the condition accentuates any optical defects the eye may already have. It also tends to produce an uncomfortable amount of dazzling. The phenomenon of *micropsia* is also evident. It is the reverse of the *macropsia* which occurs in accommodative spasm. Objects appear smaller than they really are owing to a delusion of distance induced by the accommodative anomaly. To see an object distinctly necessitates a great effort, and thus we take it to be nearer than it actually is, and consequently, judged from this standpoint, we believe it to be unnaturally small.

It is seen that paralysis of the accommodation is a symptom of general disease, and with these the refractionist should be acquainted. The ocular lesion may form the most prominent symptom and the patient may come to him first for advice. A progressive paresis should suggest incipient glaucoma. A sudden paralysis should suggest the presence of diabetes, or lead to an inquiry into a history of a sore throat that had received no attention, or to mild influenza or fever that may have been an encephalitis. On the other hand, contamination with an ointment containing atropine very frequently explains an occurrence which at first sight appears potentially serious.

Many systemic medications may interfere with accommodative activity. Although this effect is frequently transitory and may not be profound, a knowledge of those which are particularly liable to behave in this way is clearly essential both for the ophthalmologist and for those in general medical practice. While total paralysis of accommodation is uncommon as a side effect of systemic medication given for general disease, some impairment may occur with the use of any drug which has a parasympatholytic effect. Those involved include anti-hypertensive medication, antidepressants of the phenothiazine type and medication used to combat gastro-intestinal spasm.

The treatment of these conditions resolves itself primarily into a treatment of the cause. In paralysis of central nervous origin, as for example in cerebral syphilis or tabes, the prognosis is bad. In encephalitis lethargica the condition may be transient or may persist indefinitely into the post-encephalitic stage. In the toxic varieties the prognosis is favourable provided the toxaemia can be overcome; this includes diphtheria, diabetes, and the more direct poisons. In traumatic cases the condition may be permanent and the prognosis should be guarded. With regard to the local condition, especially in those toxic states wherein the lesion is presumably not permanent, no treatment is necessary. The eyes should be rested and no near work should be attempted. Stimulation of the ciliary muscle by eserine or by electrical methods has been suggested: the former probably does harm, and the latter is useless. When, however, recovery is delayed, and in those cases wherein the prognosis is bad, presbyopic spectacles should be ordered which will allow the patient to read and work in comfort.

CYCLOPLEGIA

The use of cycloplegics

A state of paralysis of the ciliary muscle is called *cycloplegia*: it may be produced by drugs instilled into the conjunctival sac, such as atropine, homatropine, and scopolamine, which are known as *cycloplegics*. These also paralyse the sphincter muscle of the iris, causing a dilatation of the pupil; for this reason they are also called *mydriatics*. Many drugs which dilate the pupil also paralyse the accommodation in some degree; and similarly, all drugs which constrict the pupil (*miotics*, such as eserine or pilocarpine) stimulate

the ciliary muscle to contract, and induce some degree of spasm of the accommodation.

Both these properties, cycloplegia and mydriasis, are of service in the estimation of refractive errors. By paralysing the parasympathetic nerve supply all accommodation for near can be abolished and refractive errors which before were latent are rendered manifest. If the sympathetic nerve mediates an active accommodation for distance, this, of course, is unaffected and is now unopposed, but is probably negligible. The dilatation of the pupil, moreover, makes the technique of estimating the error easier, and it assists in allowing a thorough and easy examination to be made of the interior of the eye. Lastly, in cases showing symptoms of strain and asthenopia, drugs which have a prolonged period of action, such as atropine, by forcing rest upon the eye, enable it to recover from its state of fatigue and keep it from further overaction until the correcting spectacles are prepared.

The cycloplegic drugs

Atropine

Atropine is the strongest cycloplegic known. When instilled into the conjunctival sac it is absorbed into the anterior chamber and abolishes all parasympathetic activity by preventing the penetration of acetylcholine into the effector muscle cells. The muscle fibres supplied by the parasympathetic system are thus paralysed, resulting in full cycloplegia and mydriasis. It dilates the pupil in about 15 minutes, and soon afterwards begins its action upon the accommodation. This action, however, is slow, and in children it is necessary to prescribe it for 4 days before the examination in order that the paralysis should be complete. In young people whose accommodation is powerful it should be given three times a day on three successive days. The action on accommodation lasts from 7 to 12 days, and pupillary dilatation persists a day or two longer; consequently the patient is precluded from near work for a considerable time, unless myopic. This prolonged reaction makes its use in patients who are candidates for closed-angle glaucoma dangerous, the more so since no drug will easily and rapidly overcome its effects.

It is prescribed in a strength of 1.0%, in the form of either drops or ointment. The drops are usually made up in watery solution and the sulphate is used; in the ointment a 1% solution of the alkaloid is employed in soft yellow paraffin. The ointment is on the whole the more useful preparation for children; it is more easily rubbed into the eye, for they frequently object strenuously to drops. In addition, it is more slowly and continuously absorbed than drops, much of which flows down the lacrimal passages and may (although rarely) give rise to symptoms of atropine intoxication (dryness of the throat, diminution of all secretions, excitability, etc.). As exceptional rarities systemic symptoms and even fatalities have been reported after its use. Care should be taken, however, that the ointment is not administered for some hours previous to the examination, as the grease on the cornea will impair its transparency and alter the regularity of its refraction.

Homatropine

Homatropine acts more rapidly and less powerfully than atropine, while its effects pass off more quickly. Its action starts in from 5 to 15 minutes, is at its maximum in about three-quarters of an hour, and has passed off to a large extent in 24 hours. There is some residual impairment of accommodation, however, which may persist for 2 or 3 days, and for this reason any post-cycloplegic test should be postponed for such an interval. Especially when there is much latent hypermetropia, a slight insufficiency of accommodation may persist for over a week. Its action is overcome by eserine, and after the administration of this drug in a drop of 1% solution, near work should be possible within an hour or two. It may be given as a 1 or 2% solution of the hydrobromide, and its administration should be repeated two or three times at intervals of 10 minutes, and the accommodation will be found almost completely under its influence in an hour or an hour and a half.

There are other mydriatics which are less widely employed. *Hyoscine* (or *scopolamine*) *hydrobromide* in 0.5% solution has an action similar to atropine; it has the advantage of being more transitory than atropine, lasting only about 5 days, and is a suitable cycloplegic for children. Constitutional symptoms — giddiness, drowsiness, and dryness of the throat — may occur. Success has also been claimed for 0.05% hyoscine drops given 1 hour before refraction. *Hyoscyamine sulphate* (1%) has a similar action, lasting from 6 to 7 days; its action is thus intermediate between that of atropine and hyoscine.

Cyclogyl (cyclopentolate) and *Mydriacyl* (bistropamide) produce a rapid and intense mydriasis and a satisfactory cycloplegia. A drop is instilled in each eye and this is repeated in 10 minutes. Paralysis of accommodation and full dilatation of the pupil are usually complete within 1 hour and the effects have worn off within 24 hours; occasionally the duration of action is much longer, even 3 or 4 days.

In very young children these short-acting cycloplegics are sometimes irritative and may actually induce a temporary spasm of accommodation. In these cases recourse to atropine is the obvious procedure.

Although cocaine acts solely as a mydriatic, the action of the weaker cholinergic drugs, particularly homatropine, may usefully be augmented by synergists of the sympathomimetic group. Thus it has been claimed that the combination of homatropine with cocaine (2% as the hydrochloride) not only accentuates and reinforces the cycloplegia but is also followed by a quicker return to normal; this has, however, been questioned.

The quantity and type of cycloplegic, however, should not be administered by a blanket formula. Individuals vary considerably in the dosage they require to produce a satisfactory degree of ciliary paralysis. Even in the same individual the two eyes sometimes show a great variability in their response, a phenomenon called *anisocycloplegia* by Beach, who found that a difference of 0.5 D in the depth of cycloplegia is common and that a difference of as much as 10 D is found in exceptional cases. The administration of these drugs should therefore be determined on an individualistic basis and the depth of the cycloplegia tested in each case before the refractive examination is begun. This is easily done by testing the amplitude of accommodation which remains; this should not exceed 1.0 D, i.e. the line on the accommodation card should become blurred at a distance of 1 metre; if it is clearly seen a further instillation of the cycloplegic drug should be made. After the refraction has been tested, the state of the accommodation may again be verified: a +3 D sphere is added to the full correction, when the far point should be at 33 cm and the near point slightly over 25 but not over 28 cm. If this amount of cycloplegia does not remain, and if the drug has been carefully administered, excessive accommodation should be suspected, and further instillations should be given or atropine should be used.

Clinical anomalies

PART 3 Binocular vision and its anomalies

12. Binocular optical defects — anisometropia

Anisometropia ($\overset{\text{`}}{\alpha}$ privative; $\overset{\text{'}}{\iota}\sigma o\varsigma$, equal; $\mu\acute{\epsilon}\tau\rho o\nu$, measure; $\overset{\text{'}}{\omega}\psi$ eye) is the term applied to that condition wherein the refractions of the two eyes are unequal. The anomaly is found in every possible variety; one eye may be emmetropic and its fellow of any other denomination, hypermetropic, myopic, or astigmatic; or both eyes may be ametropic, the refraction differing in degree or also in kind. It is extremely common in small amount, especially where astigmatic errors are present. The condition is usually congenital, and an absolutely isometropic refraction is as rare as a perfectly symmetrical face.

Another important cause of the condition arises from unequal rates of change of the refractive state between the two eyes, especially in the early years; this applies to the way hypermetropic subjects become less so and particularly to myopes who may progress much more rapidly in one eye than the other.

Finally, anisometropia can follow surgical or non-surgical trauma as well as other diseases. The most gross example of such acquired anisometropia is, of course, surgical aphakia but intended or accidental anisometropia may also be a feature of the pseudophakic subject.

Vision in anisometropia

The vision in anisometropia may be affected in one of three ways: it may be binocular, it may be alternating, or it may be exclusively uniocular.

Binocular vision is the rule in the smaller degrees of the defect, and it has been reported with a difference as high as 6 dioptres. Each 0.25 D difference between the refraction of the two eyes causes 0.5% difference in size between the two retinal images, and a difference of 5% is probably the limit which can be tolerated. Moreover, since the power of accommodation acts equally in both eyes, and is not dissociated, the image of one eye is always blurred, but the patient, superimposing the indistinct upon the distinct image, tries to combine the two and obtain a stereoscopic effect. In these circumstances binocular vision is rarely perfect; and the attempt at fusion frequently, although by no means always, brings on symptoms of accommodative asthenopia.

With the higher grades of error, fusion is impossible and one of two alternatives offers itself.

Alternating vision may result, in which case each of the two eyes is used one at a time. This is especially apt to occur when they both have good visual acuity, and when one is emmetropic or moderately hypermetropic and the other is myopic. In these circumstances the patient falls into the easy habit of using the former for distant vision and the latter for near work; he may thus be comfortable, never having to make an effort either of accommodation or convergence.

On the other hand, if the defect in one eye is high, and more especially if its visual acuity is not good, it may be *excluded altogether from vision* at an early stage in life. The other and better eye is alone relied upon and, if it is not so already, the more ametropic eye tends to become *amblyopic*, the image from it being suppressed. This amblyopia from disuse (*amblyopia ex anopsia*) is in most cases a preventable condition, since useful vision may be retained if the error in the defective eye is recognised early enough in life and the use of the eye encouraged at that time by suitable exercises and that of the better eye discouraged if necessary by occlusion.

Anisometropia probably has an important influence on the development of squint, particularly concomitant convergent strabismus in children. The more blurred image from the one eye acts as a sensory obstacle to binocular vision. This image becomes suppressed, and it is often found that in cases of uniocular squint the deviating eye is the more ametropic. Once the eye does deviate, of course, further suppression supervenes to prevent diplopia.

The state of the vision may be determined by the use of a colour test derived from a suggestion by Snellen. The word FRIEND is hung up in illuminated letters so that the alternate letters are green and red — F, I, N are green and R, E, D are red. A green glass is placed in front of one of the patient's eyes, and a red one in front of the other, and since he can see only the green letters through the green glass and the red letters through the red, we can tell at once from what he reads whether or not he is using both together. If he reads FRIEND at once he has binocular vision; if he reads FIN or RED persistently he has uniocular vision with the eye which has the corresponding glass; if he reads now one, now the other, he has alternating vision (for distance). Worth's *four-dot test*, suitable for children, is based on the same principle.

Treatment

As anisometropia is never corrected by unequal contraction of the ciliary muscles. An optical correction is the only means of treatment. Theoretically, the ideal treatment would be the full correction of each eye in order to produce a distinct image on the retinae of both. In practice, this course is satisfactory and usually advisable when dealing with small refractive differences, but in the case of the higher grades several difficulties present themselves which require attention.

When correcting spectacles are placed at the anterior focal plane of the eye, it will be seen (p. 210) that there is no change in the size of the retinal image from that formed by the emmetropic eye. This plane is 15.7 mm in front of the cornea; and in practice, if the lenses are placed farther from the eye than this, with a convex lens the retinal image is enlarged, while with a concave lens it is diminished, the difference in size becoming considerable in the higher grades of anisometropia. If the spectacles are nearer than this point, an opposite effect will be produced. Before the correction was made the discomfort caused by the unequal images may not have been great because one of them was blurred and therefore easily neglected; but now when they are both sharply defined and still unequal, they give rise to annoyance and their fusion may become difficult or impossible. Further, whenever the patient looks to the side through the periphery of the lens, a prismatic effect will be produced (see p. 212), and when the difference between the lenses is great, since the distortion is different in the two eyes, it will materially enhance the discomfort. Finally, as we have noted, these anisometropic errors are frequently associated with manifest squint. But even if a latent muscular imbalance is present, when the images of the two eyes are made clear a temporary breakdown of binocular vision may lead to the patient experiencing double vision for the first time.

This being the case, it follows that the treatment of these patients cannot be undertaken on empirical lines. Each case must be considered separately, attention being paid to the amount of discomfort and the disability from which the patient is suffering without correction, and the amount he is likely to experience with it, always bearing in mind the advantages of binocular vision and the importance of retaining the potentialities of an eye for vision in case of future injury or disease of the other.

The following guiding principles will be found to be useful:

In children (under the age of 12) every attempt should be made to induce the full correction to be worn; the younger the child the more persistent should be the attempt, the easier it will prove, and the more successful will be the result.

In adults with small grades of anisometropia and any degree of binocular vision, certainly those with a difference of 2 D and generally up to 4 D, a determined attempt should be made to wear the full correction, and the spectacles should be used constantly when symptoms of eye-strain are present or muscular imbalance is evident; in these circumstances, after a few weeks' difficulty, the symptoms of strain will happily disappear. The differences in size of the retinal images may to some extent be compensated by varying the base curve of the two lenses (see p. 206), thus a plus lens on a −12 D base curve magnifies the size of the image 1.6% as compared with a flat lens. In older patients, however, it may be found that the correction involves headache and dizziness, so that some compromise will be necessary. It is frequently advisable to undercorrect the more ametropic eye, and a small deduction will often bring comfort; thus a patient who ought to have, but will not tolerate, a +2 D and +4 D sphere may be happy with a +2 D and +3.5 D. Failing this, both eyes can be tried with the correction of the working eye which is usually the more emmetropic (i.e. +2 D and +2 D). Similarly in myopia, the weaker eye may be corrected, and a patient with −2 and −4 D of error wearing lenses of −2 D and −2 D will use the right eye for distant vision and the left for near work.

The use of contact lenses for anisometropia is now widespread, and they have been recommended for many young subjects, sometimes quite small children, who might otherwise become amblyopic on the side of the more ametropic eye. The effects of contact lenses on the size of the image are not absolutely predictable as the result depends on the precise optical cause of the ametropia.

Attempts are made at intervals to revive the popularity of iseikonic lenses (see p. 113) which would seem ideally suited for the management of anisometropic disparity in retinal image size. They have, however, to a large extent been ousted by contact lenses in this field.

At the same time attention should be given to the correction of faults in muscle balance by prisms. In this way the occurrence of diplopia may be prevented. When the difference between the two eyes is marked, the patient should be advised to turn his head instead of his eyes in looking to the side in order to avoid the prismatic effect produced by the periphery of the lenses. This disturbance may be very evident in near work, for on looking down through the lower part of the lens, a convex lens acts as a prism base up and a concave one as a prism base down; this effect may be so marked as to result in diplopia. Where a myopic eye and a hypermetropic eye are thus associated, a certain amount of comfort in reading binocularly may sometimes be obtained in neutralising this action by cementing a correcting prism onto the lower portion of each lens; but in all of these cases it is wise to prescribe a separate pair of reading spectacles carefully centred and tilted so that the visual axes in the reading position pass normally through them (see p. 214). An alternative approach is provided by 'anisometropic spectacles' (illustrated in Fig. 12.1). Here the annoyance caused by peripheral prismatic effects is minimised by making the margin of the stronger lens weaker.

In an adult with alternating vision — one eye being hypermetropic and used for distance, and the other myopic and used for near work — or with monocular vision — one eye being used exclusively for all functions — the condition is usually best left alone and certainly in the latter case is strongly to be avoided, no attempt being made to correct both eyes. If there are symptoms of eye-strain and the patient is young, an attempt may be made to induce him to wear the full correction. If this does not succeed, he should be provided with spectacles which enable each eye to perform its separate functions comfortably; in most older cases this will be found the only useful plan to adopt.

Uniocular aphakia may be considered a special case of extreme anisometropia. Partly owing to the total lack of accommodation, and partly and in greater measure owing to the increased size of the retinal image, an aphakic eye corrected by

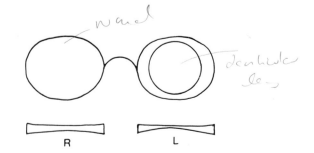

Fig. 12.1 Anisometropic spectacles.

spectacles can rarely be used in association with a normal one. In this extreme and accentuated example of anisometropia, inevitable aniseikonia makes fusion of the two images difficult or impossible and the attempt to obtain binocular vision usually results in diplopia with its attendant embarrassments, the enlarged image of the aphakic eye (a quarter or a third as large again) having a smaller central inset representing the image of the phakic eye. For this reason it was formerly the case that a patient with good visual acuity in one eye was little benefited by an extraction of a cataract from the other. Such an operation used to be advised only in special circumstances, for example where workmen or motor drivers and others were to be helped simply by an increase in the visual field on the blind side; the other indication was where it was advisable in order to prevent a cataractous lens from proceeding to hypermaturity or the Morgagnian state.

Some of the optical difficulties of uniocular aphakia can be overcome by wearing a contact lens and the success of modern varieties of extended-wear soft lenses or of gas-permeable lenses certainly encourages earlier surgery in this condition. The situation has however been completely altered with the widespread practice of intra-ocular lens implantation. It is now commonplace to advise early surgery of this type in cases of even quite minor degree of lens opacity occurring in one eye only. Furthermore, longstanding uniocular aphakics who never became tolerant of a contact lens or became progressively intolerant of such device can be offered secondary intra-ocular lens implantation in many instances.

A rational but still experimental treatment of anisometropia has been the operation of keratomileusis (see p. 62), whereby a portion of the patient's cornea is removed, frozen, ground to a new shape and then re-applied. Claims have been made that following this some recovery from even quite longstanding amblyopia has occurred.

13. Binocular optical defects — aniseikonia

Aniseikonia ($\dot{\alpha}$, privative; $\overset{\text{`}}{\iota}\sigma o\varsigma$, equal; $\overset{\text{`}}{\epsilon}\acute{\iota}\kappa\omega\nu$, an image), a condition wherein the size and shape of the images in the two eyes are unequal, is a common occurrence and probably can give rise to distressing symptoms. Its importance in the causation of eye-strain is difficult to assess; but it is significant that, after the initial enthusiasm which marked the introduction of the concept four decades ago had died down, comparatively little attention has been devoted to it.

The inequality of the images may depend on two distinct factors; it may be an optical phenomenon depending on a difference in the size of the dioptric images formed on the retinae, or it may be anatomically determined by a difference in the distribution of the retinal elements. With regard to the first factor, the difference between the dioptric images may depend on a difference between the refraction of the two eyes, and is therefore present in some degree in most cases of anisometropia. The size of the image is governed essentially by the distance of the second nodal point from the retina, and consequently a further degree of aniseikonia may be determined by differences in the magnification effectivity of the correcting lenses worn, and is varied by their power, shape, and the position at which they are worn. Especially if the anisometropia is astigmatic, therefore, the correction of the refractive error may increase the aniseikonia. With regard to the second factor, it is quite obvious that, even if dioptric images of exactly the same size were formed on the retinae, they would be appreciated as such only if the distribution of rods and cones were identical; if, for example, the visual elements were more widely separated in one eye than the

other, the image received by the brain would appear to be smaller in the first since fewer end-organs were stimulated. Presumably it is this which explains the occurrence of aniseikonia in cases wherein the dioptric mechanism cannot account for the phenomenon.

Slight changes in the size and shape of the ocular images are of constant occurrence and are responsible for stereoscopic interpretation, but these are of a very small order. A noticeable degree of aniseikonia, however, occurs in from 20 to 30% of people who wear spectacles. The usual differences which occur in binocular single vision do not exceed 5%; most commonly these occur in anisometropia. In cases of squint, however, differences of from 5 to 15% have been found, in which case the aniseikonia has an important bearing on the treatment and prognosis of the condition. But the greatest degree is seen in corrected uniocular aphakia wherein a difference of as much as 30% may exist when, as we have seen, the optical condition is intolerable.

The differences in the images may be classified as follows:

1. Symmetrical, one image being larger than the other, either in all dimensions (Fig. 13.1A), or in one meridian (Fig. 13.1B). This meridional difference may be oblique.

2. Asymmetrical, the image being distorted in some degree. It may, for example, be progressively larger in one direction and smaller in another, the effect resembling that produced by a prism (Fig. 13.1C); or its shape may be progressively distorted (Fig. 13.1D) (see p. 218). It is to be

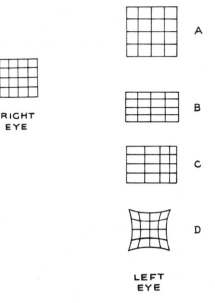

RIGHT EYE

A

B

C

D

LEFT EYE

Fig. 13.1 See text.

remembered that retinal images usually increase progressively in size across the visual field, being smaller on the nasal side and larger on the temporal, a condition which shows itself in the Hering–Hillebrand horopter deviation.

Symptoms

The symptoms caused by this inequality of retinal images, like the symptoms caused by refractive errors, are many and various. They include visual disturbances, such as blurred vision, difficulty of fixation, a tendency to diplopia and probably even a tendency to the development of squint. Complaint is sometimes made of photophobia and general ocular discomfort, as well as headaches and the general nervous manifestations associated with eye-strain. The symptoms are frequently aggravated by reading, the cinema, and especially by moving objects as when travelling.

The most interesting and important symptoms, however, are concerned with binocular vision and spatial perception. Small differences in size (under 0.25%) are not generally appreciated, and it would seem likely that these do not impair binocular vision. As a general rule differences up

to 5% can be compensated by the plasticity of the visuo-perceptive processes. When the difference is in excess of this, binocular vision becomes difficult or impossible. Ordinarily, escape from such a situation is attained by suppression of one eye at an early stage in life, and comfort is obtained in uniocularity; but if bimacular vision has already been well established and a sudden marked aniseikonia is introduced (as occurs typically in aphakia), diplopia results. It is significant that in cases of strabismus differences of the order of 5 to 15% have been found, and it is probable that the difficulty of fusion in such circumstances may have much to do with the causation and the perpetuation of the deformity and the difficulties of treatment in such cases.

Many of our perceptions of space are based on the stereoscopic effect derived from the slightly dissimilar images received by the two eyes on account of their lateral separation. It is obvious that, if normal binocular spatial localisation is based on a system of normal incongruity of the

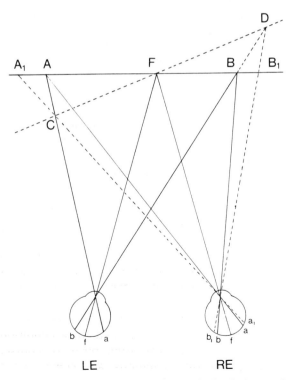

Fig. 13.2 The distortion of space in aniseikonia (see text).

visual images, when their incongruity differs from normal, anomalous spatial localisation must necessarily occur, involving apparent changes in the environment.

Figure 13.2 will make this clear wherein a meridional size lens magnifying the image in the horizontal meridian is placed before the right eye. Before such a lens is placed in position, if the eyes are converged on an object F, two objects A and B on the horopter will be imaged on corresponding retinal points a and b. After the size lens has been placed before the right eye, all sizes in the horizontal meridian will be magnified so that AB will appear as A_1B_1 and the retinal image in the right eye will be represented by $a'b'$, while that in the left eye has remained unaltered. We have already seen that an object is located in space along the apparent direction of rays of light as they enter the eye (p. 13); and this direction is obtained by a projection of the line from the retinal image through the nodal point of the eye (p. 31). The image of A seen by the left eye will therefore be projected along the line aA and that seen by the right eye along the line $a'A_1$. Seen binocularly the object will necessarily be located where these two lines meet. Since therefore the only object which can simultaneously stimulate the two retinal points a in the left eye and a' in the right is C, A will appear to have moved forwards to C. Since the only object which can stimulate the two retinal points b in the left eye and b_1 in the right is D, B will appear to have moved backwards to D. The horizontal disparity thus created results in a stereoscopic effect and the plane AB appears to be rotated around the fixation point F to CD.

If the horizontal disparity of the retinal images which is responsible for stereoscopic vision is disorientated in this way, well-defined effects are produced. Objects in the right half of the field appear larger and further away than objects of the same size and at the same distance in the left field. A flat surface such as a table slants down on the right and up on the left, and the ground seems to show the same tilt to the observer who feels as if he were walking on a hill. Objects will be correspondingly distorted; the right hand is larger than the left, the face is asymmetrical with the right side protruding, squares become rectangular, circles ellipses and the top of the table a trapezoid. In a condition which has been present from birth, of course, these spatial disorientations are compensated perceptually, but if the patient becomes fatigued

or if he is transposed to surroundings in which there is a minimum of uniocular perspective clues, such as occur in aviation or, in certain circumstances, in motoring, distortions in space may become evident with resulting errors in the judgement of distances. This condition of instability is comparable to a heterophoria (Ch. 15) becoming manifest when fusion is lost; in both cases the defect is present all the time but is only elicited in special circumstances.

Clinical investigation

The standard method for measuring the disparity in size of the retinal images depends upon the presentation to the two eyes of dissimilar objects of the same size of such a design that discrepancies between them can be readily assessed. The most accurate method depends upon the anomalous localisation in space which results from the disparity in size of the images presented to the two eyes in the *space eikonometer* of Ogle and Ames.

The principle of the space eikonometer is seen in Figure 13.3. It consists of four vertical plumb lines (A, B, C, D), two in front and two behind a cross consisting of two cords at right angles (F, G). A fifth vertical plumb line (E) passes through the centre of the cross. The whole is viewed through a test lens unit against a uniform background. When no anomalous incongruity of the visual images is present, the elements of the eikonometer appear in their normal relationships, all of them lying in planes normal to the binocular line of sight; if an anomalous incongruity exists the elements will appear to be displaced by an amount proportional to the degree and in a direction corresponding to the type of incongruence, and this can be measured by neutralising the displacement by the appropriate iseikonic lenses set in the trial test unit.

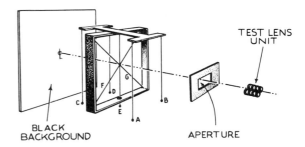

Fig. 13.3 The structure of the space eikonometer.

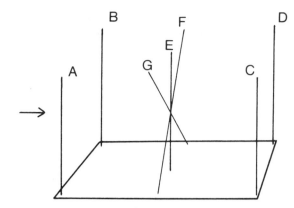

Fig. 13.4 The normal appearance.

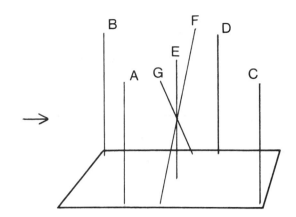

Fig. 13.7 The appearance with an overall size difference.

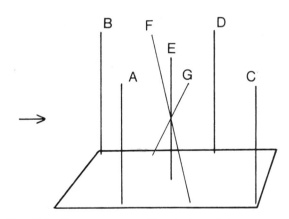

Fig. 13.5 The appearance with a horizontal size difference.

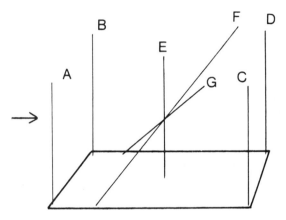

Fig. 13.8 The appearance with a meridional size difference.

Figs 13.4 to **13.8**   The appearances seen with the space eikonometer.
(In each case the arrow indicates the direction of the incident light.)

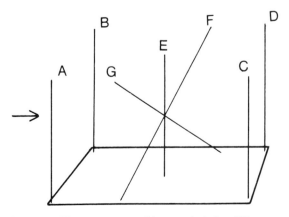

Fig. 13.6 The appearance with a vertical size difference.

Thus while the normal appearance is as in Figure 13.4, with a horizontal size difference there is an apparent displacement of the front and back vertical cords and the cross seems turned around a vertical axis in the same direction (Fig. 13.5). A rotation of the cross with correct orientation of the vertical cords indicates incongruence in the vertical direction (Fig. 13.6). Rotation of the vertical elements and not the cross indicates overall discrepancies (Fig. 13.7), and tilting of the cross indicates meridional discrepancies (Fig. 13.8).

A modified technique derived by Ruben for use with the major amblyoscope is of particular value in the assessment of binocular function and uniocular aphakia. The target slides are based on Ames's

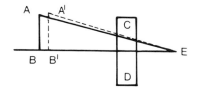

Fig. 13.9 If an object AB is regarded through a glass plate CD, held before the eye, E, the image is displaced towards the plate to A'B', producing a magnification increasing with the thickness of the plate. This is applicable to virtually parallel rays (cf. Fig. 20.1).

cross and verticals. The subject fuses two slides and the synoptophore arms are slowly diverged. From the manner in which the slides split apart, size differences of the order of 0.5% can be detected.

Treatment

The treatment of aniseikonia is the correction of the disparity in size of the retinal images with iseikonic lenses, that is lenses which cause magnification without introducing any appreciable refractive power by changing the direction of the pencils of light passing through them. Viewed through a plane parallel glass plate an image is displaced towards the plate by an amount approximating one-third the thickness of the plate; it follows that the image will suffer a corresponding angular magnification which, however, is small (Fig. 13.9). If, in addition, the glass plate is curved, the magnification, which depends on the refractive power of the front surface (and the thickness of the plate), can be much increased. The refractive power of the front surface is neutralised by an appropriate refractive power of the back surface so that the image of the object is situated at the location of the object itself — that is the lens becomes of zero refractive power. Magnifications in one or all meridians can be incorporated in the lens to suit the regular types of aniseikonia.

Using such 'size' lenses several writers have reported considerable success in the relief of patients with visual troubles; on average it would appear that some 50 to 60% of aniseikonic patients are relieved of their symptoms and a further 10 to 15% experience considerable improvement. It has been argued that the extreme care lavished upon the visual correction may account for the successful results in some cases, and that the psychological effect of a prolonged, impressive and expensive examination is the determining factor in others, the 'cure' being essentially by suggestion. However that may be, iseikonic correction has relieved of distressing symptoms some patients who have been able to obtain relief by no other means, and it would seem that, although the technique of correction is unfortunately elaborate, time-consuming and expensive, the correction of a visual fault which can be shown to cause considerable visual disability cannot be completely unsound; but sufficient clinical evidence has not yet accumulated whereon to base an authoritative estimate of its value or to lay down precise rules for its application.

In conclusion it must be said that the subject of aniseikonia, as well as some of the problems of anisometropia, have become to a certain degree eclipsed since the more widespread use of contact lenses.

14. Binocular muscular co-ordination — orthophoria

Ideally, when the eyes are at rest and are regarding a distant object situated straight in front of them, the visual axes are parallel. This is called the *primary position*. When they are so disposed, rays of light on entering fall upon corresponding points on the retina of each, so that the two images can be fused psychologically into one and binocular vision is possible. If the direction of vision is changed so that the eyes occupy any other (*secondary*) position, they must move in complete co-ordination if this psychological blending of the two sets of visual impressions is to be retained. Not only must *conjugate movements* be accurately balanced in this way, but *disjunctive movements* such as convergence and divergence must be delicately graded, so that when the two eyes fix an object at any distance they are so orientated that the macula of each comes into the direct line of vision. When we remember the free mobility of the eyes and their complicated control by six pairs of muscles, it does not seem surprising that an adjustment as delicate as the ideal conditions demand is not invariably maintained.

The condition wherein the actions of the muscles are normally balanced so as to allow fusion without effort is called *orthophoria*, while conditions of imbalance are known as *squint* or *strabismus*. When this imbalance is overcome so that the proper alignment of the eyes is maintained under duress, the condition is known as *heterophoria* (*latent strabismus*). But when this is found to be impossible, either because the muscular imbalance is too great or the desire for fusion too weak or because the vision in the two eyes is unequal, one of the eyes deviates out of its proper direction and the condition of *heterotropia* (*manifest strabismus*) is produced.

Binocular vision

There are three essentials necessary for the attainment of binocular vision. Firstly, there must be a healthy macula in each eye subserved by an efficient focusing mechanism so that two clear and approximately equally distinct images can be formed. The visual acuity at the macula must be higher than at any other region of the retina in order that a sufficiently strong reflex stimulus can be sent to the extrinsic muscles to orientate the eyes so that the image of the object of attention will be formed there. The second essential, therefore, is a normally functioning set of ocular muscles which are competent to bring about the fine adjustment which is necessary. The last essential is an efficiently working nervous mechanism which can receive the two impressions and blend them psychologically into one.

Although in normal circumstances the two eyes work in close association and are treated as one by the brain, the two retinal images are not identical. When looking at an object, the right eye sees more on the right and the left eye more on the left. These two images are fused psychologically, and their slight diversity, together with other factors derived from experience, permits an appreciation of solidity and depth and assists in the judgment of distance. The slight amount of diplopia which should theoretically be produced in this way is suppressed, but at the same time both sets of impressions reach the brain, and their combination results in an appreciation of the third dimension in stereoscopic vision. We are thus enabled to project the mosaic of retinal images in their proper perspective in space and to orientate ourselves in regard to them.

The optical adjustment, therefore, is not necessarily mathematically exact; indeed, the central co-ordination permits a considerable amount of elasticity. When the two images differ by virtue of a failure in equilibrium between the two eyes, provided the disparity is not too great, the oculomotor apparatus first places the eyes in their most favourable relative positions, and then the fusion reflexes fill in the gaps.

Binocular vision may be present in varying degrees. One person may be able to see objects clearly with each eye, and when the visual axes are in proper alignment the two images are superimposed so as to form one, but when any disturbing influence comes into play so that the axes are disorientated, there is no attempt to maintain fusion and diplopia is produced. This has been called *simultaneous perception*. A second person, however, will not only fuse the two images, but will make a considerable effort to maintain this fusion; while a third, who not only sees binocularly but blends the two so as to obtain a stereoscopic effect, will have so great a tendency to maintain fusion that it is only with the greatest difficulty that he will abandon the advantages of binocular vision. These three grades of binocular vision were first differentiated by Claud Worth, and are usually known as grade I, simultaneous macular perception; grade II, fusion with some amplitude; grade III, stereoscopic vision.

These grades may be detected most simply by the stereoscope, or its more adaptable development, the amblyoscope. The latter in its simplest form consists of two adjustable tubes, each of which carries a picture which is presented to one eye; a more sophisticated form is the synoptophore seen in Figure 14.1. If object slides as illustrated in Figure 14.2 are presented, and both eyes are able to see adequately, the cow and the moon are both seen. This represents simultaneous perception. If the instrument is adjusted for parallelism of the visual axes and a composite picture is presented so that each half of it is incomplete, as in Figure 14.3, the

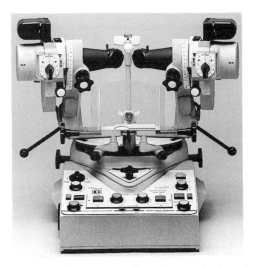

Fig. 14.1 A modern synoptophore for examination of binocular vision, the capacity for fusion and the muscle balance (Clement Clarke).

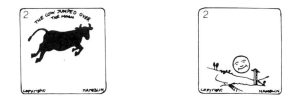

Fig. 14.2 To illustrate simultaneous perception.

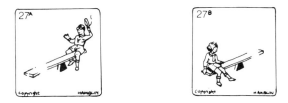

Fig. 14.3 To illustrate the capacity of fusion.

parts missing in the image formed by the one eye are accurately superimposed by the other; when fusion is present the picture appears as one complete whole. Where there is no attempt to maintain fusion, as soon as the axes are moved from the position of parallelism, the picture becomes broken up, and the extent to which the tubes may be separated or brought together, while still retaining the grouping of the figure intact, may be taken as a measurement of the development of the fusion faculty. If the pictures shown in Figure

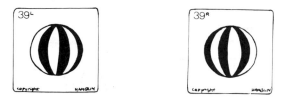

Fig. 14.4 To illustrate stereoscopic vision.

Figs 14.2 to **14.4** Amblyoscopic pictures.

14.4 are presented and the axes of the instrument moved, a person with the second grade, with binocular but no true stereoscopic vision, will either suppress one of the figures or see the two unintelligibly mixed up; but if true stereoscopic vision is present the two balls will be blended into one, giving a stereoscopic effect of almost 'hitting one in the eye', an appearance so vivid that even young children will at once remark on it.

The amount of effort which can be put forth to maintain fusion can be measured by prisms, or more easily with the amblyoscope; the underlying principles however, are the same.

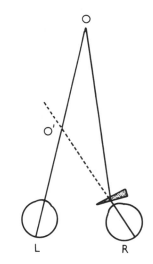
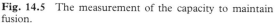

Fig. 14.5 The measurement of the capacity to maintain fusion.

If the two eyes look at an object, O, and a prism, P, with its base outwards is placed before the right, this eye will be turned inwards so that the rays of light deviated by the prism still fall upon the macula. O therefore appears to the right eye to be displaced to O', and double vision should be produced. This tendency to diplopia is overcome within limits by the power of fusion.

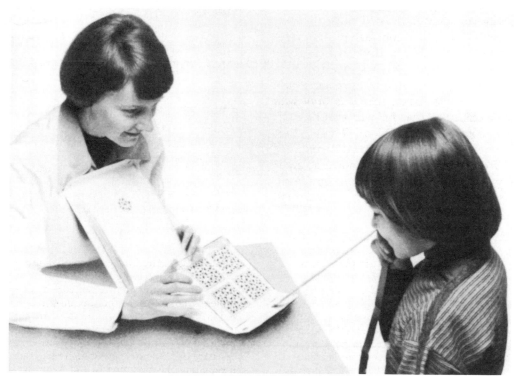

Fig. 14.6 The Frisby test.

If in Figure 14.5 the two eyes are directed towards an object (O), and a prism (P) is interposed before one with its base directed outwards, the rays from O will be deflected outwards so that they strike the retina to the outer side of the fovea. In this case, since the rays still impinge upon the macula of the other eye, double vision would be produced. Consequently the first eye is turned inwards until the deflected rays fall upon the macula once more and binocular vision is again possible. In this case the rays appear to come from O′, and to maintain fusion an excessive convergence is produced. The maximum effort which can be put out this way is measured by the strongest prism with which diplopia is not produced. It is found that very large prisms, up to 30 Δ or even 60 Δ, can be overcome by *convergence*. Weaker ones from 10 Δ to 15 Δ can be overcome by *divergence*: and only still weaker ones of 2 Δ or 4 Δ by vertical deviation of the eyes (or *sursumvergence*). This power suppressing an artificially produced diplopia is called the *verging power*, and its estimation is of importance in deciding upon the appropriate treatment indicated in cases wherein muscular imbalance exists.

Other clinical tests commonly used for assessing stereo-acuity are the Frisby, the Wirt test and the TNO.

In the TNO test, probably the most widely used, coloured random dots are viewed wearing red and green glasses. Geometrical patterns, circles, crosses, etc. appear out of the random dots if stereopsis is present.

The Frisby test (Fig. 14.6) consists of a series of transparent perspex plates, several patterns on one side only and one particular pattern on the other side. The odd one is identified by the subject if stereoscopic vision is possible. A series of progressively thinning plates gives a measure of the stereoscopic function.

For the Wirt test the subject wears polarised spectacles with the right and left lenses of different orientation of polarisation. Subjective summation of the two views of the test object (such as a large fly) give a stereoscopic view if the subject's binocularity is normal.

15. Binocular muscular anomalies — heterophoria

We have seen that when the ocular muscles are not properly balanced so that the visual axes do not normally lie in alignment, the desire for binocular vision may act as a stimulus and force the eyes into a suitable position in order that the two images may be fused into one. This condition of imbalance is called *heterophoria*, or latent squint. The cause may be a relative functional insufficiency of one or other of the muscles. It follows that in order to produce the parallelism which binocular vision demands, if there is a particularly weak muscle it will have to supplement its normal tone by a continuous active contraction, and will consequently never be at rest throughout the waking hours. The result of this constant activity is a liability to fatigue and eye-strain which, depending upon the constitution and nervous condition of the individual, may protrude itself into consciousness and produce symptoms. Thus, although a squint is potentially present, it is masked by this active correction and remains latent. If, however, the muscular coordination required for correction is inadequate, as may occur in states of debility or if the stimulus for fusion is not sufficiently strong, as may happen if the vision of one eye is much inferior or if the neurological pathways subserving the coordination of the two sets of visual impressions have not been developed, an obvious deviation results: the latent squint becomes manifest, the heterophoria becomes a heterotropia.

The causes of imbalance

The state of normal muscular equipoise may be upset by several conditions.

(1) The muscle may itself be weak, the deficiency being of congenital origin or involving a lack of normal postural tone. Such a condition may be the result of illness or general weakness, anaemia or nervous debility, and corresponds to some extent to the similar condition which results in postural deformities, for example as affecting the back in scoliosis. At times when the vitality is good no trouble may be experienced, and the deviation may be evident only in states of bodily fatigue. The heterophoria may thus be rhythmic; it may tend to appear in the evening when the patient is tired, or it may cause distress during a period of overwork or anxiety and worry, and completely disappear when a rest or holiday is secured.

(2) Alternatively, spasm of the opposing muscle or an augmentation of its postural tone may be the cause of the condition.

(3) Errors of refraction and disturbances of accommodation with the associated convergence may upset the muscle balance; thus trouble frequently commences when school or office work is started and an unaccustomed amount of near work becomes a necessity.

(4) The anatomical arrangement of the muscles or the configuration of the orbits may be an aetiological factor.

(5) Finally, disturbances of innervation may be responsible.

VARIETIES OF HETEROPHORIA

Depending on the muscle which is at fault, latent

deviation may occur in several directions. These are classified thus:

Exophoria: the eyes tend to deviate outwards, there being a relative insufficiency of the medial recti.

Esophoria: the eyes tend to deviate inwards, there being a relative insufficiency of the lateral recti.

Hyperphoria: one eye tends to deviate upwards or downwards relative to the other. A combination of deviations is sometimes spoken of as *hyperexophoria* (up and out) and *hyperesophoria* (up and in); while a condition of oblique disorientation, frequently due to inadequacy of an oblique muscle, is called *cyclophoria*.

Exophoria

Exophoria (Fig. 15.1), the condition wherein the visual axes tend to deviate outwards, is the most common anomaly of the muscle balance, for, as we have seen, the position of rest is most usually one of slight divergence. Moreover, when the eyes are converged for near vision the tendency for them to diverge by some 3 to 5 Δ from the fixation point is so constant as to be considered physiological. When, however, the divergence is actually in excess the defect is greater for distant vision than for near vision. On the other hand, it may be associated with an insufficiency of convergence, in which case, as we have seen, it is frequently associated with an insufficiency of accommodation. It thus occurs most usually in those who make little use of their accommodation, that is in myopes; it also occurs in those who put on hypermetropic or presbyopic correcting glasses for the first time and therefore are suddenly relieved of an accommodative strain.

Esophoria

Esophoria (Fig. 15.2), is also a common condition wherein the visual axes tend to deviate inwards. It may be the result of a divergence insufficiency, in which case it is more marked for distant vision than for near. Usually it is caused by an excess of convergence, in which case it is most pronounced for near vision. As such, it tends to give rise to few symptoms; in fact it may be in some respects an advantage, for in our civilisation most visual activities are undertaken for near work when an increase of convergence is sometimes a good thing. As a rule it is associated with excessive accommodation and thus accompanies hypermetropic states of refraction. It is also found in those whose vision is rendered difficult by reason of poor illumination, opacities in the media, or other causes.

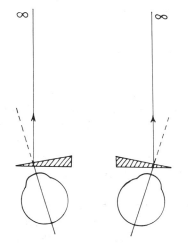

Fig. 15.1 Exophoria and its correction by prisms.

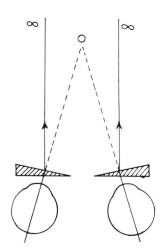

Fig. 15.2 Esophoria and its correction by prisms.

Hyperphoria

In hyperphoria the visual axis of one eye tends to be directed to a higher level than that of the other. It is impossible to be sure whether one eye is raised or the other lowered since the condition is relative. There is thus a deficiency of either the superior rectus and the inferior oblique, or of the inferior rectus and the superior oblique. In order to force the visual axes into the correct position it is therefore necessary to call more than one muscle into activity, and the adjustment in the different positions of the eyes becomes a complex matter. It will be readily understood, therefore, that a very small divergence of this nature will give rise to considerable discomfort, and that the symptoms will be more pronounced than in the more simple anomalies of convergence and divergence.

Cyclophoria

In cyclophoria the eye is twisted about an antero-posterior axis so that the vertical meridian of the cornea is deviated from the normal. When the upper end of this meridian leans towards the temple the movement is called *extorsion*, and the muscle which is primarily involved is the inferior oblique. A leaning of the upper end of the meridian in the opposite direction, that is towards the nose, is called *intorsion*, a movement which is accomplished mainly by the superior oblique.

A considerable amount of 'pseudocyclophoria' is frequently associated with astigmatism, wherein the principal axes are not vertical and horizontal. When a patient suffering from this condition looks at a vertical or horizontal line, the image formed on the retina will lean in the direction of the maximal corneal meridian. To bring the image into its proper alignment, one or other of the obliques will be called into play. A corrective torsion of this nature therefore tends to become a life habit in such cases of uncorrected astigmatism, and it probably explains to some extent the distressing symptoms which this refractive condition so frequently causes. It also explains the great discomfort which may result from an error in the direction of the axis of a cylinder in spectacles. With the proper correction of oblique astigmatism, of course, all symptoms of this nature disappear.

Another common type of cyclophoria occurs with near work when the lower part of the visual field is used: indeed, Meissner has shown that if the object is very close to the eye such a condition is physiological. In these circumstances the eyes are converged and rotated downwards; the first movement is accomplished by the medial recti, the second mainly by the inferior recti. With the downward pull of these latter muscles there is associated a certain amount of extorsion which must be counterbalanced by the intorting action of the superior obliques. When this neutralising action does not act efficiently, a certain amount of cyclophoria results; but in this case the defect rarely gives rise to symptoms or requires treatment.

Essential cyclophoria, like the other types of heterophoria, is due to pathological muscular imbalance, either muscular or innervational in origin. When the superior obliques are deficient or the inferior obliques overact, extorsion is the result; when the reverse is the case, intorsion ensues. The circumstances which determine this insufficiency or overaction are analogous to those which we have already studied as affecting the other ocular muscles. In its lower degrees the defect is common, and as a rule does not give rise to urgent symptoms; in its higher degrees it is rare. It is fortunate that this is so, for the disturbances which it may cause may be very distressing and are unfortunately not readily amenable to treatment.

Symptoms of heterophoria

The smaller degrees of eso- and exophoria are extremely common, and as a rule they give rise to no symptoms; only when the deviation is great, over 6 Δ, is there usually marked distress. Hyperphoria, however, may cause considerable trouble even when present in very small amount; and the symptoms arising from cyclophoria may be still more marked.

Visual symptoms may be evident. Vision becomes blurred on occasion, especially at times of fatigue. There is difficulty in gazing steadily at any object, and the discomfort is increased on any attempt to follow a moving body. Sudden bewilderments are thus apt to occur, when objects, especially moving things, become jumbled up. In all cases vision is improved and relief is obtained by closing one of the eyes. There is frequently a tendency towards adopting eccentric poses of the head, while an associated blepharospasm or a wrinkling of the forehead is characteristic. The most acute distress is associated with high degrees of cyclophoria; vertical lines appear deviated, the houses on either side of the street, for example, appearing to fall down upon the unfortunate patient, a sensation sometimes associated with pronounced reflex and labyrinthine disturbances.

The reflex symptoms may be marked. Headache of any kind is common and may come on a few minutes after near work is commenced, making its continuation difficult or impossible. An associated labyrinthine upset gives rise to vertigo, which may lead to nausea and, on occasion, result in vomiting. Restlessness is frequently apparent in children, and in adults of unstable temperament. Muscular imbalance, especially when associated with an error of refraction, may thus give rise to a host of varying symptoms; but, like the effects of errors of refraction, it is to be remembered that the subject has not been exempt from unfortunate exaggeration.

Treatment

Orthophoria, like emmetropia, is rare. The smaller errors of muscular balance which give rise to no symptoms require no treatment; this is so especially in the horizontal deviations, but, as we have seen, is less applicable to hyperphoria.

Two matters must first receive attention, and when they are adequately dealt with small degrees of heterophoria frequently give rise to no more trouble. The *general health* must be considered. The lack of muscle balance is frequently the expression less of a local defect than of a general neurosis, of physical debility, or of excessive work or worry; and when this is the case, optical treatment should not be adopted but a vacation or a change of occupation may be advised, accompanied by a graduated amount of suitable exercise and outdoor sport. Secondly, *errors of refraction* should be corrected fully by spectacles, which should be worn constantly, for it frequently happens that when an optical fault is removed the muscular balance returns spontaneously. The importance of the careful correction of oblique astigmatism in cyclophoria is evident.

If these measures should fail, recourse may be had to *orthoptic exercises*, which may be of value when the symptoms are labile, when the deviation is relatively small, and when it is not determined by relatively gross and static organic factors such as anatomical configuration or weakness of a muscle. The exercises should be practised not only for distant vision but also for vision at the near point; these, as in cases of convergence insufficiency, are most successful in exophoria. They must be done with *adverse prisms*, that is exercises are practised against prisms with their bases turned towards the direction of deviation, the same technique being employed as was described in cases of convergence insufficiency. With the head maintaining its original position, the object is then carried to the sides and the exercises repeated until the patient can secure a single image in all parts of the room in spite of the action of the prisms. In more recalcitrant cases a course of orthoptic treatment with the synoptophore or some such modified and adjustable amblyoscope under the guidance of an expert may be well worth while.

In cyclophoria the torsion of the eye is exercised by using two Maddox rods placed perpendicularly, one in front of either eye (p. 190); in this case two red lines are seen, and instead of running horizontally they are inclined at an angle the size of which varies with the degree of the defect. One of the rods is then rotated until the two lines are fused, and then it is moved alternately backwards and forwards in the direction which will exercise the muscle, the patient meantime trying to keep the line of light from doubling. To exercise the superior obliques the rods should be rotated toward the upper nasal quadrants; to exercise the inferior obliques they should be rotated in the upper temporal quadrants. According to the same principles, exercises may be carried out with two lines drawn on stereoscopic cards and inserted into an amblyoscope so that they can be rotated the one against the other. Both these procedures the patient can practise at home.

To be of value, these exercises must be continued for a considerable period, and even then their results are often disappointing. They may succeed, however, in relieving the symptoms, although they leave the amount of heterophoria substantially unchanged. They are particularly good in exophoria, especially when associated with convergence insufficiency, a condition which, as we have seen, plays a very large part indeed in visual troubles, especially in reading. In esophoria they are usually less successful, although the use of diverging prisms at the near point in cases of convergence excess is frequently useful. In cases of hyperphoria such exercises are generally useless. In cyclophoria, although little can be promised from them, they do on occasion relieve the symptoms. In all cases, however, they should be given a persistent trial, if only because optical methods of treatment are rarely practicable and are seldom successful.

While the rational treatment is undoubtedly to strengthen the inadequate muscles with graded exercises against adverse prisms, relief of the symptoms may be obtained by the *prescription of relieving prisms* which correct the defect optically. The base of the prism is placed in the direction of action of the muscle which is to be aided, and its apex towards that of the antagonistic muscle which is to be neutralised.

Not only may these compensate for the imbalance but, by relieving strain and producing relaxation, they may stimulate fusion and aid in establishing normal habits of binocularity. In their use, however, care should be taken to distinguish between essential deviations due to anatomical anomalies and dynamic deviations; in the first case prisms do little harm, in the second case the prisms, by removing the stimulus to function and encouraging a muscular deficiency, may perpetuate and even increase the error. It follows that, while the whole error can legitimately be corrected in the first case, the deviation should only be reduced to a comfortable margin in the second, and every endeavour should be made to weaken the prismatic correction gradually. Thus in the horizontal deviations a full prismatic correction should rarely be given, the correction of about half the error being usually sufficient; but in

hyperphoria, which is frequently determined by anatomical factors, a full correction is more happily borne. Further, when the deviation is mixed, the correction of the vertical error frequently allows the normal reflexes to deal with the horizontal error, so that prismatic correction of the vertical element may be effective in providing complete relief; conversely, an attempt to correct a horizontal in the presence of an uncorrected vertical deviation will almost certainly result in failure. In all cases prisms are combined with lenses to correct the optical error and should be divided equally between the two eyes; when the deviation is small the same effect may be produced by the cheaper expedient of decentring the lenses. Little can be done for the distressing condition of cyclophoria, for no optical device can correct the deviation.

Owing to their weight and the distortion which they produce, it is not usually advisable to prescribe prisms stronger than 6 Δ for each eye; the introduction of prisms of plastic material and Fresnel design (see Chapter 26) which can be stuck on to ordinary spectacle lenses has extended the practical range of strength that can be employed.

Where much higher degrees of deviation are present, the condition may require to be relieved by operative measures such as a muscular recession or an advancement, but the necessity or advisability of this procedure is rare. The technique of these operations is outside the scope of the refractionist as such except to note that an excess of power in a muscle should usually be corrected by recession, and a deficiency of power by resection. Moreover, if operative treatment is to be undertaken, it is essential that a similar deviation should exist for all distances, lest, for example, a pronounced esophoria for close work is treated only to produce as serious an exophoria for distance.

When a pronounced degree of insufficiency or excess of power in one of the horizontal muscles has been diagnosed, the operative correction of eso- and exophoria is a straightforward matter. Hyperphoria should be corrected, in the very rare cases wherein it would be advisable, by operating upon the superior or inferior recti, and cyclophoria upon the obliques.

16. Binocular muscular anomalies — heterotropia

OPTICAL ERRORS AND CONCOMITANT STRABISMUS

The condition of heterotropia, or manifest squint, does not properly come into the subject matter of this book, but it is essential for the refractionist to appreciate the bearing of refractive errors on the aetiology of some cases of *concomitant* strabismus and the importance of adequate optical correction in their treatment. Optical errors and their correction play little part in the genesis or management of *paralytic* strabismus.

We have seen that the three essentials which are necessary for perfect binocular vision are the production of two approximately equal images on two efficiently functioning maculae, muscle balance, and an adequate cerebral mechanism to co-ordinate and interpret the two sets of impressions. Whenever any of these is gravely deficient binocular vision becomes impossible and, deprived of the stimulus for fusion, the eyes tend to deviate away from their proper alignment with a resultant squint.

It cannot be said that the aetiology of all cases of squint is elucidated or is even clear, but one factor of importance in a large number of cases depends upon an upset of the accommodation–convergence synergy in cases of ametropia. The general trend in the dissociative tendency, which is particularly evident in early childhood before the binocular reflexes have become firmly established, is best understood when it is remembered that a hypermetrope has to use his accommodation in excess of his convergence; were he to employ them equally, he would be faced with the dilemma of either using too little accommodation, when he would be converging accurately but not seeing distinctly, or using too much convergence, in which case he would see clearly but double. Since the dominant desire is that of clear vision, he may adopt the latter alternative and develop a convergent squint. This is not to say that all or even the majority of hypermetropic children have convergent squints. It occurs only in subjects in whom the relationship between accommodation and convergence is particularly inflexible. Contrariwise, a myope uses his convergence in excess of his accommodation; if, therefore, he develops a squint it is likely to be an outward or divergent deviation. As a matter of fact it is not especially common for myopes to develop manifest divergent squint, a latent deviation being much more frequent. The refractive state most frequently found in association with divergence is either emmetropia or astigmatism. In any case the tendency is for only the better eye of the two to be employed, and the vision of the other is therefore sacrificed to eliminate the diplopia, this being particularly so in convergent squint with hypermetropia.

The sacrifice is made all the more easily if the vision of the other eye is in any way defective or if fusion is not fully developed. Those who have already developed binocular vision will not readily abandon its advantages, and they will undergo considerable strain in dissociating accommodation and convergence in order to retain it. These cases, as we have seen, are the subjects of heterophoria. It is when the stimulus for fusion is lacking that heterotropia results.

This can be simply seen in the following way: if an emmetrope looks at a distant object, and two

125

spheres of −4 D are placed in front of his eyes, he will still be able to see it by exercising +4 D of accommodation. His convergence is, however, unchanged, and the effort to see clearly produces a feeling of strain and giddiness; this is heterophoria. If, however, a coloured glass is now placed before one eye, thus taking away the possibility of binocular vision, diplopia is at once produced and this eye deviates; this is heterotropia.

The condition of accommodative convergent squint most frequently presents in childhood, between the ages of 2 and 6 (though it may well have commenced even earlier), before fusion is fully developed, just at the time when accommodation is first seriously called into play and the interest of the child has begun to be attracted by near objects such as picture books and toys. Its commencement may be preceded by a debilitating illness, such as measles or whooping cough, which may be expected to lower the general muscular tone. Divergent squint associated with myopia, on the other hand, is not usually met with at such an early stage, perhaps because myopia is usually not congenital but develops in the growing period of youth. Since the refractive condition does not appear until fusion is firmly established, a manifest divergent squint is unusual, but in later life when the near point recedes and convergence is still less required, the tendency to diverge increases and may then become manifest. On the other hand, in congenital or infantile myopia accommodation is not required but clear vision of near objects is attained by the exercise of convergence. Since distant objects are permanently outside the child's ken and are therefore neglected, the convergence tends to be continually exercised and, being consolidated by the reward of good binocular vision, becomes established and maintains itself as an esophoria for all distances and may eventually become a manifest internal squint. Again, if much astigmatism is present, clarity is not associated with the effort of convergence — indeed, there is relative blindness for near objects as well as distant. In contradistinction to the congenital myope who gains clear vision by dissociating his convergence from his accommodation, the congenital astigmat fails to attain this end by any expedient and therefore gives up all effort of either faculty with

the development of a habitual divergence at first for near and then for distant objects also.

It is again to be emphasised, however, that every ametrope does not by any means squint, nor is every case of strabismus associated with anomalies of refraction or disturbances of accommodation. It is therefore obvious that, although their influence is undoubtedly important, these considerations are by no means the sole factors in the aetiology; anomalies in the insertions of muscles or the relative weakness of one or other are common determining factors, as well as differences in the clarity, size or form of the images formed in the two eyes so that their fusion is difficult.

The vision in concomitant strabismus

Originating in early childhood, it is probably the case that diplopia accompanies most cases of squint. It happens occasionally that this condition persists, the patient being unable either to overcome it or evade it, and in the majority of cases it is extraordinary how well the average patient adapts himself to it and how little he is inconvenienced by a phenomenon which, appearing suddenly late in life as in paralytic squint, usually gives rise to the most distressing symptoms and involves the most extreme disorientation. In the majority of cases, however, the disadvantages of double vision are overcome either by the suppression of the image in the deviating eye or by a mental reorientation of the displaced image, so that it is projected in space in a position more nearly corresponding to that of the fixing eye (the phenomenon of *false projection*).

The *suppression of the image* of the deviating eye usually occurs at a very early stage. It is a psychological phenomenon, and after it has been practised for some time the function of the visual apparatus becomes impaired and the vision deteriorates progressively. Many of the cells in the visual cortex in the occipital lobe are associated with impulses derived from both eyes, and it has been shown in experimental animals that if the use of one eye is excluded from binocular vision shortly after birth these cells completely lose their binocular capability. A more or less pronounced degree of this condition of *amblyopia ex anopsia* is evident in most cases of accommodative squint acquired at an early age, and it may be found difficult or impossible to regain this loss of vision if it has persisted for a long time; the prevention of the development of this type of blindness to an irremediable degree is the strongest argument for the early and efficient treatment of every case of squint. Such an amblyopia is largely cerebral in origin and is essentially a *purposive* repression rather than a passive consequence of mere lack of use of the retina or facilitation of the central nervous paths. Thus in middle age a cataract may be removed after it has existed 20 years or more without any deleterious results in the functioning of the retina.

VARIETIES OF HETEROTROPIA

According to the direction of deviation of the squinting eye, a classification of heterotropia may be used similar to that employed in heterophoria. *Esotropia* implies a convergent strabismus, *exotropia* a divergent strabismus, *hypertropia* and *hypotropia* apply to vertical deviations. Since these last terms are relative, such cases may be further differentiated as *strabismus sursum-vergens*, wherein an eye is turned upwards, and *strabismus deorsum-vergens* wherein an eye is turned downwards.

Treatment

The ideal treatment of a squint is not only to correct the deformity but also *to bring about the restoration of binocular vision*. The laying down of the reflex pathways which subserve this function is difficult the older the child becomes, and may be quite impossible when adolescence has been reached. It will therefore be realised that the first essential in treatment is to commence active measures at the very earliest moment possible in every case, making no delay from the first time that the squint is noticed. It is only by adopting this policy that success can be anticipated or any improvement other than cosmetic can be gained. The popular impression, not only among the laity but also among medical practitioners, that a child will 'grow out' of the deformity cannot be too

strongly controverted for it has been responsible for the development of many functionally useless eyes. Ideally a squint can only be said to be cured when the end-result is good vision and full binocular co-operation in two eyes which are in perfect alignment.

The two procedures open to the refractionist in these cases are, first, to *determine and correct any refractive error* and, second, to maintain and encourage the vision in the squinting eye. The first should be done under full cycloplegia, atropine having been given for at least 3 days prior to the examination. If a significant error exists a full correction should be ordered, deducting for the effect of the atropine not more than 1 D, preferably about 0.5 D; and if the spectacles are tolerated with difficulty, atropine may be continued for some weeks until the child gets used to them. In determining the error, reliance should be placed upon retinoscopy rather than on any subjective results, while any astigmatic error, especially in the squinting eye, should receive minute attention. Retinoscopy can be done in most cases, for the youngest child will fixate a light, and the test lenses can be held in the hand at arm's length, thus doing away with the necessity for trial frames.

Some difficulty may be experienced in refracting a highly amblyopic eye; central fixation may be lost and it may be advisable to proceed to a period of occlusion of the fixing eye in order to try to restore central fixation of the amblyopic eye before again attempting to refract the latter under atropine.

It should be established as a ritual that the spectacles be worn constantly; they should be put on first thing in the morning and taken off last thing at night, and in young children who attempt to push them off, they should be tied on (see p. 202). Most accommodative squints develop between the ages of 2 and 6, and a child of 2 can usually be induced to wear spectacles. Under this age the most practicable course to adopt may be to keep the child mildly under the influence of atropine, prescribing it as an ointment once a day, or every second day, until the wearing of spectacles is possible.

In some cases the effect of abolishing the accommodation by atropine rectifies the squint, and in these the deformity is usually kept under control by spectacles.

As soon as the optical defect has been corrected, the *vision in the squinting eye should be encouraged* and every endeavour made to improve it. The acuity of vision is measured in the ordinary way in older children, but if the patient can neither read letters nor appreciate pictorial test types other tests (p. 149) may provide some information. The child should be seen soon after the spectacles have been given, and the vision estimated again. If the squinting eye is amblyopic or if its acuity of vision is defective, it should be forced into use by occluding the sound eye. The most satisfactory method is to cover up the good eye completely with surgical plaster, and ready prepared versions of this are available ('Opticlude'). This can be worn night and day and does not interfere with the wearing of spectacles.

An alternative method, spectacle occlusion, is to wear an occluder fixed to them or to paper over one lens, but this is less satisfactory than in the initial stages of a case with dense amblyopia. It may be sufficient once the vision has responded to total occlusion. Where total occlusion is employed it should be changed every 3 days or even less frequently so as to avoid abrading the skin areas that the plaster adheres to.

While we believe that amblyopia is due to an active inhibition and that theoretically periods without occlusion will do positive as well as negative harm, something of a 'Catch 22' situation exists if there is any remnant of binocular power, for example when a squint is intermittently present. Here total occlusion in order to improve the vision of the amblyopic eye may destroy the remnants of the binocular vision altogether. And there is certainly the prevailing view that amblyopia should not be treated by continuous total occlusion in certain cases and that intermittent total occlusion may be most appropriate for certain individuals, a decision to be taken by the orthoptist in co-operation with the ophthalmologist.

When the amblyopia is not marked, it may be sufficient to keep the better eye under the influence of atropine, so that while distant vision usually becomes indistinct with this eye, near vision becomes impossible. The defective eye is thus coerced into activity, and the continuous exercise thus forced upon it improves its efficiency to a considerable extent in many cases. At the same time a constant watch should be maintained over the progress of the case, since the deviation sometimes becomes transferred to the occluded eye and the vision in the latter may deteriorate.

The results of such treatment are very varied. The longer that amblyopia has been present, the less effective treatment is likely to be. Again, the older the child, the less promising is the outlook. The good eye should be occluded for a month, and if no improvement occurs a further month may be tried. If this too proves fruitless, all hope of ultimate functional utility may be abandoned; this is the most frequent outcome if treatment is started after the age of 7. If better vision can be elicited by the occlusion it should be continued. Provided the case is carefully supervised, there need be no hesitation in continuing this for considerable periods of time, *as long as any improvement is obtained*. The ideal to be aimed at is to persist until the vision in the two eyes is approximately equal or until further improvement ceases. At this stage, in the most favourable cases, true equality of vision may be obtained, the squint becoming alternating, one or other eye being used indiscriminately for fixation.

As soon as adequate vision in the two eyes is secured, an attempt should be made to develop binocular vision by *orthoptic treatment* by which habits of binocularity are practised with a view to training and facilitating binocular vision of a degree sufficiently potent to maintain the eyes in alignment. In those cases wherein the vision in the squinting eye is useful when first seen, this should, of course, be inaugurated from the first. Unfortunately the application of such treatment by itself is limited and if the deviation is large and has been present for some time it will almost certainly be found to be ineffective.

In this event, preferably as soon as a desire for fusion has been initiated orthoptically, operative treatment should be undertaken. With the eyes approximately in alignment, the subsequent training of binocular vision is greatly facilitated, and if orthoptic exercises are started a few days after the operation and the habit of binocular vision maintained the risk of subsequent deviation is small.

It is to be remembered, however, that in all cases of accommodative squint operation should be postponed until correcting spectacles have been worn for some months and the deviation has been stabilised. Thus if the original squint is of 20 degrees, and with spectacles the deformity is reduced to 15 degrees, the operation should be planned to relieve the latter degree of deformity only, as otherwise, when the lenses are worn, the eyes will be overcorrected and the opposite condition produced. In squints due to other causes such as congenital or infantile neuromuscular anomalies the refractionist plays no part except perhaps to ensure the maintenance of good vision in both eyes until they are surgically realigned.

17. Binocular muscular co-ordination — convergence

Voluntary and reflex convergence

Convergence can be initiated in two ways — voluntarily and involuntarily. Voluntary convergence — the volitional rotation of the two eyes nasalwards — is initiated in the frontal lobe of the cerebrum, a faculty which is not universally present but can be acquired by training to a remarkable degree. Involuntary convergence, on the other hand, is a psycho-optical reflex centred, like the movements of fixation and accommodation, in the peristriate area of the occipital cortex. In normal circumstances it is a fusion movement carried out synergically with accommodation. It is the latter type of convergence with which we are essentially concerned here, but it is important that if voluntary convergence is well developed the reflex type usually acts more efficiently and automatically.

Reflex convergence

When the eyes are at rest and looking in the distance, the visual axes are parallel and no effort of accommodation is made; in order to see something clearly near at hand, not only must the eyes accommodate, but the visual axes must also be turned inwards so that they are both directed upon the object of attention. If an object is gradually brought nearer to the eyes, they converge more and more upon it, but ultimately a point is reached when the limit of convergence is attained. At this point the image appears double, and, giving up the sustained effort, the eyes usually diverge slightly outwards. Normally it should be possible to maintain convergence when the object is about 8 cm away. The nearest point for which convergence is possible, is called the *near point (punctum proximum) of convergence*.

The near point of convergence is found by moving a small object, such as a wire stretched vertically in a frame, or a luminous slit, or a line drawn on a card, towards the eyes until it appears double. Care should be taken to distinguish the near point of accommodation from the near point of convergence; at the former the test object appears blurred and indistinct, but is not necessarily double. Although the two points may coincide, this does not by any means always occur. Theoretically the distance should be measured from the line joining the centre of rotation of the two eyes (the *base line*), but in practice it is measured from the anterior principal focus, and an average correction of 25 mm is added on to the measurement found.

The relative position of the eyes when they are completely at rest is called the *far point (punctum remotum) of convergence*. We have already seen that as a rule the visual and the optic axes do not coincide (p. 34), but that in the position of rest there is generally (although not always) a slight deviation of the visual axes outwards. The far point, instead of being at infinity, is thus situated 'beyond infinity' and, corresponding to the far point of accommodation in the hypermetropic eye, can be found mathematically by producing the axes backwards so as to meet at a point behind the eye. On the other hand, in those cases wherein there is an apparent convergence of the eyes in the position of rest, the far point will be situated at a finite distance. Corresponding to the terminology used in accommodation, the distance between the far point and the near point is called the *range of convergence*, and the difference in converging power required to maintain the eyes in each position is called the *amplitude of convergence*. That part of the range of convergence between the eye and infinity is described as *positive*: that part 'beyond infinity', that is behind the eye and in reality a *divergence*, is spoken of as *negative* convergence.

The measurement of convergence

A convenient method for measuring convergence was proposed by Nagel, the unit of which is called the *metre angle* (m.a.). Let us imagine that when the eyes are at rest the visual axes are directed straight forwards in parallel lines (Fig. 17.1). If they are converged upon an object situated 1 metre away on the median line between the two eyes, then the angle which the line joining the object to the centre of rotation of either eye makes with the median line is called 1 metre angle. The angular displacement will necessarily vary with the distance between the

two eyes. With an inter-pupillary distance of 60 mm, this angle is about 2 degrees (see Table 2, Appendix I). If the object is 2 metres away, the angle will be halved (0.5 m.a.); if it is brought nearer, say to 0.5 metre, the angle will be doubled (2 m.a.). The normal amplitude of convergence may be taken to be 10.5 metre angles, which is made up of 9.5 m.a. of positive and 1 m.a. of negative convergence, but it may exceed this and equal 15 or 17 m.a. It will be remembered that the amount of accommodation used by an emmetrope to see an object 1 metre away is 1 dioptre, so that the amount of accommodation expressed in dioptres is the same as the amount of convergence expressed in metre angles.

A second method of measuring convergence is by means of *prisms*. If an adducting prism be placed before one eye (that is a prism with its base directed outwards), the rays of light entering the eye will be deviated outwards by an amount depending on the strength of the prism (Fig. 17.2), and diplopia will tend to be produced. Consequently, if binocular vision is to be maintained, the eye must be turned inwards by a corresponding amount. The strongest adducting prism through which binocular vision can still be retained is therefore the measure of the power of convergence. Conversely, if an abducting prism be placed before the eye (that is

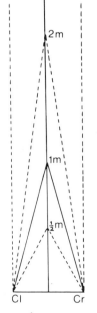

Fig. 17.1 The metre angle.
Cl and *Cr*, the centres of rotation of the two eyes. When the object is 1 metre away, the angle which *mCl* makes with the median line is 1 metre angle. Similarly at 0.5 metre, the corresponding angle is 2 metre angles, and at 2 metres, the corresponding angle is 0.5 metre angle.

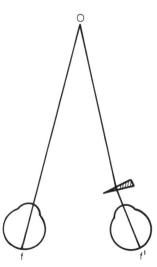

Fig. 17.2 The effect of an adducting prism before the eye.

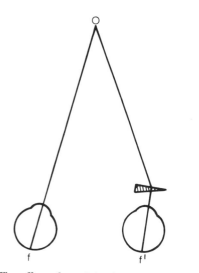

Fig. 17.3 The effect of an abducting prism before the eye.

a prism with its base inwards), the rays of light will be converged inwards and, in order to compensate for this, the eye will have to be deviated outwards (Fig. 17.3). The strongest prism which can be borne without producing diplopia is thus a measure of the negative convergence (or divergence). In all these cases the amount of convergence is shared equally between the two eyes, so that the effect is the same whether one prism is used before one eye, or two prisms, each of half the strength, are placed one before each eye. The positive portion of convergence is much larger than the negative; each varies within wide limits, but on average, with prisms gradually applied, the former can amount to about 55 to 60 Δ, and the latter varies between 3 and 7 Δ. Again, for an inter-pupillary distance of 60 mm, 3 Δ corresponds to 1 metre angle of convergence, and this allows one to express convergence measured by prisms in the metre angle notation.

The relation between accommodation and convergence

We have seen that the two synkinetic functions of accommodation and convergence are normally closely inter-related so that accommodation in

dioptres is numerically equal to convergence in metre angles. The relation between them, however, is quite elastic, and either can be exercised separately. For example, if we look at an object with both eyes and then, while still looking at it, place weak concave or convex lenses in front of the eyes, we can overcome the effect of the lenses by an effort of accommodation and still see the object binocularly; in this case we are making an effort of accommodation without employing convergence. Conversely, if we repeat the experiment, this time placing prisms in front of the eyes, we can still see the object distinctly, thus demonstrating that convergence can be called upon without involving accommodation. When accommodation fails in middle age, convergence is retained, and when the ciliary muscle is paralysed by atropine, convergence is still possible. It is indeed fortunate that this is so, for a dissociation of the two is necessary in ametropia. Thus an emmetrope who wishes to look at an object 25 cm away exercises 4 dioptres of accommodation and 4 metre angles of convergence; but a hypermetrope of 2 D must employ 6 D of accommodation, and a myope of 2 D will require only 2 D, while the amount of convergence remains the same. The hypermetrope, therefore, has to use his accommodation in excess of his convergence, and the myope his convergence in excess of his accommodation. The amount of dissociation which is possible is not, however, unlimited; it can be increased by practice, and it varies with different individuals and in the same individual at different times. The effort to dissociate the two may give rise to no trouble, while, on the other hand, it may be the cause of considerable distress; indeed, the necessary amount of dissociation may on occasion be impossible to attain, and since a clear image is of more immediate advantage than the retention of binocular vision, one eye may eventually deviate and a squint develop.

The amount of accommodation which it is thus possible to exert while the convergence remains fixed is called the *relative accommodation*: the amount in excess of the convergence is called *positive*, that below, *negative*. The relation between these will be made clear from Figure 17.4.

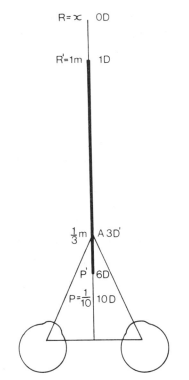

Fig. 17.4 Relative accommodation.
For convergence upon an object, A, $\frac{1}{3}$ metre away, the
relative range of accommodation is R'P' (i.e. 100 − 17, or
83 cm). The relative amplitude of accommodation is
6 D − 1 D, or 5 D. AP' represents positive relative
accommodation; R'A represents negative relative
accommodation.

The subject is emmetropic, and has his far point
(R) at infinity and his near point (P) at 10 cm.
Suppose he looks at an object (A) situated 33 cm
away, he will then be exercising 3 D of
accommodation and 3 m.a. of convergence.
Concave lenses are now placed in front of his eyes
until the object begins to be blurred; if this occurs
with −3 D lenses he has augmented his
accommodation from 3 to 6 D, and his relative near
point (P') is at a distance equivalent to 6 D, that is
at 17 cm. Convex lenses are now substituted for the
concave lenses, and it is found that the image
begins to be blurred when lenses of +2 D are
presented. He has thus relaxed his accommodation
by 2 D, that is from 3 to 1 D, and his relative far
point (R') is at a distance from the eye equivalent
to 1 D, that is 1 metre. For 3 m.a. of convergence,
therefore, the relative far point is at 1 metre, the
relative near point is at 17 cm, the relative range of
accommodation is 83 cm (R'P'), of which 67 cm
(R'A) is negative and 16 cm (AP') positive, and the
relative amplitude is 5 D (i.e. 6 D — 1 D), of
which 2 D is negative and 3 D is positive.

It is obvious that the nearer the object is to
the eye, the smaller will be the positive and the
larger the negative range of accommodation. In
the ultimate, if the eyes are emmetropic, when
the object of fixation is at infinity, there will be
no negative accommodation, and it will be found
that no convex lens can be tolerated and at the
same time good vision obtained. Similarly, if the
object is at the near point the positive moiety will
have become *nil*, for here no concave lens can be
tolerated since it requires all the accommodative
effort possible to see an object at this distance.
Thus, while there is one absolute far point, one
absolute near point, and one absolute range of
accommodation, there is a different relative far
point, near point, and range for every degree of
convergence.

Accommodation is thus one of the most
important factors which may stimulate
convergence; this is termed *accommodative
convergence*. The relation between the two, that
is the magnitude of the change in convergence
in prism dioptres caused by an increase in
accommodation expressed in dioptres, *the
accommodative convergence/accommodation ratio*
(AC/A), is remarkably constant for each
individual, being about 3.5 Δ/D. It is, however,
upset if the tone of the ciliary muscle is changed
(as in cycloplegia) or in presbyopia.

In practice, it is only necessary to measure the
amount of relative accommodation at the working
distance — usually 33 cm, that is with a
convergence of 3 m.a. The patient is first
rendered emmetropic with lenses, and small type
is held at this distance from the eye. Concave
lenses are then put up until the strongest is found
which enables him to see readily; this is a
measure of the amount by which he can augment
his accommodation, i.e. of the positive accommodation. A similar procedure is carried out with
convex lenses; this is a measure of the amount
by which he can relax his accommodation, i.e. of
the negative accommodation: and the sum of the
two gives the total relative accommodation.

The importance of this relationship is that *it is
essential for comfort that the positive portion of the
relative accommodation should be as large as possible*;
it should be at least as great as the negative
portion. When it is large, the patient has a
correspondingly large amount of accommodation

in reserve, but in the opposite case he will be working too near the limit of his capacity for comfort, for, like all other muscles, the ciliary muscle becomes fatigued if it is called upon to contract to its utmost for any length of time. Landolt estimated that in such circumstances two-thirds of the accommodation could be made available, and that about one-third of the total accommodative power must be held in reserve. If for any reason the amplitude of accommodation is diminished, and the near point recedes to the region of the working distance so that the positive accommodation becomes small, prolonged near work can be undertaken without distress only if convex lenses are provided which bring the range of accommodation nearer to the eye.

In a similar manner, if the accommodation is kept constant, the convergence may be made to vary. The amount of convergence which can thus be exerted or relaxed is called the *relative convergence*. This can be measured in a manner similar to that described for relative accommodation by accommodating for a fixed object and varying the convergence by prisms (Fig. 17.5). The strongest prism, base outwards,

which can be tolerated without producing diplopia is a measure of the positive portion (*Ba*) of the relative convergence (*ab*), or the amount by which the normal convergence can be augmented. Similarly, the strongest prism, base inwards, which can be borne is a measure of the negative portion (*Bb*) of the relative convergence, and is the amount by which the convergence can be relaxed. Again, it is preferable for comfort that *the positive portion should be the greater* and, if it is not so, it may be advisable to prescribe prisms, bases in, to assist the convergence of those who are doing much continuous near work. Percival found that it is the rule for patients to be able to exercise only the middle third of their relative convergence for any length of time without fatigue. This he called the 'area of comfort'. If, in his near work, a patient has habitually to go outside this limit, in either a positive or negative direction, he should be provided with prisms so that his work is kept within his area of comfort, or, alternatively, he should undergo a course of exercises to stimulate his converging power. Such a weakness is a prolific cause of visual discomfort and will be spoken of again.

Binocular accommodation

Not only are convergence and accommodation closely related, they also have a mutual effect the one upon the other. This is most readily seen in the fact that when both eyes are being used the power of accommodation is notably increased, the increase being due to the stimulus which the act of convergence gives to its related function. The excess of binocular over uniocular accommodation averages about one-half a dioptre, although individual variations are large, and it may be as high as 1.5 D. Duane gave the following figures:

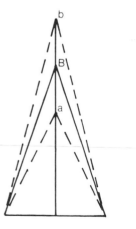

Fig. 17.5 Relative convergence.
O and O represent the centres of rotation of the two eyes. The eyes look at B, and keep this amount of accommodation constant. Prisms, base out, are then placed before the eyes until the limit of single vision is reached: the deviation produced (*Ba*) is the positive portion of the relative convergence. Similarly prisms, base in, are used, and the negative portion (*Bb*) of the relative convergence for the accommodation required for B is found. The total relative convergence is *ab*.

Below 17 years, excess averages	0.6 D
18 to 31 years, excess averages	0.5 D
32 to 53 years, excess averages	0.4 D
Above 53 years, excess averages	0.3 D

It appears to be definitely established that this additional accommodative efficiency is due to the stimulus derived from convergence. It is not a result of the accompanying pupillary contraction, for it occurs independently of this. Nor is it due to an increase in visual acuity depending upon the fusion of the two images from both eyes, for the increase is as notable in patients in whom one eye is amblyopic or who have a diverging squint which allows an effort of convergence but does not permit a fusion of the two images. The two functions are closely interwoven physiologically, and it appears that their maximum efficiency can be attained only if, by working with and supplementing each other, their synkinetic action is retained.

Fatigue of convergence

The study of the development of fatigue of convergence can be carried out in the same way as of accommodative fatigue by means of an ophthalmic ergograph. By repeatedly approximating a target towards the eyes until a fine line thereon appears double, the maximum excursion attained and the length of time during which such repeated efforts can be maintained can be studied. These may be recorded mechanically by the ergograph of Berens so that records can be made of the rate of development of fatigue and the individual capacity of resistance to fatigue.

18. Binocular muscular anomalies — anomalies of convergence and other reading difficulties

Insufficiency of convergence

An insufficiency of convergence is a common condition, the clinical importance of which has been recognised from the time of von Graefe (1862), and, since convergence is constantly called into play and is indispensable for the maintenance of single binocular vision for all distances optically nearer than infinity, its failure is of great clinical importance. A condition of *absolute insufficiency* may be said to exist when the near point (in the absence of presbyopia) is greater than 11 cm from the intra-ocular baseline (9.5 cm from the apex of the cornea) or when there is difficulty in attaining 30 degrees of convergence. These criteria, of course, measure involuntary convergence. In such cases voluntary convergence is frequently impossible. As we have just seen, however, a condition of *relative insufficiency* for the particular working distance employed is of more clinical importance. The frequency of insufficiency of the involuntary convergence associated with fixation has been variously estimated, but there is no doubt that it is a common condition. Its prevalence shows no significant correlation with age or the refractive error. Failure of voluntary convergence (that is converging to order without a specific point of fixation) is more common.

The aetiology of convergence insufficiency is not thoroughly understood but is certainly varied. Among local causes anatomical conditions such as a wide inter-pupillary distance may make convergence difficult, but the basis of the anomaly may well be the delayed development of a lately acquired function. The greater frequency of insufficiency in the more highly evolved voluntary faculty compared with the reflex points in this direction, and the occurrence of deficiency in otherwise normal individuals, which rarely gives rise to symptoms until excessive close work is undertaken, and its ready cure by facilitation with training can receive no other likely explanation. Accommodative difficulties are also a common cause. Normally accommodation and convergence are synergic and are equally expended; if accommodation is not ordinarily employed, convergence tends to suffer from disuse, and its insufficiency therefore occurs typically in uncorrected myopes, and is seen in hypermetropes and presbyopes when their refractive error is corrected for the first time and in those suffering from accommodative insufficiency. An insufficiency from disuse may also be seen in those who cannot see clearly at close distances and therefore do not call upon convergence habitually, such as marked hypermetropes, anisometropes or presbyopes. At all ages, but particularly in the elderly, the binocular stimulus to converge will be interfered with by defective vision in one or both eyes. This is seen typically in a subject with some degree of senile cataract more marked in one eye than the other.

General disease or debility due to illness, toxic conditions, or metabolic or endocrine disorders may also be the cause of insufficiency, while intra-nasal disease is given a prominent aetiological place by some writers. Stress is undoubtedly a factor of importance in many cases. Paresis or weakness of the medial rectus muscles is a rare cause; a typical example of the latter occurs in myasthenia gravis.

The *symptoms* of convergence insufficiency

are essentially those of 'eye-strain', particularly intensified in attempting close work which may be rendered impossible owing to blurring, diplopia and headaches. Many patients suffer no discomfort, and a large proportion are worried only when an unusual amount of near work is attempted or when they are fatigued or unwell; others, again, complain bitterly and continuously, although their defect is small. Where defective vision of one or other eye is the precipitating factor the complaint may be of having to close one eye when reading. Such subjects often have such gross failure of attempted convergence that a manifest divergence of the worst seeing eye appears on close work.

The *diagnosis* is based on the presence of orthophoria for distance, the periodic increase of relative divergence as the near point is approached, the remoteness of the near point (beyond 9.5 cm), the low prism convergence (below 15 Δ) and normal prism divergence.

If the vision of both eyes is good *treatment* is usually eminently satisfactory provided any physical or physiological basis can be adequately dealt with, provided the patient is well or can be made well, and provided he is psychologically balanced and not working under poor hygienic conditions or under strain. Orthoptic training appears at its best in the treatment of this condition, partly because the fusion amplitude is large and partly because the reflexes concerned are unusually plastic, and because voluntary effort can be enlisted to aid their facilitation. Such training may devolve along two lines, and to be most effective both should be used — the facilitation of the reflexes mediating involuntary convergence (the deficiency of which is responsible for the symptoms) and the encouragement of this process by enlisting the aid of voluntary convergence.

Involuntary convergence should be exercised by increasing the power of stereopsis by the study of stereograms of increasing difficulty to build up an adequate fusional reserve and by duction exercises placing prisms, base out, of gradually increasing strength in front of one or both eyes in order to produce convergence in the distance.

The patient is asked to look at an object and, while his gaze is still fixed, prisms initially weak and gradually increasing in strength are placed before the eyes at intervals of 5 seconds, the patient being encouraged to fuse the two images into one. These exercises may be continued at home. The patient is given a 4 Δ prism with which to practise for a week, and this may well be augmented by 2 Δ at weekly intervals. These exercises are done for distant vision, and then the object is brought nearer and exercises at the near point and far point are alternated. In more recalcitrant cases a course of orthoptic treatment including vergence exercises with the amblyoscope may be worth while. These, which are frequently rapidly effective, can be supplemented by simple exercises of convergence carried out at home whereby the patient attempts to approximate the near point by fixing an object (the finger or a pencil) as it approaches his eyes until it appears double. In cases wherein temperament or stupidity does not hamper co-operation, fusion up to 50 or 60 degrees and abolition of the symptoms are usually attained in from 2 to 6 weeks.

In the training of voluntary convergence the patient must first be taught to recognise and then control the position of his eyes. In the first place he is taught to demonstrate to himself physiological diplopia. Holding a pencil in front of his eyes he sees two pencils while fixing a distant object; looking at the pencil he then sees two objects, and as the pencil is moved backwards and forwards the objects separate and approximate. While this is being done the pencil is removed and the patient, without moving his eyes, tries to retain the two objects apart as long as possible. The exercise is completed by doubling the objects without the aid of the pencil. Exercises with the stereoscope follow, and, finally, fusion of stereoscopic pictures by convergence without the aid of the stereoscope. If this is attained a fusion amplitude of some 70 degrees will have been consolidated and cure with the relief of symptoms will have been complete.

So far as spectacles are concerned — if they are required — hypermetropes should be given an undercorrection and myopes should be fully corrected, particularly for reading, in order to stimulate accommodation and with it convergence.

It is only when these and exercises fail that relieving prisms, base in, should be prescribed in spectacles for near work, in which case sufficient prismatic correction should be incorporated to bring the convergence just within the area of comfort (the middle third of the total relative convergence) for the particular distance required. These are most usually needed for presbyopes who have insufficient converging power for near vision, and for the elderly in whom the practicalities of formal orthoptic exercises or more extensive treatment are precluded. In cases of uncomplicated convergence insufficiency, in the absence of a divergent squint, operation (advancement or resection of the medial recti) is usually inadvisable since the deficiency at the near point is corrected at the cost of an equally serious esophoria for distance.

Convergence excess

A habitual excessive convergence or even spasm of convergence due to innervational influences of a hyperkinetic type is not very uncommon: White and Brown (1939) found a measurable degree of excess in 16.6% of ophthalmic patients. Aetiologically three types occur.

An increase of convergence associated with an increase in accommodation is the most common clinical picture, for being habitually synergic in their activities the two functions tend to vary in parallel. It is thus found typically in uncorrected hypermetropes in whom excessive accommodation becomes a life habit, and less frequently in recently corrected myopes who are using accommodation for the first time, or in an early presbyope. It also occurs when the desire for clear vision in spite of difficulties, either ocular or environmental, calls for unusually accentuated accommodation. For the same reason but to a less dramatic degree, it may occur in the child starting near work for the first time or the young clerical or industrial worker starting a sedentary life of concentration. Less commonly a primary type of convergence excess may arise in irritative

conditions of the central nervous system, such as meningeal irritation or increased labyrinthine pressure. In many cases an unstable neurotic temperament always favours the development of reflex hyperkinesia and may itself determine its origin.

The *symptoms* of convergence excess may be merely annoying or completely incapacitating. In its milder degrees reading and close work are difficult — the print rapidly becomes blurred and fatigue and headaches follow any attempt at concentration thereon. These symptoms are frequently variable in their incidence, disappearing when the patient is well and reappearing when he is ill or fatigued, thus serving as a barometer of his general condition. At other times, particularly when the convergence (usually with the accommodation) goes into spasm, near work becomes impossible and diplopia occurs.

The *treatment* of excessive convergence should be directed in the first place to the elimination of the causal factor. Refractive errors should be corrected along with any significant heterophoria, and at the same time near work should be reduced and every care taken that the book be held well away from the eyes. In all cases the amount of near work must be curtailed to the capacity of the patient and it should be done in the best conditions of illumination and posture. Orthoptic exercises may be tried but they are rarely effective, although considerable help may be gained by exercises inducing voluntary relaxation: the patient looks at a distant object through two transparent slides and is taught to obtain physiological diplopia of markings on the transparencies, a feat which necessitates relaxation of accommodation and convergence; this may be followed by divergence exercises with the amblyoscope.

The ophthalmologist and the reading ability of children

It is no part of this work to provide an extensive review of the vexed question of 'dyslexia'. Even the definition of this term is controversial and all that will be referred to here is the ophthalmological aspect of reading disability that may be relevant in certain cases.

Those children labelled dyslexic or perhaps more acceptably those having 'specific learning disability' are not a homogeneous group, and whatever putative aetiologies are proposed are multiple and have therefore spawned their own appropriate therapies.

There is no evidence that visual acuity or accommodative abnormalities are particular features of dyslexic children. It goes without saying that in any child having reading difficulties exclusion of such abnormalities must be a first task for the ophthalmologist.

Oculo-motor anomalies are said to be a feature of some dyslexics and they often complain that print does not stay still but jumps around. Indeed one form of treatment involves isolating words or letters to train recognition.

The concept of a binocular defect has been promulgated by evidence that ocular dominance may be found to be variable. In particular orthoptists have been widely employed applying the Dunlop test. Two synoptophore slides are presented, a house with a big tree to one eye and a house with a small tree to the other. Initially the subject sees one house and both trees; the tubes of the instrument are then slightly diverged and the subject says which tree moved first. The eye opposite the other slide is taken as a *fixed reference eye*. A test is repeated 10 times and eight or more consistent results indicate fixed reference. Dyslexics are said to have less than 8 out of 10 consistency and may only give the same response on 5 out of 10 occasions. It is said, but has not been confirmed, that part-time occlusion of the less preferred eye for tasks such as reading, homework and mathematics fixes reference and improves reading ability; orthoptic exercises of some type are also said to be helpful.

Other binocular defects are said to include inappropriate eye movement during reading and more than the average number of verifications (leftward eye movements) of the text. Dyslexics are said to have difficulty following a sequence of illuminated light sources, and treatment based on this has been advised, but independent confirmation of the technique's helpfulness is wanting.

Reduced contrast sensitivity in the lower spatial frequencies is said to be present in some dyslexics, giving a basis to therapies involving filtering of the higher spatial frequencies. Other treatments with a putative neuro-ophthalmic basis include the provision of tinted lenses (the Irlen technique), but the basis of such an approach has yet to find sound scientific validity.

All in all it seems that the ophthalmologist's main duty in the sphere of dyslexia is examination of and attention to the standard refraction and oculo-motor anomalies combined with reassurance and sympathy to the subject and parents.

It is recognised nevertheless that faced with a subject who appears to be typical of one sub group of dyslexics, a young male with a family history of the condition and perhaps a past history of hyperactivity, the ophthalmic findings are likely to be completely negative. And while in all cases of childhood reading difficulty the possibility exists of some serious even remediable organic neuro-ophthalmic disability, such as cone dystrophy of the retina, or cerebral neoplasm, such a finding is very uncommon indeed.

Clinical investigation

19. The place of refraction in general ophthalmological examination

It cannot be too strongly emphasised that the estimation of a patient's refractive state is not a complete examination of the eyes. Indeed, as a physician, the ophthalmologist will need not only to take note of objective abnormalities found on ophthalmic examination but to pay particular attention to the history of the patient and the story of his complaint, for these will frequently provide most important information. His habits should be inquired into, since it is to suit the necessities of these that he has come for advice. His general condition should also be assessed, since an ophthalmic complaint may be the indication of a constitutional disturbance, and it is useless to correct the ocular error alone leaving the underlying cause untreated. Such a course, it is true, may provide some temporary relief, but ultimately can only result in the development of further and more serious manifestations of the basic condition.

The general aspect of the face and eyes should be noted — the position of the head, the symmetry of the face, the shape of the orbits, and the size of the eyes. Suggestive features may give some slight but, of course, far from conclusive indication of what the full examination is to reveal. Thus a flat-looking face is sometimes suggestive of hypermetropia, a head elongated in its antero-posterior diameter is often associated with myopia, and a markedly asymmetrical face may indicate astigmatism. An abnormal head posture may be ocular torticollis, perhaps giving a clue to a state of muscular imbalance. A small eye is usually hypermetropic, a large and prominent eye myopic. Small pupils are suggestive of hypermetropia, large ones of myopia.

The state of the lids and conjunctivae should be examined, the occurrence of blepharitis, styes, and conjunctivitis should be noted, and the ocular congestion which may denote refractive errors discriminated from the injection of inflammatory disease. The lacrimal puncta and sacs should receive attention, especially where weeping is one of the symptoms giving rise to complaint.

The anterior segments should now be examined under focal illumination and ideally with magnification, using the slit-lamp microscope; failing this a 'lens and loupe' inspection may suffice. The cornea should be examined, its transparency verified, keratic deposits looked for, and the nature of its reflex investigated. The depth of the anterior chamber should be assessed, and the clarity of its contents verified; the appearance of the iris, the shape and reactions of the pupils, and the presence of synechiae should be noted; and in all cases an estimate should be made of the ocular tension. The presence or absence of a squint should be assessed by examination of the corneal reflections, by a cover test and by testing the ocular movements. A rapid estimate should be made of the extent of the visual field.

The examination with the ophthalmoscope should now be undertaken in the dark room. It should be the routine when using the direct ophthalmoscope to commence with sufficient optical power to focus objects at the level of the lens of the eye. One then adjusts progressively, decreasing the convex or increasing the concave power until one has proceeded through all the ocular media before finally focusing on the retina. The fundus should be examined throughout its entire extent, particular attention being paid to the condition of the macula and the optic disc, the state of the vascular system, and the retinal periphery. If this examination offers difficulty it should be repeated under mydriasis.

All this is to be done as a matter of routine, and any pathological condition which is found should receive its appropriate treatment and the patient advised accordingly. When it does become a routine, it occupies a surprisingly small space of time and works out much less formidably in practice than it may appear on paper.

Where in this routine should the refraction therefore take place? The answer to this will depend very much upon the nature of the patient's complaint and upon the possible relevance to it of the optical state. It will also depend to some extent on the temperament of the examiner. One oculist may like to complete the general examination first, the other prefers to assess the refraction at an early stage, usually at the beginning, as a direct sequel to an estimation of the visual acuity. Indeed, most would agree that, whatever the complaint and whatever the subsequent order of events, every ophthalmic examination should begin with an estimation of the visual acuity, and with this subject we begin our account of the clinical methods of refraction.

20. Visual acuity

A patient's visual acuity is, of course, a function not only of the dioptric apparatus of the eye but also of the retina, the nerve paths, and the central nervous mechanism. It is only with the defects of vision which are due to anomalies in the first of these that we are concerned at the moment.

In differentiating between an impairment of vision due to an abnormality of the dioptric apparatus and one due to retinal or neurological disease, some help may be given by the pin-hole test. When an opaque disc perforated by a small hole is held in front of the eye, only a small pencil of rays gets through which passes through the axis of the dioptric system and is therefore unaffected by it. It follows that if the hole were small enough all refraction would be eliminated, and a clear image would thus be formed in the same manner as is seen in the pin-hole camera (see p. 36).

A patient complaining of defective vision is asked to look at a distant object (the test types), and then an opaque disc perforated with a small central hole is placed in front of his eye. He is then asked whether his vision is better or worse or unchanged.

In evaluating the result of the test we must remind ourselves that abnormalities of the dioptric apparatus take two principal forms, firstly refractive errors and secondly organic diseases of the media associated with a greater or less degree of opacity. A substantial improvement of visual acuity with the pin-hole test is found when refractive errors or minor degrees of opacification of the media are present. No improvement, indeed some worsening of vision, may be found in retinal or neuro-ophthalmic diseases and in cases having substantial opacification of the media. The effect of the pin-hole on refractive errors is easily explained on purely optical grounds. In minor degrees of opacification of the media its action seems to be to allow the patient to take notice of and, indeed, perhaps to select a narrow pencil of rays passing through some path which is still optically clear and regular. A good standard of illumination is essential in carrying out the test and the hole in the disc should be opposite the centre of the pupil. The test also has therapeutic implications and these will be discussed later.

The acuity of vision is determined by the smallest retinal image the form of which can be appreciated, and it is measured by the smallest object which can be clearly seen at a certain distance. In order to discriminate the form of an object its several parts must be differentiated; and if two separate points are to be distinguished by the retina, it is probably necessary that two individual cones should be stimulated while the one between them remains unstimulated. Histological measurement has shown that the average diameter of a cone in the macular region is 0.004 mm; this therefore represents the smallest distance between two cones. It thus appears that a normal eye should be able to appreciate a retinal image of this size, and although the standard varies very markedly between individuals, this estimate has on the whole been corroborated by subjective experiments.

We have seen that the further away an object is from the eye, the smaller will be the image formed on the retina; that is, the size of the latter is a function not only of the size of the object but also of its distance away (Fig. 20.1). Consequently, combining these two factors, the most convenient standard to adopt in estimating the acuity of vision is the size of the visual angle, that is the size of the angle formed by two lines drawn from the extremities of the object through the nodal point of the eye. It is found that in order to produce an image of the minimal size of 0.004 mm, the object must subtend a visual

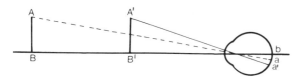

Fig. 20.1 The size of the retinal image varies with the distance of the object from the eye.
AB and A′B′ are of the same size. If A′B′ is one-half of the distance of AB from the eye, the image *a′b* will necessarily be twice the size of the image *ab*.

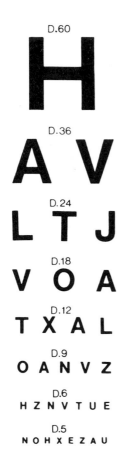

Fig. 20.2 Snellen's test types.

the lines composing the letter. The size of these squares, that is, the breadth of the lines, is such that their edges subtend a visual angle of 1 minute when they are a certain specified distance away. Each entire letter therefore subtends an angle of 5 minutes at this distance, but in order to analyse its form completely and see its constituent parts the eye must be able to resolve them down to the standard limit of 1 minute. The first line of type is so constructed that this angle is formed at a distance of 60 metres, the second at 36 metres, the third at 24, the fourth at 18, the fifth at 12, the sixth at 9, the seventh at 6, while additional lines are usually inserted which subtend the same angle at 5 and at 4 metres (Fig. 20.3). These letters should thus be read by a person with standard vision at these distances away. Consequently, if a patient is placed at a convenient distance, which is usually taken as 6 metres, he should be able to read easily down to the line with a theoretical viewpoint 9 metres away, while the 6 metre line should just be distinct. If he cannot reach this limit, his distant vision is defective; and if he can exceed it, it is above the standard. In practice it will be found that the standard is a liberal one, for the acuity of the vision of the great majority of people can readily be raised above it.

The results of the test are expressed as a fraction, the numerator of which denotes the distance at which the patient is from the type, and the denominator the line he sees at this distance. Thus if his vision is 'normal' and he sees the line which ought to be read at 6 metres when he is 6 metres distant, his visual acuity is 6/6; if, when he is at this distance, he can only see the line which a person with standard vision should see at 24 metres, his visual acuity is 6/24; while if he reads still further and reaches the line constructed to subtend the normal visual angle at 4 metres, his acuity is 6/4. These fractions

angle of 1 minute. This then, is taken as the standard of the normal visual acuity.

These principles have been embodied in *Snellen's Test Types*, which are now used almost universally in testing the acuity of vision. The types consist of a series of letters of diminishing size, as is seen in Figure 20.2. Each letter is of such a shape that it can be enclosed in a square the size of which is five times the thickness of

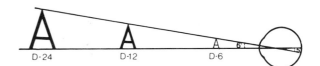

Fig. 20.3 The formation of Snellen's test types.

denoting visual acuity should not be reduced since they are conventions giving an accurate numerical estimate in special conditions. In their original form they indicate the actual types used and the actual distance away from the test types.

In the United States of America the metric system is not usually employed but the fraction is written in terms of feet (6 metres $\triangleq$ 20 feet): vision of 6/6 is therefore 20/20; of 6/60, 20/200; of 1/60, 3/200 (approx.), etc.

Notations other than the original suggestion of Snellen are widely used. On the continent of Europe many employ Monoyer's scale in arithmetical progression wherein the relative sizes of the test types are 10/10, 10/9, 10/8 . . . giving a relative visual acuity of 1.0, 0.9, 0.8 . . . 0.1.

The following table gives the approximate equivalence in Snellen's notation of metres and feet and in the decimal system; there are added the corresponding visual angles in minutes and the generally accepted percentages of visual efficiency and percentage loss of vision.

Snellen's notation		Decimal notation	Visual angle (1′)	Visual efficiency (%)	Visual loss (%)
Metres	Feet				
6/6	20/20	1.0	1.0	100.0	0.0
6/9	20/30	0.7	1.5	91.4	8.6
6/12	20/40	0.5	2.0	83.6	16.4
6/18	20/60	0.3	3.0	69.9	30.1
6/24	20/80	0.25	4.0	58.5	41.5
6/60	20/200	0.1	10.0	20.0	80.0

It is obvious that the visual acuity will vary in the corrected and uncorrected eye. The efficiency of the eye without correction may be called the *unaided visual acuity*. In contradistinction, the theoretical ideal of a comparable standard is attained by determining the acuity when accommodation is relaxed and when the refractive error is corrected by a spectacle lens situated at the anterior focal point of the eye (15.7 mm in front of the cornea); this is the *absolute visual acuity*. Since, however, spectacle lenses are not usually worn at this distance, the *relative visual acuity* is more usually determined, that is the visual acuity of the eye with its refraction fully corrected by spectacle lenses worn in the ordinary position; this is referred to as the *corrected visual acuity*.

THE ROUTINE TESTING OF THE VISUAL ACUITY

The *test types* should be clearly printed and legible, and should not, as sometimes is the case, be obscured by the outlines of the squares upon which they are constructed. It is essential that they be well and uniformly illuminated (Fig. 20.4). The amount of illumination has a considerable effect on the visual acuity. In the normal eye, below 2 lumens per square foot the efficiency falls very rapidly, and above this value it rises slowly and by a small amount until an illumination of about 50 lumen/sq. ft. is attained, above which the improvement is negligible. This forms the ideal standard, and in practice, since an illumination of 100 lumen./sq. ft. is easy to attain with modern strip lighting, it is well to install an illumination of the latter standard where external illumination is employed so that, as its efficiency decreases with time, it will still remain effective. Internally illuminated types are now standard as well as projection types.

The *distance* at which the test types are placed should preferably be 6 metres or 20 feet; 5 metres is the shortest which should be allowed. If 6 metres, or at least 5, are not obtainable, the required distance should be made up by using reversed test types placed above the patient's head, and making him look at their reflection in a mirror hung on the opposite wall. In this case the light from the types travels to the mirror and then from the mirror to the patient's eyes, and thus an available room space of 3 metres can be converted optically into one of 6. The distance between infinity and 6 metres represents approximately the depth of focus of the eye; and at this distance the rays of light in the small bundle which enters the pupil suffer so little divergence that for most purposes they may be taken as parallel, that is as coming from infinity. In actual fact the divergence

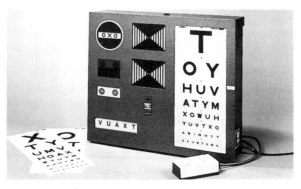

Fig. 20.4 An internally illuminated test type for clinical use (combined with other subjective tests, see Ch. 21)(Keeler).

at this distance is equivalent to about one-sixth of a dioptre, and in the final adjustment of glasses this divergence should be recognised and an allowance made for it.

The right eye should always be tested first, except where the patient's complaint is particularly of defective left vision, in which case the left is assessed first. The patient reads down the chart as far as he can and then this is repeated with the other eye. Both eyes are then tested together. If the visual acuities (V) of the two eyes are about equal it is usually found that they reinforce each other so that the binocular vision is slightly better than the uniocular. The result is usually recorded thus:

$$\left.\begin{array}{l} V_R = 6/6, \text{ or whatever the case may be} \\ V_L = 6/6, \text{ or whatever the case may be} \end{array}\right\} = 6/5$$

As testing may be done with or without glasses in place we record this fact by using the letters s (sine) if the acuity is unaided, and c (cum) if with correction — thus 6/6c or 6/12s.

The matter sounds straightforward but may not be. Many patients will hesitate as they get lower down the chart and the exact line to record as the visual acuity may not be obvious. Some authorities require the last completed correct line as the level to be taken; but this is probably too strict an application of the theory of test types. With increasing experience most examiners feel happy to compromise by using such modifications as 6/9+, 6/18 pt. (partly), 6/24-- or by actual specification of the defect as in 6/12 (–2 letters). The difficulties are often worst in cases of astigmatism where the patient may get some letters right and some wrong over even three or four lines of the chart. Myopes, known or assumed, should be discouraged from screwing up their eyes so that the examiner can get a truly unaided visual acuity.

If the subject cannot read the largest letter he is asked to walk towards the types and at a certain distance he may be able to see the largest. Having thus made sure that he understands exactly where to look and what to look for, he should then be moved back a little, and the longest distance is determined at which the top letter is seen. For example, if he sees the top letter at a distance of 2 metres, then $V = 2/60$. If this is found to be impossible, the surgeon holds out the fingers of his hand against a dark background (such as his coat) and asks him to count them. The vision is

then recorded as at the farthest point at which the fingers are distinguishable, thus: $V = $ CF (counts fingers) at 1 metre. If this is not possible, the surgeon then moves his hand in front of the patient's eye against a light, such as the window; vision of this meagre degree is recorded as: $V = $ HM (hand movements). Even this may be beyond the patient's power, in which case the room is darkened, and a light is thrown into his eye by the ophthalmoscope; if he can recognise the presence of the light and tell when it is thrown into his eye and when it is not, the vision is recorded as: $V = $ PL (perception of light). If, on the contrary, no light is recognised, the vision is recorded as: $V = $ no PL; this is total blindness. Where bare perception of light exists the light is thrown into his eye from different directions, and he is asked to point to the place from which he imagines it is coming, and in this way an indication is obtained of any area of the retina which is totally blind; this faculty is spoken of as *projection* and a note is made of the extent to which it is good or bad.

The ordinary test as thus undertaken is dependent entirely upon the patient's co-operation, and in this way fails in the case of malingerers, illiterates, or young children. Illiterates may be tested by *Landolt's broken ring test* (Fig. 20.5). This test, which was

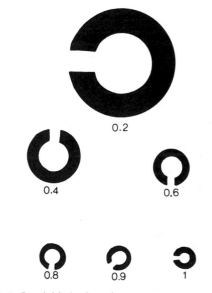

Fig. 20.5 Landolt's broken ring test types.

recommended by the International Congress in 1909, has the advantage that it is applicable to subjects of any nationality, while it does away with the assistance in reading which a knowledge of the forms of the letters of the alphabet gives to those who know them. The rings are constructed on the same basis as regards size and visual angle as the letters of Snellen's types, and the patient is instructed to indicate by a motion of the hand at which point each one is broken.

In children who do not yet know their letters, familiar figures of varying sizes, such as a ship, a cow, a doll, etc., may be used, their constituent parts being constructed as far as possible on Snellen's principles, and from the child's description of these a very good, although perhaps not a scientifically accurate, knowledge of the visual acuity is gained. A useful alternative is the '*E test*' wherein a printed E of varying sizes on a card or a plastic cube with different sizes of E on its various faces (Fig. 20.6) is held in various directions before the child (preferably at the regulation distance of 6 metres), and the child is cajoled into putting a wooden E held in his hand in the same direction. The graded 'hand-test' wherein a hand is held up with the fingers outstretched can be similarly used. It is surprising how very small children can be persuaded to co-operate in this if it is played as a game.

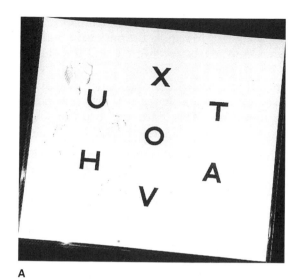

A

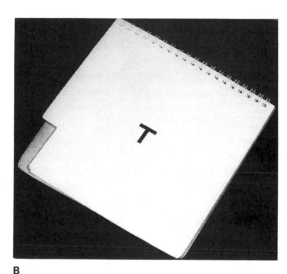

B

Fig. 20.7 (A and B) The Sheridan–Gardiner test.

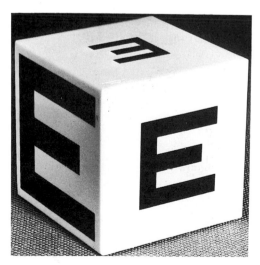

Fig. 20.6 The E test. The various sizes of E are on different faces of a cube.

Of established popularity, and deservedly so, is the Sheridan–Gardiner test which requires the recognition of certain letters but only by their shape. The child holds a card (Fig. 20.7) which has on it a small range of letters. The examiner holds at 6 metres various Snellen-graded sizes of these. The child points at the one on the card held which is identical to the one the examiner shows.

With still younger children, such as may require to be tested for amblyopia in squint,

Worth's *ivory ball test* may be employed. The child is allowed to handle the balls with both eyes open. One eye is then covered, and the balls are thrown on the floor at a distance of 6 or 7 yards. They are thrown with a slight spin so that they 'break' on touching the carpet, and thus change their direction. There are five balls of graded sizes, varying in diameter from $\frac{1}{2}$ to $1\frac{1}{2}$ inches. They are thrown one by one beginning with the largest, and the child is encouraged to run after them. In this way a rough estimate of the visual acuity can be made from the size of the smallest ball which the child can see.

Visual acuity of very young subjects

Although rarely part of routine clinical practice it is possible to assess the visual potential of very young infants. The methods used are sophisticated and fall into three groups.

In the first optokinetic nystagmus is generated and its presence noted by observation, or objectively by using the electro-oculogram to record the eye movements. A useful clinical instrument is the Catford drum.

Another means of assessing visual acuity depends on the recording of the visual evoked potential in response to pattern stimulation.

The third technique derived from experimental psychology is that of Forced Preferential Looking (FPL). An observer, unseen by the infant, watches the way the head or eyes move towards one or other of two test objects: one plain, the other with gratings or stripes upon it. A series of test objects in which the stripe width progressively narrows is then shown randomly to the right or to the left of the plain test object. The observer assesses which way the infant looks on a number of occasions and the degree to which the assessment correlates with the actual side of the interesting 'test object' allows a reliable calculation of the visual acuity.

The original method of carrying out FPL involved quite complex and space-occupying apparatus in order to accord with stringent psychological criteria. So much so that set-ups of this nature have been somewhat eschewed by paediatric ophthalmologists. However, simpler versions considered by many to be equally reliable are now available. The acuity card procedure using the Teller acuity cards has now become a more commonly employed methodology for assessing forced preferential looking.

THE TESTING OF NEAR VISION

When the distant vision has been tested, the visual acuity at reading distance is investigated; for this, test types are also employed. Snellen constructed a set of letters of graded sizes and thicknesses on the same principles as his distant types, and this is the most scientifically accurate test. The unusual configuration of letters of this construction, however, is not reproduced in the ordinary printers' founts, and the requirements can only be attained by a photographic reduction of the standard Snellen types to approximately 1/17th of their normal size (Fig. 20.8). In this event the letters in the 6/6 line subtend an angle of 5 minutes at an average reading distance (35 cm or 14 in). This may be called the 'Snellen equivalent' for near vision.

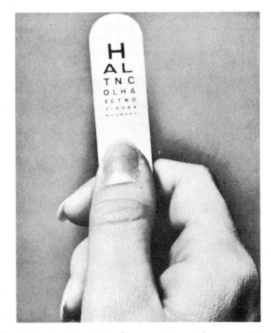

Fig. 20.8 A reduced Snellen type for testing near vision (Clement Clarke).

Such a test, however, has never become popular and graded sizes of letters of pleasing types have been habitually employed. The first test of this kind was suggested by Jaeger in 1867; these were simply the ordinary printers' founts of type of varying sizes as used at that time (non-pareil, minion, etc.). Unfortunately, however, printers' founts have changed considerably since then, and it is now the general custom to use various sizes of modern types on test cards which approximate Jaeger's original choice; these are traditionally called J.1, J.2, etc.,

and although they deviate considerably from the original standard they are probably sufficiently accurate for all practical purposes.

To overcome this difficulty the Faculty of Ophthalmologists of Great Britain in 1952 put forward suggestions for a more consistent standard (Fig. 20.9). In this, Times Roman type face is used with 'standard' spacing, and specimens of printing are given in sizes 5 pt, 6 pt, 8 pt, 10 pt, 12 pt, 14 pt, 18 pt, 24 pt, 36 pt and 48 pt upon dead-white matt-surface cartridge paper. In addition to passages from literature,

N.5.

The streets of London are better paved and better lighted than those of any metropolis in Europe: there are lamps on both sides of every street, in the mean proportion of one lamp to three doors. The effect pro-

cave   acorn   veneer   succour

N.8.

Water Cresses are sold in small bunches, one penny each, or three bunches for twopence. The crier of Water Cresses frequently travels seven or eight miles

rose   sauce   cannon   reverse

N.10.

Hearth Brooms, Brushes, Sieves, Bowls, Clothes-horses, and Lines, and almost every household article of turnery, are cried in the

neon   verse   runner   caravan

N.12.

Strawberries, brought fresh gathered to the market in the height of their season, both morning and afternoon,

nuns   score   severe   careers

N.18.

Door-mats of all kinds, rush and rope, from sixpence to four shillings

crave   savour   concern

Fig. 20.9 Test types for near vision.
A sample of the different sizes of printing in Times Roman type face with 'standard' spacing advised by the Faculty of Ophthalmologists (Hamblin's arrangement). N.5. is printed in 5 point type; N.8. in 8 point, etc.

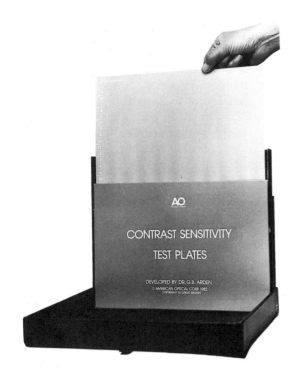

Fig. 20.10

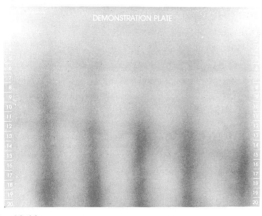

Fig. 20.11

Figs 20.10 and **20.11** The Arden contrast sensitivity plates. Each plate is slowly raised from the housing and the patient indicates immediately a grating pattern is recognisable.

in the reading of which the sense helps the interpretation, a few isolated words consisting only of lower-case letters without ascenders or descenders are also printed in each size. In this test the near acuity is recorded by the letter N

(near vision) followed by a number indicating the typeface size, e.g. N.5, N.8, etc.

In testing, the patient remains seated in the chair and, with a good light thrown over the left shoulder, he is given the card with the test types to hold and asked to read them. The near vision is recorded as the smallest type which he can comfortably read with a note of the approximate distance at which the card is held; thus NV = J.1 at 30 cm in Jaeger's notation or N.5 at 30 cm in the Faculty's notation.

CONTRAST SENSITIVITY

It is claimed that the high contrast of Snellen acuity charts may fail to differentiate certain types of visual defects occurring in eyes with pathological conditions. While it would be out of place here to detail the arguments for and against more recherché methods of assessing visual

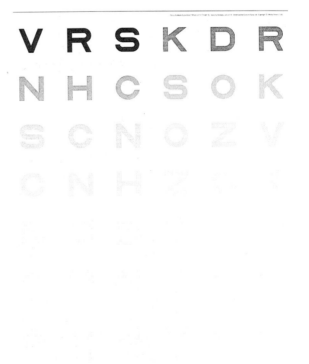

Fig. 20.12 The Pelli–Robson chart.

function, contrast sensitivity assessment has now an established place in clinical ophthalmology. In particular fields where it has been most widely employed it is suggested that the contrast sensitivity function may be significantly impaired in the presence of relatively unaffected Snellen visual acuity. The conditions most frequently assessed are:

Possible glaucoma in those with intra-ocular pressures considered outside the normal range, in diabetic retinopathy, in the amblyopia of squint, in optic nerve affections and in the pre-operative investigation of potential subjects for cataract surgery, and in their post-operative assessment.

The original technique based on the generation of sinusoidal gratings on cathode-ray tubes is not applicable to routine clinical practice, but several charts are now available for this purpose.

One of the first of these was the Arden gratings (Fig. 20.10): a pattern of stripes is exposed from low to high contrast, and an arbitrary scale figure is read off from the side of the test plate at the level where the grating bars become visible (Fig. 20.11). There are six plates, studied at 57 cm, with spatial frequency increasing from 0.2 cycles/degree to 6.4 cycles/degree, each being double the frequency of the previous one. The scale readings for recognition level of all the plates are summated, and a higher sum represents poorer contrast sensitivity.

The Vistech chart (used at 3 m from the subject) and the Cambridge chart (at 6 m from the subject) are more recent versions of such techniques. In the former contrast is assessed at several spatial frequencies (distance of separation of the grating bars) and the subject has to identify the orientation of the grating, i.e. whether vertical or 15 degrees clockwise, or anti-clockwise. In the latter only one spatial frequency is used and the subject simply identifies whether one of two charts has a visible grating on it.

A more recent introduction uses letters rather than bars. The Pelli–Robson letter sensitivity chart (Fig. 20.12) has eight rows of six upper-case letters all of the same size but decreasing in contrast every group of 3. The test is carried out at 0.5 metre and the limit of sensitivity is determined when two or more errors are made in a group of three letters.

21. Objective methods of refraction

RETINOSCOPY

The most valuable method of estimating the optical state of the eye is the technique of *retinoscopy*. Its popularity derives from both its usefulness and its accuracy which, when the technique is mastered, can give results correct to within 0.25 D.

The optics of retinoscopy

In retinoscopy an illuminated area of the retina serves as an object, and the image at the far point of the eye is located by moving the illumination across the fundus and noting the behaviour of the luminous reflex in the pupil. The observer does not see the illuminated area of the patient's fundus, but only the rays emanating from it to form an illuminated area of the pupil. If the image is formed between the patient and the observer, the movements of the reflex and the external light are in opposite directions; if it falls outside this region, either behind the patient's eye or behind the observer's, the two move in the same direction. When the far point of the patient's eye corresponds to the nodal point of the observer's eye, a *neutral point* (the *point of reversal* or *end point*) occurs. If the eyes are separated by the convenient distance of, say, $\frac{2}{3}$ of a metre (the 'working distance'), the far point of the patient must be $\frac{2}{3}$ of a metre away, and therefore he must have −1.5 D of myopia. The rationale of the method is therefore to add lenses to the dioptric system of the patient's eye until the point of reversal is seen by the observer; at that point the patient's refractive error is measured by the added lenses less the dioptric

value of the working distance (i.e. 1.5 D assuming patient and observer are $\frac{2}{3}$ of a metre apart).

If the patient and the observer are separated by 2 metres, the point of reversal would be when the patient was corrected to −0.5 D; if they were only 0.5 metre apart, the point of reversal would be at −2 D; and so on. The farther away the surgeon is the more theoretically accurate are the results obtained, but in practice this is counterbalanced by the difficulty in seeing clearly the play of lights in the pupil.

The detailed optics is most easily considered in three stages: first, the illumination of the subject's retina; second, the reflex imagery of this illuminated area formed by the subject's dioptric apparatus; and finally, the projection of the image by the observer. A crucial element in retinoscopy as a diagnostic procedure is the second stage wherein an image is formed of the illuminated retina and is therefore situated at the subject's far point. The most convenient exposition is an examination of the conditions obtaining in the three principal refractive states. We shall first examine retinoscopy using a plane mirror and also assume that the illumination is by a point source.

Retinoscopy in emmetropia

In the accompanying figures the observer, to the left, rotates a plane mirror so that the image, S_1 of a point source, S_0, moves as indicated. S_1, is referred to as the 'immediate source', S_0 being the 'original source'. In the first condition (Fig. 21.1) no light enters the subject's eye, but with

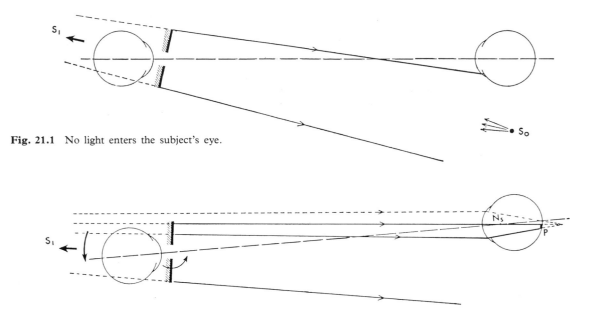

Fig. 21.1 No light enters the subject's eye.

Fig. 21.2 The illumination stage in emmetropia.

rotation of the mirror in the direction of the arrow (Fig. 21.2) some light enters through the subject's pupil and illuminates a patch of retina, P (the *illumination stage*). The site of this patch is determined by the line from S_1, through the nodal point, N_s, of the subject's eye. As S_1 is a finite distance from the subject and the eye is emmetropic, an image of S_1 will be formed behind the retina.

The illuminated patch can now be considered as an object in its own right and will form an image at the far point of the eye, which in emmetropia is at infinity (the *reflex stage* — so called because the light is actually reflected from the fundus) (Fig. 21.3).

Even although the subject's retina is illuminated, the observer will not be able to see the reflex unless light enters the sight hole of the mirror. In Figure 21.3 the determining ray, R, is that from the upper margin of P which just strikes the lower margin of the subject's pupil. With further rotation of the mirror, P moves upwards towards the principal axis of the eye. The ray R subtends a progressively smaller angle with the axis until it just enters the sight hole (Fig. 21.4). At this point the reflex is seen by the observer.

Its position is determined by projecting it in relation to the subject's pupil. It will be recalled that the ray R is one of a series of parallel rays formed by the dioptric apparatus of the subject's eye from the top edge of the illuminated patch, P. A ray parallel to R passing through the observer's nodal point will therefore strike the observer's retina at P_0 where the parallel rays will be focused, presuming the observer to be emmetropic. As can be appreciated from the figure, the observer will project this to the lower border of the subject's pupil (the *projection stage*) (Fig. 21.4). As the mirror rotates further, P will move up and P_0 move downwards. The reflex seen by the observer appears as a light area with a shadow above it. These travel apparently upwards across the pupil in the *same* direction as the light moving across the eye externally. Thus in emmetropia a 'with' movement is obtained.

Finally, the reflex disappears, the last ray to enter the observer's eye coming from the lower margin of the patch, P, which emerges close to the upper border of the subject's pupil and just passes the lower border of the sight hole. The observer sees the reflex move as from Figure 21.8 to Figure 21.9.

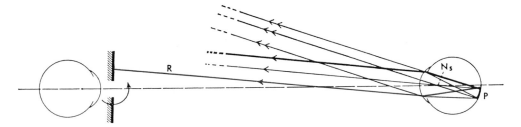

Fig. 21.3 The reflex stage in emmetropia.

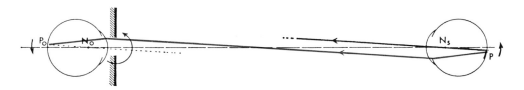

Fig. 21.4 The projection stage in emmetropia.

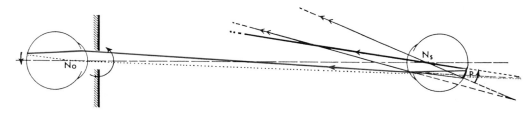

Fig. 21.5 The reflex and projection stages in hypermetropia.

Retinoscopy in hypermetropia

The illumination stage is similar to that in emmetropia. The reflex stage differs because the patch of illuminated retina, P, forms a virtual image at the far point behind the subject's eye (Fig. 21.5). Again, it is the ray from the upper margin of P emerging close to the lower border of the pupil that subtends the smallest angle with the principal axis, and as the mirror continues to rotate it will be the first to strike the sight hole. The projection stage is the same as in emmetropia and therefore a 'with' movement of the reflex is obtained.

Retinoscopy in myopia

The illumination stage is again similar to that in emmetropia and hypermetropia. There is a slight difference since in high myopia the image of the immediate source may be in front of the retina (see Fig. 21.7), but the illuminated blur patch moves in the same way as in the other refractive conditions — in the *opposite* sense to the immediate source.

In the reflex stage a real image of the illuminated patch, P, is formed at the far point in front of the subject's eye. Two situations must be considered. In the first (Fig. 21.6) the far point is behind the observer — again, the determining ray is that from the upper edge of the area, P, which just passes the sight hole and a 'with' movement of the reflex is obtained as in emmetropia and hypermetropia. In the second situation (Fig. 21.7) the degree of myopia is higher and the image of the illuminated patch, P, is formed between the observer and the subject. As can be appreciated from the figure,

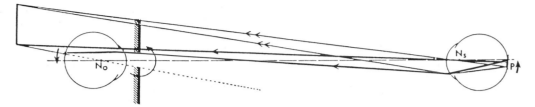

Fig. 21.6 The reflex and projection stages in myopia less than 1.5 D.

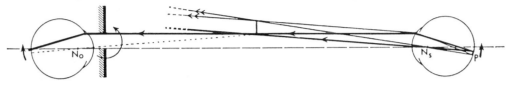

Fig. 21.7 The reflex and projection stages in myopia greater than 1.5 D.

the movement of the reflex is 'against' that of the external movement of light across the subject's eye. The determining ray (shown in red) is that from the upper border of the patch, P, emerging through the upper border of the pupil, and this is the first to strike the sight hole and therefore to be visible to the observer, who consequently projects the reflex as if coming from the upper border of the subject's pupil, even though the light from the source strikes the lower border of the pupil first, thus giving rise to an 'against' movement. The object of retinoscopy is to place lenses in front of the subject's eye so as to find the point of neutralisation at which the direction of movement of the reflex is indeterminate. This occurs when the subject's eye is made myopic by lenses so that the image in the reflex stage is at the observer's nodal point — the situation obtaining somewhere between Figures 21.6 and 21.7.

In practice the illuminated area of the pupil is not so readily observed as its border with the unilluminated area, for on movement this appears as a sharp contrast of advancing or receding light and shadow (Figs 21.8 and 21.9). Moreover, the greater the degree of ametropia the shorter the excursion and the slower the speed of movement (Figs 21.10 and 21.11); as the refractive error is being corrected, the area of the light pencil becomes progressively smaller, and a small movement of the source makes it flit more rapidly

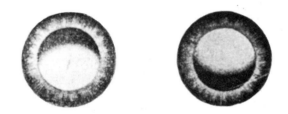

Figs 21.8 and 21.9 Retinoscopy shadows.

across the pupillary aperture; at the neutral point the area of an image element on the retina is so small that when it passes the aperture it passes entirely, so that the pupil appears at one moment uniformly light (but not brightly so), at the next uniformly dark. The accuracy of retinoscopy depends on the sharpness of this neutralisation, but there is often no clearly defined neutral point but rather a *neutral zone*, since optical aberrations and irregularities of the retinal surface cause the conjugate focus to be formed not on a plane but in depth. Moreover, the issue is sometimes further confused by the appearance of irregular and scissor-like shadows as the neutral region is being approached.

THE METHODS OF RETINOSCOPY

Retinoscopes

In the practice of retinoscopy a patch upon the retina is illuminated by a retinoscope.

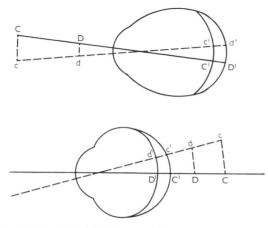

Figs 21.10 and **21.11** The rate of movement of the illuminated retinal area. The movement is referred to the remote point. In hypermetropia (L) and myopia (R) the greater the refractive error the slower the movement.

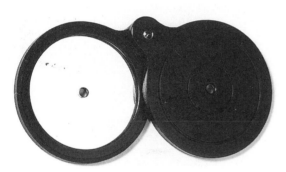

Fig. 21.12 The reflecting retinoscope: here, combined plane and concave mirrors.

The classical combination is a separate source of light and a *reflecting retinoscope* (Fig. 21.12): this consists of a perforated mirror by which the beam is reflected into the patient's eye and through a central hole in which the emergent rays enter the observer's eye. Movements of the illuminated retinal area are produced by tilting the mirror. Either a plane or a concave mirror can be used; with the former when the mirror is tilted, the image (the immediate source of light) moves in the opposite direction and the illuminated retinal area in the same direction as the tilt of the mirror; with a concave mirror, on the other hand, the illuminated area moves in a direction which depends on the focal length of the mirror in relation to the working distance.

When a plane mirror is employed, more accurate results are obtained than with a concave one. Its

central opening should be at least 4 mm in diameter so that an abundance of light can enter the observer's eye. The advantages of a hole of this size are counterbalanced by the appearance of a circular dark patch in the centre of the reflection corresponding to the hole, which reduces the illumination in the pupillary area and confuses the retinoscopy. This difficulty is overcome by using a very slightly concave mirror wherein the focal length is greater than the distance between the surgeon and the patient, that is at least 150 cm. This, as will be more clearly understood from the previous explanation, for the purposes of retinoscopy acts in the same manner as a plane mirror. At the same time, the rays are made to converge slightly upon the pupil, increasing the illumination there and eliminating the shadow of the central hole. Since its action is identical to that of a plane mirror, it will be referred to as such in the following pages. The hole should be pierced and not be formed by a defect in the silvering of an imperforate mirror, as the glass reflects an appreciable fraction of the light which should enter the eye. If it is pierced, annoying reflexes may be formed at the edges, but these are avoided if the sides of the hole are blackened and are made to widen out posteriorly so that it is narrowest at the mirror end. The source of light used should be small, bright and enclosed; a Pointolite is ideal.

The *luminous retinoscope* (Fig. 21.13), in which both light source and mirror are incorporated, is the standard modern instrument. It is easily manipulated, with the advantage that the intensity and type of the beam can be readily controlled. The optical principles, of course, are

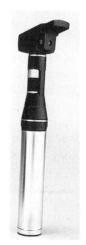

Fig. 21.13 The electric retinoscope (Keeler).

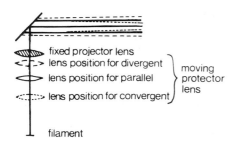

fixed projector lens
lens position for divergent
lens position for parallel   moving
                                    protector
lens position for convergent   lens

filament

Fig. 21.14 Optical construction of the electric retinoscope.

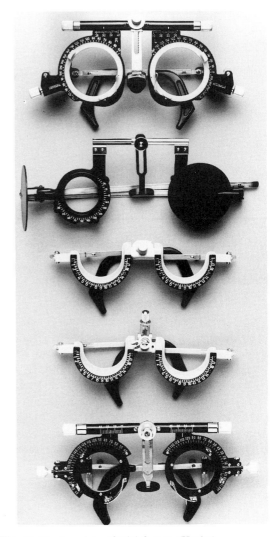

Fig. 21.15 A variety of trial frames (Keeler).

identical (Fig. 21.14) to those described above; in the portable instrument a strong convex lens and a mirror at 45 degrees project the light onto the patient's eye. Both types of mirror effect can be provided by altering the distance between the light and the condensing lens to vary the angularity of the light leaving the mirror, so that at one extreme the rays converge at a point close to the instrument (concave mirror) and at the other the rays are parallel (plane mirror). Deservedly the most popular luminous retinoscope in use today is the *streak retinoscope*. The reflexes this produces in practice are easier to recognise, and allow the axes of the meridian of any astigmatism to be more readily identified. Even greater efficiency is obtained from modern retinoscopes by the use of halogen bulbs and mains or rechargeable electrical sources.

Trial frames

A trial frame (Fig. 21.15) is used to carry test lenses during retinoscopy or during subjective examination of refraction. It should be light and readily adaptable, allowing adjustments for each eye separately. These are necessary so that the trial lenses when in place are a standard distance from the eye and are accurately centred. Antero-posterior adjustment must therefore be possible as well as lateral and vertical. It must also be ensured that the dial indicating the orientation of the frame is truly positioned, otherwise mistakes may occur in the reading of the axis of any cylindrical correction. Simplicity to ensure lightness and a comfortable-fitting nose rest are the greatest essentials, for many patients are very sensitive to the weight, and will express

annoyance and dissatisfaction with the lenses which are put up for trial, complaining that they make their eyes ache or give rise to a headache, when the trouble lies in the irritation caused by heavy and oppressive frames. An aluminium alloy is a suitable material and a weight of more than 30 grams is unnecessary.

Each eye should be fitted with at least three cells: one situated next to the eye to hold a spherical lens, one in the middle for a cylindrical lens, and one furthest from the eye for a prism, Maddox rod, etc. The compartment for the cylinder should be capable of smooth and accurate rotation, so that no trouble is experienced in arriving at the correct direction of the axis. The lenses should be carried close to the eye so that they occupy as nearly as possible the same position as the spectacle lenses when in use. It is very advisable, also, that the compartments should be as close together as is compatible with holding lenses, for, as will be pointed out, errors arise when any considerable distance is allowed to intervene between the constituent lenses. Finally, the frame should have its side-pieces jointed so that, when the near vision is being tested by reading, the glasses can be angled so that their optic axes correspond to the downward inclination of the line of vision.

Test lenses

A sufficiency of test lenses should be at hand so that any reasonable combination of sphere, cylinder and prism can be put before the patient's eyes. A typical *trial set* of test lenses will have spheres every quarter of a dioptre to 4 D and every half to 6 D, thereafter every dioptre to 14 D and every 2 dioptres to 20 D and cylinders every quarter to 2 and every half to 6. Many refined versions have one-eighth dioptre subdivisions up to 1 dioptre and higher powers at the other end of the range of spheres and cylinders. This division into eighths is, of course, curious insofar as the dioptre is a typically metric measurement and a tenth might be a more appropriate subdivision; it might be that those who go so far as to flatter themselves that their retinoscopy is accurate to within an eighth of a dioptre would be pushing things beyond credibility if they claimed they needed a standard involving tenths! In practice, most of us are happy with an accuracy of one-quarter of a dioptre. By a combination of spheres and cylinders an excellent range of possible optical effects can be produced.

For a complete examination, prisms up to 10, with an additional two of 15 and 20 prism dioptres are also required, and accessories such as plano lenses, opaque discs, pin-hole and stenopaeic discs, Maddox rods, red and green glasses, and so on. All these are enclosed in a trial case (Fig. 21.16).

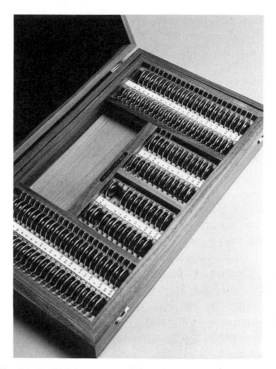

Fig. 21.16 Trial case containing the necessary lenses, prisms.

The type of test lenses employed does not usually receive the attention its importance warrants. In the interest of practical accuracy the effective power of the trial lenses should conform as closely as possible, particularly in the higher powers, to the type of lens which is to be used in the spectacles. It is obvious that this ideal cannot be attained, but practical convenience should involve as few departures from theoretical accuracy as possible.

We have already seen that in combination with the optical system of the eye the effect of a spectacle lens is determined by its *back vertex power*, and this varies with its position in front of the eye, its thickness and its form. If the ophthalmic lens is to duplicate the effect of the spectacle lens to be prescribed, the former should correspond in these respects to the latter. When the lenses are of low power these discrepancies may not matter much, but if they are of high power the possible error may be considerable. This matter will be gone into more fully at a later stage but so far as the immediate argument is concerned every endeavour should be made to reduce these errors to the minimum.

Thus the back lens in the trial frames should occupy as nearly as possible the position of a spectacle lens, and this position — the spectacle plane — is usually chosen just to clear the lashes, averaging about 12 mm in front of the cornea. Obviously several lenses cannot stand at the same distance from the eye; the ideal test lenses should therefore not be calibrated accurately as individual lenses, but should indicate the effectivity of a lens in this plane so that the effective power of a combination of lenses in the trial frame will correspond additively to that of a single lens located in this plane. If the lenses are not compensated additively in this way, significant errors arise when two or more trial lenses are used. For this purpose, of course, a set of trial lenses must be used in specific compartments of a correspondingly designed trial frame which must be placed in a designated position.

The test lenses should also conform so far as possible in form and thickness to the spectacle lenses subsequently to be worn. This may of course be impracticable, but the best approximation is obtained by the use of thin lenses of relatively small size (reduced aperture lenses, Fig. 21.17) of approximately 25 mm diameter. These should preferably be in plano-convex and plano-concave form, not biconvex or biconcave (Figs 21.18 and 21.19) and in the trial frame the plane surfaces of a

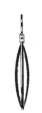

Fig. 21.18 Biconvex lens of unsuitable type.

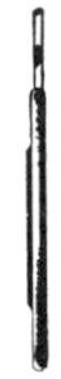

Fig. 21.19 Plano-convex lens of suitable type.

convex lens and a concave lens should, when possible, be next to the eye, but when more than one lens is used, the plane surfaces of two component lenses should preferably be in apposition; to allow close apposition, the rim of the lens should be mounted so that it is as nearly as practicable in the plane of the plano surface.

These desiderata are not always compatible; and it will readily be understood that with the use of the old-fashioned large-aperture biconvex and biconcave lenses set in a trial frame not designed for their use large inaccuracies arise. The least compromise that should be accepted is the use of reduced-aperture lenses positioned as normally worn and marked according to the back vertex measurement, in a trial frame designed for their use. But even so, errors arise in the higher powers, particularly if combinations of lenses are used, and in all cases when a strength of over 5 dioptres in any meridian is involved the back vertex power of the combination should be determined and the prescription modified accordingly (p. 217).

It has been suggested that ease of manipulation may be attained and time be saved if many of the various pieces of apparatus used in the testing of vision and muscle balance were combined in a single instrument. Such an instrument is called an *optical unit*, an example of which is illustrated in Figure 21.20. The instruments supplied by

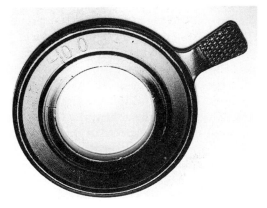

Fig. 21.17 Reduced-aperture test lens (Keeler).

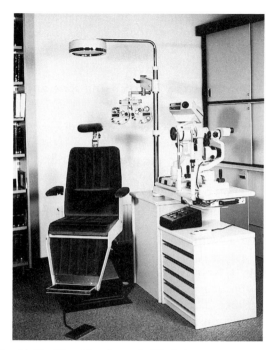

Fig. 21.20 The refracting unit (Keeler).

different makers vary, but most of them comprise a spirit level for horizontal adjustment, a lever adjustment for inter-pupillary distance, large batteries of plus and minus spherical and cylindrical lenses, multiple Maddox rods (p. 190), a Stevens phorometer (p. 192) for measuring right and left hyperphoria, esophoria and exophoria, rotary prisms for measuring prismatic deviation and for duction testing and prism exercising, a septum for use in stereoscopic work, a drum calibrated in centimetres and dioptres for reading and muscle testing at close range, cross cylinders, prisms giving a vertical separation for testing muscle balance, and complementary red and blue filters. Most modern instruments incorporate projection test-types. Sophisticated electronic controls and displays are recent developments.

Such instruments reflect more than ordinary ingenuity, and theoretically approaches the ideal. In practice, however, it is somewhat complicated for use for a simple refraction with an orthophoric patient, especially for the beginner, for in such a patient the correction should be known to within a very small margin indeed by objective retinoscopy; but there is no doubt that when

heterophoria exists or when the relationship of accommodation to convergence has gone astray, a wide range of tests can be made easily, accurately and more rapidly than if each individual test has to be performed by a separate piece of apparatus. The technique of the various tests described in the following pages applies, of course, whether they are performed separately or on such a unit.

Before commencing the retinoscopy the trial frames must be accurately centred so that the optical centre of any lens inserted into them lies upon the patient's visual axis. This can only be done roughly by mere inspection, adjusting the trial frames to the middle of the pupil; indeed, most accept this as being of adequate accuracy. However, we have noted previously that this point may not be on the visual axis and, if there is reason to suspect this, a more accurate centration may be found by inserting in the frames in front of each eye a glass with two cross-markings meeting in the centre (Fig. 21.21). The patient looks straight forward at a light in the distance, and the surgeon notes its reflection upon the cornea. The frames are then adjusted so that the cross-lines meet in the centre of the reflection.

THE PRACTICE OF RETINOSCOPY

The optical conditions in which retinoscopy is undertaken are important, particularly if a

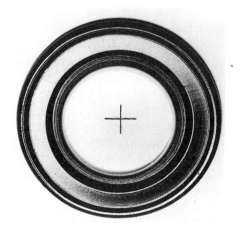

Fig. 21.21 Centring device (Keeler).

cycloplegic is not employed. The room should be long and darkened, otherwise it is impossible for the majority of patients to relax their accommodation. Where a cycloplegic is not used, it is difficult in most cases to refract the macular region itself since the pupil contracts and the view is obscured by reflexes. A *slightly* eccentric position is therefore chosen, and the patient is instructed to look past the surgeon's head on the side opposite to that which corresponds to the eye under examination. Obviously, the less eccentric the gaze the better, for it is important to get as near to the macula as possible and, essentially, the accommodation must be inactive. The best way to ensure these two desiderata is to have two small spotlights fixed to the opposite wall at least 6 metres away, at which the patient can look steadily in the appropriate direction; or, alternatively, one light exactly opposite the patient can be employed, and the surgeon can orientate himself slightly to one side or other when the opposite eye is being refracted. If no fixation lights are available the subject is asked to gaze into the distance just past the examiner's ear but as close as possible to it. In either event, in cases of squint, one or other eye should be occluded. Ideally, the examiner should use his right eye for the patient's right, his left for the patient's left so that the eccentricity is minimal. When a cycloplegic is used the patient may look directly at the retinoscope. It is customary to set the projector lens of the retinoscope so as to produce a slightly convergent beam.

The surgeon fits the trial frame on the patient's face with the trial lenses near at hand, sits at his chosen distance in front of the patient, usually at arm's length which is equivalent to a working distance of $\frac{2}{3}$ metre, and directs the light from the retinoscope into the patient's pupil. He then slowly tilts the retinoscope from one side to the other, and notes the appearance and movement of the light and shadow (Figs 21.8 and 21.9).

The principal features to be looked for are two. First, whether the movement of the reflex obtained is seen to be in a direction the same as or opposite to that of the external movement of the light across the pupil; in other words, is a 'with' or 'against' movement found? Secondly, does the plane of movement (whether with or against) parallel that of the external movement? The speed of movement of the reflex, its intensity and shape are also noted.

The power of the neutralising lens and the meridian of the astigmatism

The great majority of refractions are cases either without astigmatism or if any astigmatism is present it is regular, the principal meridians being at right angles to one another. In the former case the retinoscopy will show a neutralisation point which is the same in all meridians and what is determined is that power of lens which produces neither a 'with' nor an 'against' movement.

In astigmatism the situation is not quite so simple. The refractionist has to determine not only the neutralisation points of the major and minor meridians but also the orientation of these. The relationship of the direction of external movement to that of the reflex has an important bearing on this last matter.

The initial examinations with the retinoscope are therefore always exploratory. A start is made with vertical and horizontal movements and lenses are put up to determine a neutralisation point provided the direction of the reflexes indicates these to be the correct meridian. If the same lens neutralises both horizontal and vertical meridians, then no astigmatism is present.

If this is not so then, close to the neutralisation point, the reflex may alter its plane of movement indicating that the astigmatism present is not with its principal axis horizontal and vertical. In this case the examiner must again explore different planes of external movement of his light until they correspond to those of the retinoscopy reflexes. Neutralising lenses are now found in these new meridians, starting with the less emmetropic.

It should be emphasised that the selection of the appropriate meridian and the determination of the lens required for neutralisation are not separate manoeuvres. The two are interlinked and, as the refraction proceeds, the closer the lens interposed is to the one required for neutralisation, the easier will it be to ensure the correctness of the meridian.

Whether a 'with' or 'against' movement is

obtained initially depends on the optical power of the eye. With the surgeon at arm's length away from the patient ($\frac{2}{3}$ metre), and using a slightly convergent beam, a 'with' movement is obtained in any meridian which is hypermetropic, emmetropic or myopic less than −1.5 D. If such a movement is obtained, convex spheres of increasing strength are interposed until neutralisation, or 'reversal' as it is also known, is obtained. If an against movement is found, concave lenses are used to the same end. If neutralisation is obtained with no lens then the meridian tested is −1.5 D myopic.

Neutralisation itself is confirmed by the pupil filling with light or becoming totally dark and in such a way that it is impossible to say whether the reflex moves with or against. In practice, rather than agonising about the exact power at which this occurs, it is simplest to aim for the lens which *just* gives a 'with' movement.

The approach of neutralisation as the trial lenses are changed is heralded by an increase in the speed of movement of the reflex. Consequently if the lens tried is a long way from the one required for neutralisation, the reflex will be slow. Furthermore in very high ametropia the reflex without lenses interposed may be extremely faint and may be made recognisable only by the interposition of a strong lens.

Neutralisation can also be verified by altering the working distance. If the refractionist bends forward from a distance at which a neutralisation is obtained, a 'with' movement should be seen and conversely on increasing the working distance.

We have already noted the importance of choosing the appropriate meridian in which to move the light across the eye. If marked oblique astigmatism is present then horizontal and vertical movement of the retinoscope will produce obliquely moving reflexes and furthermore, when the external movement is adjusted to correspond to these meridians, a characteristic form of neutralisation may be seen. The illumination of the pupil assumes a band shape (Fig. 21.22) and, on tilting the mirror parallel to this band, a shadow appears coming from both edges of the pupil at once to meet in the centre, leaving the peripheral parts of the

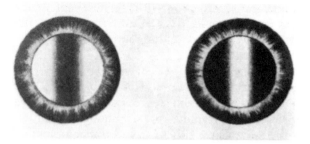

Fig. 21.22 Retinoscopy shadows in astigmatism: the band-shaped shadow.

pupil illuminated. This appearance is coincident with the exact neutralisation of the meridian corresponding to the band, the effect being due to the conversion of the retinal images into the form of lines.

To sum up, the practitioner will explore the retinoscopy reflex found by horizontal and vertical movement of the external light; from this he will note whether a 'with' or 'against' movement is present and also whether the appearance and movement indicate that he is exploring a meridian which corresponds to the patient's astigmatism if this be present. Should the latter not be the case, other meridians are explored both without and with lenses in place until it is so, and then the lenses are altered until neutralisation is found in the two principal meridians, i.e. those of greatest and least refractive power.

The value of sphero-cylindrical combinations in retinoscopy

Spherical lenses may be used throughout the examination and the final correcting lens found from the powers of the two principal meridians, the direction of the axis of the cylinder being assessed. It is more accurate (and ultimately saves time), however, if the first meridian is corrected with spherical lenses and the second with the addition of a cylindrical lens.

The strength of the combination can be further verified if the technique mentioned above is employed, wherein the examiner moves closer or further from the patient as a means of confirming neutralisation, using a sphero-cylindrical correction; the effect of such movement should be identical in each of the principal meridians if the combination is of the correct strength.

A further advantage of using sphere plus cylinder is in *verifying* the position of the axis. For this purpose the appropriate sphere and a slight undercorrecting cylinder should be put up. If the neutralising sphero-cylindrical combination is, for example, +3 D sphere and + 4.00 cylinder, a +3 D sphere and a +3.5 D cylinder should be placed in the trial frame. In this case, on rotating the mirror at right angles to the axis of the cylinder, a shadow (representing the +0.5 D of uncorrected hypermetropia) should move exactly at right angles to the axis of the cylinder. If the cylinder is not in the proper direction this shadow will not move at right angles to the cylinder, but obliquely, and the direction of its obliquity will be considerably exaggerated. If the discrepancy in the strength is 0.5 D, it can be shown mathematically that the error in direction is multiplied six times. If the cylinder is undercorrected by 1 D, a stronger shadow will be obtained, but the error in direction will only be magnified four times. It is immaterial to the test whether the cylinder is undercorrected or overcorrected: thus, in the above example, the same effect would be produced by using a cylinder of +4.5 D, but the shadow, of course, would move in the reverse direction.

Since the obliquity of the shadow multiplies any error in the direction of the axis to such an enormous extent, a very small deviation from the true axis is easily detected. The angle which the shadow makes with the axis of the cylinder can be roughly assessed and the cylinder should be rotated through an angle one-sixth of this. The test should be again repeated when any remaining error is as easily seen and corrected, until the final and correct position is attained. Such a test in practice takes very little time and is exceedingly valuable and delicate, being especially useful where, for one reason or another, the subjective verification of the axis of the cylinder by the patient is not to be relied upon, as in children.

For example, if in the above case where the correction is a +3 D sph. +4 D cyl. axis 85 degrees, a +3 D sph. + 3.5 D cyl., is put up. Suppose the surgeon wrongly estimates that the direction of the axis is 90 degrees, and he puts the cylinder vertically. On tilting the mirror in the horizontal direction, he will find that the shadow does not move horizontally, as it should, but that it runs obliquely at about 150 degrees, as indicated on the trial frame. This shows that the cylinder is not set correctly, and, since the shadow is diverted 30 degrees from the horizontal, he must rotate the cylinder through one-sixth of this angle in the corresponding direction. He must, therefore, rotate it through 5 degrees and change the axis from 90 to 85 degrees.

The calculation of the final refraction

This is obtained by deducting a dioptric value corresponding to the working distance. Thus for a working distance of $\frac{2}{3}$ metre, arm's length, we would deduct 1.5 D. Suppose that one meridian neutralises with a +4 D and the meridian at right angles with a +6 D we would consider that the patient's refractive error was +2.5 D sphere, +2 D cylinder.

As another example, suppose that one meridian neutralised at +4.50 D and the other at −1.00 D, the refractive error would be +3.00 D sphere, −5.50 D cylinder, or −2.50 D sphere and +5.50 D cylinder, with the axis of the cylinder in this last ('transposed') form being at right angles to that in the former version. In the event that the two meridians were not at right angles, it is possible to calculate trigonometrically a suitable sphero-cylindrical optical equivalent. This, however, is such a rare occurrence as to be outside the scope of this book.

The recording of retinoscopic results is usually done in the form of a cross which indicates the neutralisation point of the two main meridians and also their orientation (Fig. 21.23).

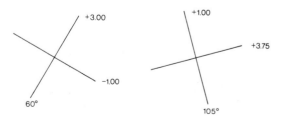

Fig. 21.23 Records of retinoscopy results. The right eye is recorded on the left half of the page and vice versa.

Streak retinoscopy

The classical source of light used in retinoscopy is circular, giving a cone-shaped beam and a circular image with spherical refractions and an elongated image in astigmatism. There are, however, considerable optical advantages to be gained from using a linear image. Such an image can be obtained from an ordinary circular light source which is made to produce a linear image by a plano-cylindrical retinoscopy mirror or a slit-shaped retinoscope or, more easily, by suitably adjusting the optical system of the electric retinoscope. With this type of illumination the refraction is done in the usual way, a band of light appearing in the pupillary aperture and moving 'with' or 'against' the band of light outside the pupil (Figs 21.24 to 21.26). The first meridian is neutralised, at which point the streak disappears and the pupil becomes completely filled with light or completely dark (Fig. 21.27). If all meridians are similarly neutralised there is no astigmatism; if a band-shaped reflex appears in any other meridian, astigmatism is present.

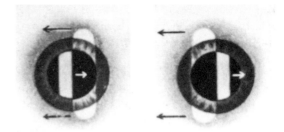

Fig. 21.26 'Against' movement.

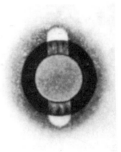

Fig. 21.27 The neutralisation point.

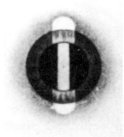

Fig. 21.24 The typical appearance of the streak.

Figs 21.24 to 21.28 Streak retinoscopy.

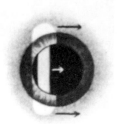
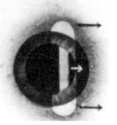

Fig. 21.25 'With' movement.

When the first meridian is neutralised, therefore, the streak is turned through 90 degrees; if it passes exactly through the axis of astigmatism, a sharply defined reflex band is seen which moves exactly parallel to the band of light outside the pupil, either 'with' or 'against'. If it does not pass exactly through the astigmatic axis, the reflex becomes more poorly defined and tends to remain fixed in the astigmatic meridian, producing a break in the alignment between the reflex in the pupil and the band outside it and tending to lie in a position intermediate between that of the latter and the true axis of astigmatism (Fig. 21.28). The axis, even in the case of low astigmatic errors, can thus be determined by rotating the streak until it moves parallel with the reflex. The astigmatic meridian is then similarly neutralised.

The great advantage of streak retinoscopy lies in the last facility; it allows the examiner to resolve quickly and more easily than with conventional illumination the problem of the orientation of the principal meridian of the refraction. For this reason it has for many

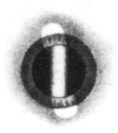

Fig. 21.28 Appearance when the streak is not in the axis of astigmatism.

refractionists superseded the other methods of retinoscopy.

Difficulties in retinoscopy

Some refractions are easy; some are extremely difficult. It is an art which requires much painstaking practice and cannot be learned in a day; and it is only after the surgeon has done many retinoscopies that he can justifiably rely on his findings with any degree of safety. It is essentially practical and cannot be learned from textbooks, but only under careful supervision. The problems usually encountered fall into two classes. In the first are those resulting from poor technique.

Inadequacies of technique

Here the results of the retinoscopy, which may itself not appear to be technically difficult, appear incorrect when related to the lenses the patient accepts when subjective examination is carried out. Such a state of affairs commonly results from the mistakes of an inexperienced refractionist. We shall therefore recapitulate several points of particular note.

It is important to keep to a definite working distance and to ensure that the retinoscopic examination is performed close to the visual axis in order to refract at the macula. In this respect not only is the horizontal orientation to be noted but also the vertical. Failure to observe this may falsely introduce or exaggerate a cylindrical element in the result.

The next matter is that of the relaxation of the subject's accommodation. It can usually be recognised that the accommodation is not being kept inactive by the fact that the retinoscopic results are changing during the course of the examination. Before recourse to cycloplegia it is worth trying several simple manoeuvres.

First, *fogging* retinoscopy can be attempted. With the trial frames in place, high plus lenses — higher, that is, than the highest presumed retinoscopic meridian of either eye — are put before both eyes. The subject is told to gaze into the distance and to make no attempt to see clearly, simply to let everything stay blurred. Replacement of the lenses in the trial frames as the retinoscopy proceeds is always done so that neither eye is ever exposed without a lens before it; in other words, the replac*ing* lens is inserted before the replac*ed* lens is removed.

A further trick in these cases is to get the subject to close then open the eyes, inspecting the reflex as the eye opens again.

If these fail, and this is particularly liable to happen in the younger subject and in those whose symptoms otherwise might be due to some irregular overactivity of accommodation, then resort is made to cycloplegia.

Cycloplegia

The advantages of a cycloplegic are these: that the accommodation is paralysed, that the pupil is dilated, and that the macular refraction can be estimated.

The use of these drugs, however, is not an unmixed blessing or without disadvantages. The eye with its accommodation paralysed is a pathological eye, and cannot be legitimately compared with the normal organ. The dilatation of the pupil considerably alters the optical properties of its refractive apparatus and intensifies the physical errors due to aberration through the peripheral parts of the refractive media. Further, the periphery of the pupillary aperture frequently has a refraction different from the central part, which is alone employed in the normal circumstances of life. Moreover, when the parasympathetic nerve is paralysed, the lens capsule is in a considerable state of tension, but when the ciliary muscle once more becomes active it allows a relaxation of the capsule, and the lens becomes more spherical. This is at its maximum in states of spasm of the ciliary muscle, but is present in some degree under the influence of its normal physiological tone.

It is excessively pedantic to insist, as some do, that the refraction should be estimated under cycloplegics in all cases below 40 or 45 years of age, that is in all cases wherein a considerable accommodative activity may be assumed to exist; and equally unnecessary to suggest that the smallest error, particularly the smallest astigmatic error, which is found in these conditions should be neutralised by correcting lenses which should be forced upon the patient even although they do not improve his vision. The question of the wholesale correction of minute astigmatic errors has been dealt with elsewhere (p. 68), but apart from the advisability or otherwise of this principle it would seem undoubted that the practice is physiologically wrong. If 0.25 dioptre of astigmatism exists under cycloplegia and mydriasis, then, when the pupil has assumed its normal dimensions and the action of the normal ciliary tone has altered the shape of the lens, it will not necessarily follow that the same 0.25 dioptre will still exist. The refraction we set out to correct is not the abnormal refraction of the eye in a pathological state, but the refraction which determines the images cast upon the retina of the patient in his everyday life.

Apart from this, cycloplegia frequently involves certain economic disadvantages. During the period of its activity near work is impossible, and this the patient may not be willing or able to put up with unless he is assured that it is essential. To some extent this is obviated by the employment of shorter acting cycloplegics. Even so, however, there is the economic disadvantage to the patient of the necessity for a further consultation if a post-cycloplegic test is thought to be necessary. We suggest below a method of getting round this difficulty in certain cases.

Further, it must always be remembered that in the routine use of mydriatics the danger of producing glaucoma in an eye with a narrow angle of the anterior chamber is by no means negligible. Before these drugs are used the possibility of such a complication should always

be excluded, and when doubt is felt a milder mydriatic than atropine should be employed and the patient kept under observation until the pupil is fully contracted by the subsequent instillation of a miotic such as 2% pilocarpine. This last is a precaution which should always be adopted in patients over 40 years of age.

It thus appears that the use of cycloplegics has definite indications and contra-indications which should be borne in mind whenever one is prompted to make use of them. Having said this, it must be stated that the age of the patient plays the most important part in the decision. Guidelines only can be given, most refractionists having their own ideas as to when and what to use.

In the young child, nothing is so effective as atropine given as 1% drops or ointment twice daily for a week or thrice daily for 4 days prior to the examination. We feel this is mandatory in all children under 7 and even older if there is any possible anomaly of the muscle balance in which accommodation may be implicated.

In some older children, however, cycloplegia may not be indicated in follow-up examinations. We have in mind here the young myope. Habitual underuse of accommodation is a feature of the condition itself. It may therefore reasonably be expected that they would be able to relax their accommodation easily, and such is indeed often the case. At the initial examination we have found it perfectly acceptable to refract the child without cycloplegia and to carry out a subjective test in confirmation of the retinoscopic findings. Elimination of the possibility of accommodative spasm causing pseudo-myopia can be made by instilling a short-acting cycloplegic such as cyclopentolate after the initial retinoscopy and subjective test. If the post-cycloplegic retinoscopy corresponds, as it usually does in a myope, to that previously performed, spectacles can be ordered on the basis of the subjective test already carried out. A further visit is thus obviated, and at follow-up examinations a cycloplegic may not be necessary.

In hypermetropia the pre-cycloplegic retinoscopy may be shown to be a considerable underestimate once cycloplegia is induced. It could however be the case that the patient will not accept even the lower hypermetropic correction indicated, the plus lenses blurring the vision both for far and for near. In such a case a careful reappraisal of the patient's complaint would be needed in relation to the relevance, if any, of the hypermetropia.

We have found 1% cyclopentolate quite acceptable as the alternative to atropine and the other longer acting cycloplegics and use it for cycloplegia at all ages where the latter are no longer required.

In older patients, certainly those over 20, the routine use of cycloplegics is to be frowned upon. They should not be employed unless there is a suspicion that the accommodation is abnormally active, unless the objective findings by retinoscopy do not agree with the patient's subjective desires, unless definite symptoms of accommodative asthenopia are present which do not seem to be explained by the error found without a cycloplegic, or unless the pupil is small and the refraction presents difficulties. It may also be advisable to use cycloplegia in cases of disputed refraction, as for example when a patient presents with several corrections none of which are subjectively satisfactory. Sometimes a mydriatic is necessary in order to obtain the refraction at the macula, for example in cases of high myopia when this region of the retina is involved in a posterior staphyloma. A mydriatic may also be indicated for ophthalmological purposes, in order to see the macula or the periphery of the fundus. It is to be remembered, however, as has been pointed out already, that the refraction under cycloplegia is pathological, and after the lens has assumed its normal shape minute errors cannot reasonably be transposed to the dioptric system in the ordinary conditions of use; a post-cycloplegic test is therefore advisable in most cases. This may never, of course, be necessary where direct ordering of spectacles from a cycloplegic retinoscopy is the usual practice, as in squinting children under atropine.

Nevertheless in the general run of cases, when the optical conditions are good and the room large, when the surgeon is an expert and is prepared to spend a little time, and when the patient is reasonably intelligent and is an adult not suffering from accommodative disturbances, the ideal refraction is undoubtedly that estimated in the absence of a cycloplegic.

Special difficulties in retinoscopy

Some difficulties are not related to faults in technique. The initial retinoscopic reflex may be too faint to be recognisable. There are two possible causes for this. The first is that the ocular media may be opaque; ophthalmoscopic examination will settle this matter. Secondly, a very high refractive error may be present and there may be some indication of this, in a follow-up examination, from any spectacles the patient already has. It might be added here that a knowledge of the lenses the patient is wearing can be a great help in deciding the suitable lens for starting the retinoscopy. In the first examination of a high ametrope, when the reflex is not recognisable, try a 7.0 lens first convex and then, if still unrecognisable, concave. If neither of these gives a recognisable reflex, proceed to even higher powers, 15 or 20 D, until in the range of a discernible reflex and proceed from there.

Some special difficulties may be mentioned. It sometimes happens that the refraction varies in different parts of the pupil, the central part being different from the periphery. Such differences, of course, are accentuated with a mydriatic. Thus spherical aberrations tend to cause an increase of brightness at the centre or the periphery of the pupillary reflex depending on whether the aberrations are negative or positive (Figs 21.29 and 21.30). These aberrations may be considerable even in the normal eye, but in pathological conditions, such as lenticular sclerosis, the difference between the two zones may be as much

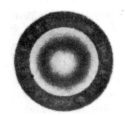

Fig. 21.29 Positive aberration.

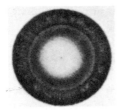

Fig. 21.30 Negative aberration.

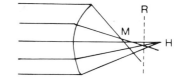

Fig. 21.33 The optics of scissor shadows wherein at the plane of observation (R), one part of the aperture is relatively myopic (M), the other relatively hypermetropic (H).

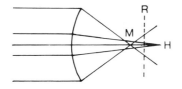

Fig. 21.31 The optics of positive aberration. Two foci are indicated, and at the plane of observation (R) the appearance in Figure 21.29 is seen wherein the peripheral zone is more myopic than the central.

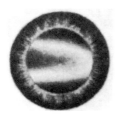

Fig. 21.32 Scissor shadows.

as 14 D. The optics of these appearances can be seen from Figure 21.31.

When a mixed aberration occurs so that one half of the reflex differs in its refractivity considerably in character from the other, two band reflexes appear which move towards and away from each other like the blades of scissors (*scissor shadows*) (Fig. 21.32). The optics of this phenomenon wherein one part of the aperture is relatively myopic and the other hypermetropic is seen in Figure 21.33. Such an appearance may present itself only in the neighbourhood of the point of reversal; it is common with corneal scarring, the blades of the scissors pointing in the direction of the cicatrix. The best way to arrive at the approximate correction in this case is to find the lens which causes the two portions to meet in the centre of the pupil, attention being

directed to the central part of the shadow to the exclusion of the periphery, for it is through this part of the pupil that vision is conducted. An irregular astigmatism or a tilting of the lens sometimes appears to give rise to the same condition.

In children retinoscopy may turn out to be of any degree of difficulty. While older children may be co-operative both looking in the distance and in a satisfactory direction without cycloplegia, in younger children cycloplegia is mandatory, and here it is advisable to ask the child to look straight at the light. Trial lenses may be put up in a trial frame or hand held; in the United States it is said that the lenses of the phoropter type machine are well tolerated by some children.

There are horses for courses, and what works well in one child may not work well in another. Very young infants are often more co-operative than those in the 18-month- to 3-year-old group. Particular difficulty may arise with a squinting eye that has lost central fixation, and as mentioned elsewhere it may be necessary to repeat the retinoscopy always under atropine, after a period of occlusion of the fixing eye. When it is felt to be of clinical importance to examine the fundi as well as the refraction in a totally unco-operative child an examination under a light general anaesthetic or heavy sedation with prior cycloplegia should be carried out.

In immature cataract very confused reflexes are often obtained. Even here, however, an experienced retinoscopist may get some rough guide to the patient's subjective requirements. It may even be the case that a neutralisation of the reflex can be obtained in only one particular meridian, the one at right angles, or indeed any other, being too abnormal. Even so this may serve as a guide to a spherical correction onto which cylinders, with their axes along this known meridian, may be superimposed in subjective testing.

In conical cornea the shadow is frequently triangular with its apex at the centre of the cone, and it appears to swirl round as the mirror is moved. In irregular astigmatism all sorts of distorted shadows may be apparent, which may move about in the most confusing manner. In such cases an approximate correction can often only be guessed, and in many greatest reliance should be placed upon subjective tests.

ALTERNATIVE METHODS FOR THE OBJECTIVE ESTIMATION OF THE REFRACTION

Ophthalmoscopy and refraction

Ophthalmoscopic examination is primarily a means of investigating the state of the fundus and of detecting opacities of the ocular media. However, it also provides incidental useful information as to the nature of the refraction, although this information is by no means exact and cannot be relied upon as a final estimation. There are two methods of ophthalmoscopy, indirect and direct.

Indirect ophthalmoscopy

The principle of the indirect method of ophthalmoscopy is to make the eye highly myopic by placing a strong convex lens in front of it. This, as we have already seen, forms a real inverted image of the fundus in the air between the lens and the observer, which can be studied. Such an image is always magnified; with a +13 D condensing lens the retina of the emmetropic eye is magnified about five times. If a stronger condensing lens is employed the image is smaller and brighter; if a weaker lens is employed the magnification is greater and the illumination less.

In classical (uniocular) indirect ophthalmoscopy the observer remains seated before the patient 1 metre away, and throws the light into his eye from the large concave mirror of the reflecting ophthalmoscope or from the electric ophthalmoscope suitably adjusted. Keeping his eye on the red reflex, he interposes the condensing lens (about +13 D) in the path of the beam of light close up to the patient's eye, and slowly moves the lens from the eye towards himself until the image of the retina is seen clearly. In order to bring the optic disc into view when the patient's left eye is being examined, he is asked to look at the surgeon's left ear, and when his right eye is being examined a convenient point of fixation is the little finger of the surgeon's right hand, which is extended as he holds the ophthalmoscope up to his right eye.

For the beginner this requires practice, and some difficulties may be encountered. One of these is the formation of reflexes by the surface observer can look between them. The first can also be eliminated by holding the condensing lens at a distance equal to its focal length from the anterior focus of the eye, that is about 9 cm away. In this case the tilting of the lens moves the corneal reflex and the image of the fundus in opposite directions so that the view is unimpaired. The tilting should not be overdone as otherwise a false astigmatic effect will be produced.

Finally, it is to be remembered that the observer must remain a metre away from the eye he is examining, for, although he seems to be looking at the pupil, he is in reality studying an image in the air between the condensing lens and himself; consequently, if he approaches too closely it will become indistinct. If he finds it difficult to maintain a distance suitable for his accommodation, he will be aided if he puts up a +1 or +2 D lens behind the mirror in the ophthalmoscope.

The illumination of the retina in indirect ophthalmoscopy is seen in Figure 21.34.

The path of the rays of light to the eye is seen in Figure 21.34. In the emmetropic eye rays coming from the fundus are parallel, and are therefore brought to a focus by the condensing lens. It will be seen from Figure 21.35 that an inverted image of the retina is therefore formed in the air at the principal focus of the lens, between it and the observer's eye. In hypermetropia the emerging rays will diverge, and they will thus appear to come from an

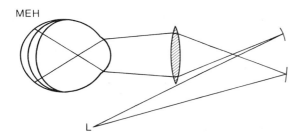

Fig. 21.34 The path of the rays of light to the eye in the indirect method of ophthalmoscopy with the concave mirror.

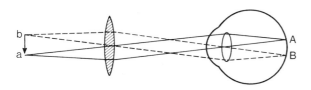

Fig. 21.35 Path of the rays of light from the eye in the indirect method of ophthalmoscopy in emmetropia.
AB, the illuminated area on the retina, gives an image, *ab*, in the air on the side of the condensing lens farthest from the eye.

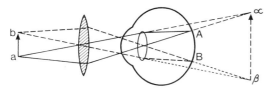

Fig. 21.36 Path of the rays of light from the eye in indirect ophthalmoscopy in hypermetropia.
AB, the illuminated area on the retina, gives an imaginary image αβ behind the eye. This is focused in a final image at *ab* by the condensing lens.

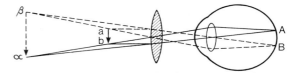

Fig. 21.37 Path of the rays of light from the eye in indirect ophthalmoscopy in myopia.
AB, the illuminated area on the retina, forms an inverted aerial image in front of the eye at αβ. The condensing lens gives a final image (*ab*) situated within its own focal length.

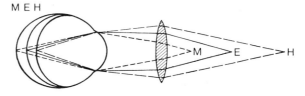

Fig. 21.38 The relative positions of the image in indirect ophthalmoscopy in emmetropia, hypermetropia, and myopia.
The lens is situated at its own focal distance from the cornea. In emmetropia the emergent rays are parallel and therefore cross at the principal focus of the lens (E). In myopia the emergent rays are convergent, and cross nearer to the lens than its principal focus, i.e. at M. In hypermetropia the emergent rays are divergent, and therefore cross farther away than the principal focus, i.e. at H.

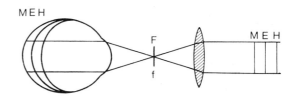

Fig. 21.39 The size of the image in different refractive states when the condensing lens is held at such a distance that its principal focus (*f*) corresponds to the anterior focus of the eye (F). The size of the image is the same in hypermetropia and myopia as in emmetropia.

imaginary enlarged upright image situated behind the eye (Fig. 21.36). The condensing lens therefore uses this as an object and forms an inverted image of it. Since the rays are divergent this final image will be situated in front of its principal focus. In the myopic eye, on the other hand, the rays coming from the fundus are convergent, and therefore an inverted image is formed in front of the eye (Fig. 21.37). The condensing lens then forms a second smaller image of this at a point within its focal length. The relative position of these images will be evident from Figure 21.38.

It follows that in the emmetropic eye, no matter what the position of the lens may be, the size of the image always remains the same and will be situated at its principal focus, because the rays issuing from such an eye are parallel. When the lens is held at such a distance that its principal focus corresponds to the anterior focus of the eye, rays parallel to the optic axis as represented in Figure 21.39 will run parallel after

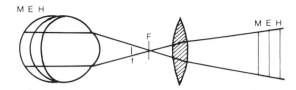

Fig. 21.40 When the principal focus of the condensing lens (*f*) is nearer than the anterior focus of the eye (F), the image of the myopic eye is smaller and that of the hypermetropic eye larger than that of the emmetropic eye.

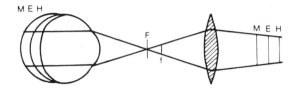

Fig. 21.41 When the principal focus of the lens (*f*) is farther away than the anterior focus of the eye (F), the image of the myopic eye is larger and that of the hypermetropic eye smaller than that of the emmetropic eye.

passing through the lens. The size of the image is therefore the same in hypermetropia and myopia as in emmetropia. If, however, the principal focus is nearer to the eye than this, such rays will leave the lens in a divergent direction. In this case it is seen from Figure 21.40 that, since the image of the myopic fundus is nearer the lens and that of the hypermetropic farther than the emmetropic, the image of the first will be smaller and that of the second larger. Conversely, when the principal focus of the lens

is farther from the eye than the anterior principal focus, these rays converge after leaving the lens, and the opposite relation will be produced (Fig. 21.41).

Consequently an idea of the refraction can be gathered from the size of the image as seen by the indirect method. When the condensing lens is held nearer to the eye than 9 cm, as is usually the case (that is, when its principal focus is nearer to the eye than the anterior focus), the image of the disc in myopia will be smaller than usual, and in hypermetropia it will be larger. In astigmatism it will be oval and will change its shape as the condensing lens is moved. When we therefore place the lens close up to the eye and slowly bring it farther away, if the image of the disc does not alter in size, the eye is emmetropic; if it decreases, the eye is hypermetropic; and if it increases, the eye is myopic.

The modern technique of binocular indirect ophthalmoscopy (Fig. 21.42) does not differ in principle but has the great advantage of 'built in' illumination and stereoscopic viewing of the retinal image.

Direct ophthalmoscopy

In this technique the image of the fundus which is obtained is much larger than that obtained in indirect ophthalmoscopy — and conversely the field of view is more restricted. Close approximation of observer and subject are

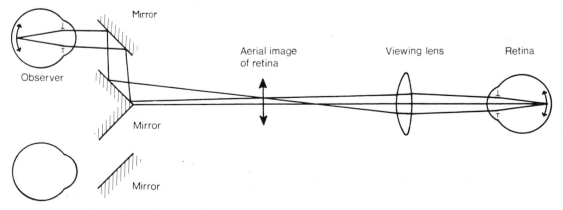

Fig. 21.42 Optics of binocular indirect ophthalmoscopy.

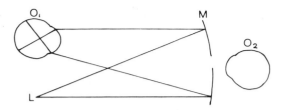

Fig. 21.43 Path of rays of light into the eye in the direct method of ophthalmoscopy.
M, the mirror of the ophthalmoscope; O₁, the patient's eye; O₂, the observer's eye; L, the source of light.

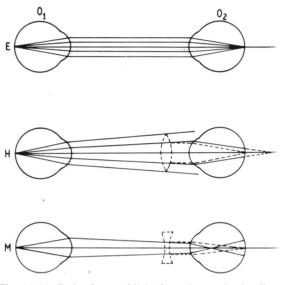

Fig. 21.44 Path of rays of light from the eye in the direct method of ophthalmoscopy.
In emmetropia (E) the emergent rays are parallel and therefore brought to a focus on the retina of the observer's eye (O₂) if he is emmetropic (or corrected) and his accommodation is at rest. In hypermetropia (H) the emergent rays are divergent, and can only be brought to a focus on the retina of O₂ by means of accommodation or a convex lens. In myopia (M) the emergent rays are convergent, and if they are to meet on the retina of O₂, they must be diverged into parallelism by a concave lens.

essential. The path of rays of light to the fundus are as seen in Figure 21.43.

Emergent rays from the fundus of the patient's eye enter the observer's eye directly. If the patient is emmetropic (Fig. 21.44, E), the issuing rays will be parallel, and will be brought to a focus on the retina of the observer. If he is hypermetropic, the emergent rays will diverge (Fig. 21.44, H), and consequently will only be

brought to a focus on the observer's retina if the latter accommodates, or by the help of a convex lens. If he is myopic, they are convergent (Fig. 21.44, M) and must be made more divergent by the interposition of a concave lens if a similar focus is to be formed. In emmetropia, therefore, the image of the retina is seen clearly without any lens in the ophthalmoscope; in ametropia, in order that the image be clearly seen, a lens corresponding to the refractive error must be used, and the strength of this lens is thus a measure of the refraction.

If this is to be correctly estimated, however, several precautions must be observed. Firstly, the accommodation of both the patient and the observer must be thoroughly relaxed, and this is not always an easy matter unless a cycloplegic is used for the patient and the surgeon is an adept at relaxing his accommodation at will. Any refractive error which the surgeon may have must be also corrected; or, failing this, his error must be known and deducted from the result obtained.

Ideally, the refraction at the macula should be estimated, but when the light is thrown upon this region the pupil contracts and the reflexes obscure the vision. The region of the optic disc is therefore usually chosen since here the sensitivity of the retina is less and in this region there are large blood vessels which form useful points upon which to focus.

When the accommodation of both parties is relaxed, and the refractive error of the surgeon is corrected, and when the mirror of the ophthalmoscope is held at the anterior focus of the eye (15.7 mm in front of the cornea), if the region of the disc is clearly seen in all directions, the eye is emmetropic. If it is not, gradually increasing convex lenses are turned in front of the observer's eye, and the strongest lens with which a clear image is obtained gives a measure of the hypermetropia. If, however, convex lenses make the blurring more marked, concave lenses are tried, and the weakest of these with which the fundus can be clearly seen gives a measure of the amount of myopia. If astigmatism exists, the lines of the blood vessels will be unequally blurred in different directions, and when spherical lenses are presented in the ophthalmoscope only those lines which are perpendicular to the meridian which is corrected are seen clearly. The lens is therefore found which makes the vessels in one meridian distinct, and then the lens which makes those at right angles to the first clear, and a combination of the two can be resolved into the sphero-cylindrical correction of the refraction.

This estimation may be made more exact by projecting a figure of radial lines onto the fundus in the beam of an electric ophthalmoscope; if some of these are blurred while others are clear, astigmatism is present, and by noting the difference in the lenses required to focus the two meridians of extreme refraction, the degree of astigmatism can be calculated.

The oval appearance of the disc in astigmatism is also apparent by the direct method, and since the image here is erect, while that in the indirect method was inverted, the long axis of the oval will be seen to run in a direction at right angles.

This method of estimating the refraction requires an immense amount of experience before it can be practised with any degree of accuracy, and even then the margin of error is always large. It is not to be recommended as a routine test on which reliance is to be placed, although it may be useful as an emergency measure when for one reason or another (for example, with a bed-ridden patient where apparatus is not available) a more efficient method is impracticable.

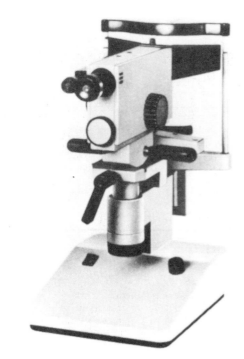

Fig. 21.45 The Rodenstock refractometer (London Williamson).

REFRACTOMETRY (OBJECTIVE OPTOMETRY)

Apart from the ophthalmoscope many special instruments have been designed which allow an observer to determine the degree of ametropia. These instruments — optometers — are based on one of two principles.

In the first, a clear retinal image of a test object is formed by an optical system and the degree of adjustment required gives a measure of the ametropia; the clarity of the retinal image is determined by ophthalmoscopic inspection. The adjustment giving maximum clarity, however, may not be easily defined. The method allows a comparison of subjective and objective findings, the observer's judgement of the clarity of the retinal image taken together with the subject's

appreciation of it. An example of this is the Rodenstock refractometer (Figs 21.45 and 21.46).

In the second group of optometers, instead of a measurable adjustment being made to the rays entering the subject's eye, the vergence of the emergent rays is primarily determined. The principle is based on the method of indirect ophthalmoscopy wherein a condensing lens in front of the eye brings the emergent rays to a focus at a convenient distance. At the principal focus of the objective lens is placed a transilluminated test object. The rays from this object are collimated by the lens, enter the pupil as a parallel beam and, if the eye is emmetropic, are focused on the retina. From this image light emerges from the pupil, again as a parallel beam, and is focused by the objective lens at the position of the test object. If the eye is myopic the emergent rays will be convergent and the image will be formed at a nearer point; if hypermetropic, the emergent rays will be divergent and the image will be formed farther away by an amount depending on the ametropia.

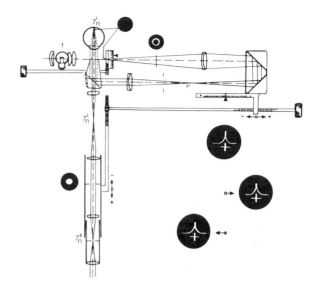

Fig. 21.46 The Rodenstock refractometer.
The principle of the refractometer depends on the uniting of two separate paths of rays. The optometric system (horizontal) projects the measuring target onto the retina; its length is altered by means of an adjustable deviating prism. The resulting image is observed through the ophthalmoscopic system (vertical). Both systems are coupled in such a way that their focusing can be continually observed through the ophthalmoscope. The control for focusing connected to a measuring scale reads off in dioptres any deviation of the eye from emmetropia in terms of vertex power of the correcting lens required to correct the ametropic condition.

Two further principles have been employed. In Henker's refractometer, displacement by parallax is the basis of the measurement, wherein the distance of the test object and that of the retinal image formed by an objective lens are compared. If the two distances are equal, the image will be superimposed on the object and will not be seen. In ametropia they are displaced to one or other side. The test object is then adjusted until coincidence is attained.

The principle of coincidence was utilised by Fincham in his coincidence optometer. In it, when the target is not in a position conjugate to the subject's retina the retinal image is displaced from the axis. The image is viewed through a system of prisms which divides the field into two; the setting is correct when the two halves are aligned.

AUTOMATED REFRACTION

Electronically automated objective optometry is now well established, and it is fair to say that the whole future of the practice of refraction will change in this direction where it has not already done so. The only serious bar to its widespread dissemination is the expense of the instruments. They are easily operated by technical staff and all now use up-to-date computer facilities, producing a printout of the refraction of both eyes within a few minutes.

One of the earliest versions of these was the Bausch & Lomb instrument of Kroll & Mohrmann, the Ophthalmetron. It uses the principle of the second group of optometers. A pair of photodetectors sense from the vergence of the emerging rays whether the movable apparatus housing them is nearer to or further from the eye than the far point. According to the position 'sensed', movement of the detector housing is automatically instigated in the appropriate direction until it is at the far point when a recording is made. The eye is scanned in numerous meridians many times and the result is given graphically.

Modern instruments produce reliable objective refraction using a variety of optical principles. Infra-red light sources are common to them all and the measurements depend on one of three optical principles: the Scheiner double pin-hole method, a retinoscopy illumination system, or a grating principle. The speed of the assessment varies between instruments being anything from 10 down to less than 1 second. The patient either fixes a target or gazes straight ahead. Most instruments will cope with refraction through contact lenses and intra-ocular lenses. Very small pupils make for difficulties, as do opacities of the media reducing vision to worse than 6/18 (20/60 or 0.3). Most instruments have some automatic method of indicating the unreliability of a result whether because of poor fixation, blinking, media opacity, etc.

The range of measurable refractive errors varies between instruments, but + or – 15 D sphere and + or – 7 D cylinder are typical. It should be remembered that these instruments do not give a visual acuity! They should be used as a preliminary to subjective verification of the refraction.

In the modern Canon Autorefractor (Fig. 21.47) the principle is again to assess the vergence of rays

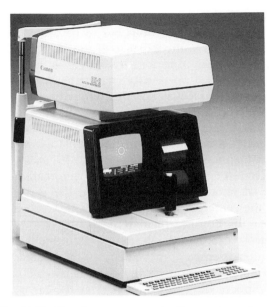

Fig. 21.47 The Canon automated refractometer and combined keratometer (Clement Clarke).

emerging from the eye. A disc with three slits in it orientated in 'Y' fashion at 120 degrees to each other is illuminated and the image of the slits is projected via the centre of an aperture mirror positioned conjugate to the subject's pupil close to the retina. The rays emerging from the illuminated slit images on the retina come out through the periphery of the pupil and then pass through three pairs of apertures in the periphery of the aperture mirror. Each pair corresponds to one slit and the rays relating to this pair are passed via a lens and prism to 3 ccds (charge coupled devices), linear image sensors which measure the distance between the beams. From these measurements the refraction can then be computed.

We must ask the question 'Is retinoscopy dying out?'. Can the newer subjective and objective optometers replace this? At present the answer is, as yet, probably 'No' in the author's view. However a situation can certainly be foreseen where economic pressure and public 'awareness' dictate that an electronic printout of anything produced by a trained technician will be considered more acceptable than a handwritten prescription. Perhaps in 20 years the advance of the electronic refractometer over the self-luminous retinoscope will be similar to that between the retinoscope itself and the candle of nineteenth century optics.

It is here pertinent to remind ourselves that even with these up-to-date devices patient alignment, relaxation of accommodation and general co-operation are just as important for accuracy as with the retinoscope.

Keratometry

This is the technique of measurement of a curvature of the anterior corneal surface. Its place in clinical refraction is predominantly in two fields, in contact lens work and in the estimation of intra-ocular lens power prior to cataract surgery. We shall discuss the various methods and instruments used (see above) in the section on contact lenses. Suffice it to note here that the keratometer is not an established method of assessing corneal astigmatism as part of routine clinical refraction. The greatest recommendation of the instrument seems to be that with its aid the estimation can be done very rapidly in the hands of an expert. The saving of time however is gained at the cost of accuracy. It is to be noted that the astigmatic error only, not the spherical one, is determined, and that of the anterior surface of the cornea alone. It is also to be remembered:

1. That the refraction of the posterior surface of the cornea is neglected. Tscherning found that this sometimes amounts to about 0.5 D of astigmatism, usually against the rule.
2. That the lenticular astigmatism is neglected; this again may amount to 0.5 D or more.
3. That the refraction of the central part of the cornea is not estimated but that of 2 points about 1.25 mm on either side, and the result may be influenced by the variability of the size of this optical zone (see Ch. 25 on contact lenses).
4. That the reading does not give the cylinder required for correcting lenses but the value of the cylinder which when placed in contact with the cornea would correct the astigmatic curvature of its surface. When the lenses are worn 13 or 15 mm away from the eye their effective value may be quite different, and significantly so if their cylindrical powers are higher.

Apart from the two very important uses mentioned above the scientific value of the keratometer is considerable but, although it gives a rough idea of the type and extent of an astigmatic error with little expenditure of trouble and time, as a clinical instrument it is both misleading and inaccurate and should never be relied upon, especially if importance is to be attached to the meticulous correction of astigmatic errors.

22. Subjective verification of the refraction, and testing of muscle balance

SUBJECTIVE VERIFICATION OF THE REFRACTION

The distant vision

In the great majority of cases the refractionist should aim at getting the vision up to the standard of 6/5, and if this is not attained he should satisfy himself that he is able to account for the visual defect ophthalmologically. It should be borne in mind, however, that this standard of acuity is usually attained only in the lower degrees of refractive error. Even in the absence of definite pathology in the media or fundus, subjects with high hypermetropia or those with marked astigmatism often do not reach this level of vision. A pin-hole test may give some indication of the best vision attainable by lenses if the condition is solely a refractive error. The standard of vision obtained with a pin-hole in a patient with opacities of the media, however, may not be attainable with lenses (see p. 145).

When the retinoscopy has been completed the test types are illuminated and the visual acuity is tested with the appropriate lenses inserted in the trial frame positioned as they are normally worn. Each eye is tested separately while an opaque disc is placed in the other compartment of the frame, and then the two are finally tested together.

The patient is asked to read the test types, and the effects of slight modifications in the lenses are tried, any small change being made which gives a marked improvement in visual acuity.

Alteration in the spheres is tried first. This can be done in various ways. Rapid changing of the spherical lens to one slightly stronger or weaker is a common method. Alternatively, a weak sphere may be held in the hand in front of the lens in the trial frame and any improvement in acuity with it is gauged. The last type of examination is made easier by having a mounted row of weak spheres (+0.25, +0.50, −0.25, −0.50) which can quickly be moved over the front of the trial lens; when the best combination is found, the strength of the sphere in the trial frame is changed, being either increased or decreased appropriately.

The verification of the cylindrical lens is not quite so straightforward. Here we have both the strength and the axis to take into account. It is usually best to check the axis first, and this can be done most simply by rotating the cylinder in steps 5 or 10 degrees in either direction and asking whether the acuity improves. Patients with lower powered cylinders may have difficulty deciding if any significant change is taking place, and here it may be helpful to change to a stronger cylinder to check the axis. When this has been settled the correct strength of the cylinder can be more definitely determined. In the lower degrees of astigmatism it is well to change the cylinder in the trial frame; in higher degrees it may be better for the examiner to hold weak cylinders in front of the trial frame; testing first with the axis parallel to that in the frame and then at right angles to it. If either of these produces an improvement, the sphero-cylindrical combination in the trial frame is adjusted appropriately.

Holding a cylindrical lens at right angles to the trial frame may sometimes necessitate a rapid application of the rules concerning the combination of lenses. Suppose first that in the trial frame we have +2 D sph. + 3.25 D cyl. axis 105°; it is found that a −0.75 D cyl. axis 15° improves the vision. We must now alter the trial

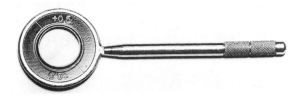

Fig. 22.1 Jackson's crossed cylinders.

frame lens to the equivalent, which is +1.25 D sph. with +4.00 D cyl. axis 105°. Alternatively, if in this case a +0.75 D cyl. axis 15° improves the vision we would alter the lenses in the frame to +2.75 D sph. with +2.50 D cyl. axis 105°.

The manoeuvres for ascertaining strength and axis of the cylinder are greatly facilitated by the use of a *crossed cylinder* (usually referred to as a cross-cylinder), a mixed cylindrical combination of various strengths in which the spherical component is one half the (opposite) power of the cylindrical with the axes at right angles (Fig. 22.1). The most convenient form is a combination of a −0.25 D sphere with a +0.5 D cylinder. To check the strength of the cylinder in the lenses, one of the two marked cylindrical axes of the cross-cylinder is first placed in the same direction as the axis of the cylinder in the trial frame and then perpendicular to it. In the first position it enhances the effect of the cylinder by 0.25 D, in the second it diminishes it by the same amount. If the visual acuity is unimproved in either of these positions, the cylinder in the trial frame is correct. If the visual acuity is improved by any of these, the change should be made unless it is specially contra-indicated, and the verification repeated with the new combination by running through the cycle again.

To check the axis of the cylinder the principles of obliquely crossed cylinders are applied. A moderately strong cross-cylinder (0.5 or 1.00 D) is held before the eye so that each axis lies alternately 45 degrees to either side of the axis of the trial cylinder. This is easily done as the cross-cylinder is always constructed so that its handle is at 45 degrees to its major and minor cylindrical axes. The examiner therefore simply holds it in front of the trial frame with its handle in the axis of the cylinder already there, testing first with one face and then twirling it through

180 degrees to assess the other position. If visual improvement is attained by one or other alternative, the correcting cylinder is turned slightly in the direction of the axis of the cylinder

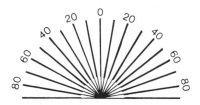

Fig. 22.2 Landolt's chart.

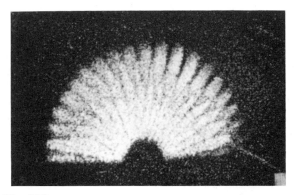

Fig. 22.3

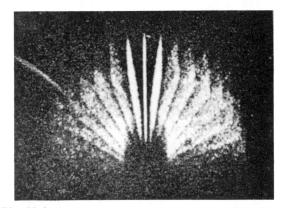

Fig. 22.4

Figs 22.3 and **22.4** The optical effect of a fan-shaped figure seen through an astigmatic lens. In Figure 22.3 the entire fan is seen equally fogged through a spherical lens. In Figure 22.4 the vertical line is most clearly defined and the others progressively ill-defined, the effect being obtained by photographing through a cylindrical lens with its axis at right angles to the sharply focused line (after Landolt).

Figs 22.2 to 22.4 The astigmatic fan.

of the same denomination in the cross-cylinder. The test is then repeated several times until the position of the trial cylinder is found at which rotation of the cross-cylinder gives no alteration in distinctness.

It is not always easy for the patient to give definite answers with the use of the test types alone, especially in cases of small degrees of astigmatism. In these the results should be confirmed by the use of some type of *astigmatic fan* (Figs 22.2 and 22.3). On looking at such a figure, if any of the lines are seen more clearly than the others, astigmatism must be present; if the vertical lines are clear, the diffusion ellipses on the retina must be vertical, that is the horizontal meridian must be more nearly emmetropic than the vertical (Fig. 22.4). A cylinder placed in front of the eye with its axis horizontal will therefore correct the vertical meridian, and when the correct glass is found all the lines will appear equally distinct. The cylinder which thus renders the outline of the whole fan equally clear is a measure of the amount of astigmatism, and the axis of the cylinder is at right angles to the line which was initially the most clearly defined.

In clinical testing a convenient pattern is the Maddox V test, or some modification of it (Fig. 22.5). It consists of a series of radiating lines arranged after the manner of the rays of a rising sun, over which the V can be rotated through 180 degrees and controlled from the part of the room where the surgeon is seated. When the cylindrical correction is removed from the trial frame and the spherical element left, the refraction in one meridian only is corrected. The line at right angles to this meridian therefore appears sharply defined and distinctly black, while the others appear blurred and grey. The V is then rotated to the neighbourhood of this line, and the exact point of maximum definition is more accurately determined by comparing the relative intensity of the oblique lines forming the limbs of the V. By rotating the V slightly in the direction of the blacker limb, an intermediate position is then reached when the two limbs appear equally distinct. This denotes the direction at right angles to the exact axis of the correcting cylinder. The points of maximum definition and maximum blurring may be more easily appreciated by observing the two discs represented below the fan on the figure, the one with lines arranged at right angles to the other, which is also rotated simultaneously with the V. If they are not equally distinct the cylinder should be slightly modified until they are. The appropriate cylinder is then inserted in the trial frame in this axis, which should correspond, or nearly so, to that already found by retinoscopy, whereupon all the lines on the chart should appear equally distinct.

As a clinical routine the test should be carried out with the patient's vision slightly fogged by an amount sufficient to overcorrect every meridian by +0.5 D, and the patient is asked to observe if any of the lines stand out more clearly than the others. If astigmatism is present he will see one of a neighbouring group of lines more sharply defined by a degree depending on the amount of the astigmatism; concave cylinders are now added, their axes lying at right angles to this until all the lines — including that at right angles to the first — are equally clear, additional convex spheres being added to maintain the fogging if necessary. In irregular astigmatism a stenopaeic slit may be placed in the trial frame and rotated into the position in which the patient sees best. This meridian is then corrected as far as possible with spherical lenses, and then the meridian at right angles is treated similarly, and the two combined in the appropriate sphero-cylindrical lens.

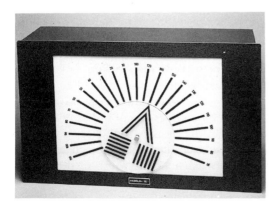

Fig. 22.5 The Maddox V test.

The duochrome test

In the verification of the correct refraction a high degree of accuracy may be obtained by making use of the phenomenon of chromatic aberration. We saw (p. 32) that the blue rays, having a short wavelength, were refracted more acutely and brought to a focus sooner than the long red waves. If the eye is corrected so that it is exactly emmetropic, a focus is formed between these two extremes; if it is myopic the red is seen more distinctly; if it is hypermetropic the blue is more sharply defined. These principles form the basis of the well-known test with cobalt blue glass, which allows only blue and red rays to pass through it; and if lines of type are employed transilluminated through two colours of glass, one red and the other blue, an alteration of one-eighth of a dioptre usually produces a change so marked as to be appreciable (duochrome test). The greatest asset of the test is its purely comparative nature, for when the two foci are presented to the eye simultaneously and are both approximately equally clear, it will not attempt to focus the one at the expense of the other; although accommodation is not abolished completely, much of the stimulus to accommodate is therefore lacking.

The test is of added value in ensuring that the two eyes are both equally corrected. The examiner usually aims in myopia, for example, to get the correction in front of each eye so that it is one-quarter dioptre 'to the red' side, a minus lens of this power added to the trial frame correction making the red and blue equally distinct. The weaker combination is ordered. Certainly in myopia a patient who reads the blue letters more easily is overcorrected. In practice most test types employ red and green illumination for the duochrome test.

The elimination of accommodation

In order to induce a relaxation of accommodation in the absence of a cycloplegic, it has long been advocated to make the eyes artificially myopic by adding convex spheres. This forms the basis of the various 'fogging' methods of the subjective estimation of the refraction. When the refraction has been measured objectively and the vision thereby determined (say 6/6, 6/6), the correcting lenses are left in place and, with both eyes uncovered, sufficient spheres (say +4 D) are added to each eye to make the acuity less than 6/60. The patient remains wearing these for some time, relaxing his accommodation by looking at the distant test objects. The strength of the added lens in one is gradually lessened by small fractions (0.5 D) until the maximum acuity is just reached; the first lens is not removed until the next is in position to prevent the accommodation from becoming active. The completely fogging lens (+4 D) is then placed in front of the first eye and the same process repeated in the second. The entire examination must be slow and leisurely, and the patient is given the strongest hypermetropic (or weakest myopic) correction with which he can attain normal vision.

Subjective testing without retinoscopic findings

In some instances it is simply impossible to obtain a satisfactory retinoscopy, usually on account of opacification of the media. Recourse here has to be to subjective testing, perhaps assessing initially the potential acuity with a pin-hole and the astigmatism with the stenopaeic slit.

Spheres are tried, and sometimes quite powerful ones may be helpful, but obviously these tests cannot be based on blind trial and error throughout the box of lenses. Some clue will be given by the nature of the visual complaint, the unaided visual acuity, the age of the patient, the spectacles previously worn, and also by the ophthalmic diagnosis. Thus a child of 12 complaining of difficulty in seeing the blackboard at school is likely to be myopic, with unaided vision of 6/18 about −1.5 D, of 6/60 about −2.5 D; a man in his 50s with previously good but now slightly impaired unaided distance vision is likely to be hypermetropic; while an elderly patient with a poor retinoscopic reflex because of cataract may benefit from a correction slightly more myopic than before.

A purely subjective technique of refraction is, of course, the diametrical opposite of that indulged in by a select few of ordering a spectacle correction on the basis of retinoscopy alone. This is unjustified save where subjective tests are impossible because of the youth of the subject, a lack of comprehension, or because spectacles are being ordered as part of the optical treatment of strabismus.

There are many other subjective tests of refraction, some applicable where recognition of letters is not required. These may be incorporated in instruments which have variable lens power and a selection of targets representing several levels of visual acuity. The result may be presented as a printout showing the refraction and the corrected visual acuity. The Humphrey vision analyser and the American optical SR IV are instruments of this type. One Dioptron instrument combines subjective and objective optometry.

The laser has provided an interesting method of subjective refraction. If a subject looks at the reflection of low-powered laser light projected onto a slowly moving surface (typically a rotating drum) a fine-grain pattern of moving speckles is perceived. Generally speaking and if no accommodation is exerted (and this may be difficult to avoid) a myope perceives the motion of this 'laser speckle' in the same direction as the movement of the drum, a hypermetrope in the opposite direction; an emmetrope sees a stationary pattern. The technique may be helpful for experimental investigation of accommodation. Its routine use perhaps for screening purposes requires relaxation of the accommodation or the subject to be focused on the drum itself while considering the motion of the speckle pattern. Either of these may be found difficult. However the method appears to be quite sensitive.

The binocular correction

When we have arrived at the final verified correction for the refraction of each eye separately, binocular vision is tested. It will usually be found that an additional +0.25 D sphere is easily tolerated and may even be an advantage. The test, however, is carried out at a distance of 6 metres instead of (theoretically) at infinity, and to allow for the small amount of error thus introduced at this distance an allowance of one-sixth of a dioptre should be deducted. The final glass therefore remains approximately the same or at most one-eighth of a dioptre only should be added. On this basis the correction for distant vision should be ordered and in all cases wherein the total refraction in any meridian exceeds 5 dioptres, the *back vertex power* of the combination at the spectacle plane

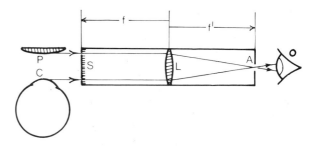

Fig. 22.6 Wessely's keratometer.
The lens (L) has a millimetre scale (S) at its first principal focus and a pin-hole aperture (A) at the second. An observer looking through the aperture reads off the distances between the patient's cornea (C) and the posterior vertex of the trial lens (P).

as determined by a focimeter (p. 217) should be ordered.

For this purpose the distance between the posterior lens in the trial frame and the cornea should be measured (the *back vertex distance*). For such a measurement several methods are available, none of which is of extreme accuracy but most of which serve the purpose. In the first place, the trial frames may be provided with a screw or a millimetre scale on the side-arm, pointing towards the temple, enabling a sight to be taken at the level of the apex of the cornea as judged visually. More elaborate instruments are the Zeiss parallax vertexometer, the Wessely 'keratometer' (Fig. 22.6), and Belgard's lenscorometer; but a useful and simple method is to insert into the cell occupied by the lens a disc with a stenopaeic slit through which a millimeter rule is passed until it touches the closed upper lid. In this measurement, of course, a correction factor must be added to allow for the thickness of the lid. Various exophthalmometers have also been used for this purpose.

The ordering of spectacles for distance

The principles underlying the final choice of lenses have already been discussed in the appropriate chapters of this book. Other things being equal, it is usually indicated that the fullest correction consistent with good vision should be ordered, and especially is this necessary when the error is small and the symptoms are those of eye-strain rather than of defective vision. It will be remembered that in very high degrees of ametropia, especially of myopia, the full correction may not be tolerated, and an undercorrection is usually necessary. The more so is this necessary (and in this case it applies also, but to less extent, to hypermetropia) in cases wherein the patient does not propose to use the spectacles constantly.

When a mydriatic has been used, a deduction must be made to allow for the normal tone of the ciliary muscle, which has been temporarily abolished (see p. 168). In most cases, especially when the error is large, it is well to have a subsequent post-cycloplegic test after the effect of the drug has passed off. In any event, this will be necessary after the presbyopic age has been reached, unless an arbitrary glass is ordered for reading — an unsatisfactory and dangerous proceeding.

THE DETERMINATION OF THE ACCOMMODATION AND THE TESTS FOR NEAR VISION

When the lenses for distance have been determined in the manner already described, attention is turned to the near vision. As an initial step the trial frames should be tilted to the appropriate angle for reading and the centring should be altered to allow for the convergence of the eyes. This latter can most easily be done by holding a light at the working distance with the centring lenses in the trial frame (see Fig. 21.20), and adjusting the latter so that the cross-wires meet in the centre of the reflection of the light on the corneae.

During these tests the full correction for distant vision should be retained in the trial frame: they form a measure of the far point. The near point is then determined.

The determination of the near point of accommodation

This may be done in a rough, but fairly efficient, manner by asking the patient to bring the reading test types close up to his eyes until the smallest print appears blurred. With print, however, it is difficult to differentiate between blurring, which marks the near point of accommodation, and

diplopia, which marks the near point of convergence. A more accurate method, which involves little additional time, is to use the *accommodation card* of Duane. This is a white card (such as a visiting card) upon which a black vertical line, 0.2 mm thick and 3.0 mm long, is drawn. It is brought up to the eye until it appears blurred.

In young subjects, in whom the accommodation is very active, a -3 D or -4 D sphere should be added to the distance correction in order to carry the near point a convenient distance away, and in presbyopes plus lenses should be added to bring it within measurable distance. These, of course, have to be added to, or deducted from, the final value. The distance at which the object appears blurred is then measured from the point at which spectacles are to be fitted, usually about 14 mm in front of the cornea. The distance is measured in centimetres or more conveniently, by means of a Prince rule, in dioptres. If it is measured in centimetres, the dioptric value of the reading on the rule is the reciprocal of the length expressed in metres: thus a distance of 25 cm represents 100/25, or 4 dioptres.

The distance is measured by a tape held at the outer canthus of the eye; looking from the side, the surgeon estimates the level of the anterior summit of the cornea and, deducting this distance plus 14 mm from the total measurement to the accommodation card, he obtains the measurement to the near point. Duane introduced a very useful *accommodation rule* to act as a measure. It is a modification of Prince's rule, and consists of a straight wooden ruler placed between the eyes with a groove cut at the end to fit the bridge of the nose. It is calibrated along the top and down the sides to serve binocular and uniocular measurements, and is marked in centimetres to register the near point, and in dioptres to register the amplitude of accommodation, the scale commencing at a distance of 14 mm in front of the cornea. As the accommodation card is approximated to the eye its distance can be read off in centimetres, and translated simultaneously into dioptres of accommodative power.

All these tests can be done with greater rapidity and ease with the refracting unit described on page 163.

The near point should be measured with each eye singly while the other is occluded by an opaque disc; then both eyes should be uncovered and the binocular accommodation estimated, the patient being asked at the same time to converge. The binocular result is usually about 0.5 D greater.

The determination of the near point of convergence

This may again be measured with the accommodation card. When the near point of convergence is reached the line appears double. The near point of convergence may be reached simultaneously with the near point of accommodation when the doubling and the blurring appear together; it may be reached first, in which case the image becomes double while yet clearly outlined; or it may be the nearer of the two to the eye, when the line becomes blurred and subsequently doubled. In any case the patient should be instructed to differentiate between the two phenomena. The surgeon can verify the observation by watching for the point at which one eye begins to deviate outwards.

The *relative* accommodation and convergence may now be investigated at the working distance, that is the amount of accommodation or convergence which can be additionally exerted or relaxed by the one function while the other remains constant. The amount of accommodation which can be thus relaxed while the patient still fixes (the negative relative accommodation) is determined by adding further plus lenses until the object becomes blurred. The positive relative accommodation (that is, the amount by which accommodation can be augmented) is similarly found by adding concave lenses to the normal reading correction. Similarly with convergence, while the patient fixes the near object, prisms are placed in front of the correcting lenses. The strongest prism, base out, which can be tolerated without producing diplopia measures the positive portion, and the strongest prism, base in, measures the negative portion of the relative convergence.

Dynamic retinoscopy

An attempt has been made to give these measurements objective accuracy by the method of dynamic retinoscopy. Here the retinoscopy is done with the patient's eyes fixed at a near distance instead of at infinity (as in 'static' retinoscopy) so that an estimate of the refraction is made while the patient is actively accommodating and converging. A self-luminous retinoscope is used projecting a slightly diverging beam of light or, alternatively, light is reflected into the eye from a plane mirror, and while it is held at the working distance the patient fixes and focuses upon a target carried in front of the instrument as the retinoscopy is done: the most effective target is probably the patient's finger held by the examiner since it is easy to fix and accommodate upon it. When the static refraction has been determined and while the correcting lenses are before the eye, the patient focuses the target binocularly; this is brought nearer and nearer to his eye until the band of light and shadow in his pupil is reversed, despite his strongest effort of accommodation for the distance of the target. The surgeon then moves closer to the patient until the reversed movement stops; this may be considered the neutral position and measures the near point of accommodation; for example, if it occurs at 0.33 metre from the eye, the total accommodation is 3 D. If the retinoscopy is done without the correcting lenses in place, the position of reversal marks the near point of accommodation.

The refraction is then measured with the retinoscope and the target maintained at the working distance (say 33 cm); the patient wears his distance correction, both eyes are uncovered and he is asked to fix and focus the target. With a plane mirror and a patient with considerable accommodative power, a 'with' movement is obtained when a plane mirror is employed. This is neutralised with the addition of convex lenses to the trial frame (+0.5 or +0.75 D are usually required) thus giving the 'low neutral point'. Further convex lenses are then added but no rapid reversal of the shadow is obtained as occurs in static retinoscopy; as accommodation gradually relaxes a wide 'neutral zone' is traversed until eventually the shadow is reversed marking the 'high neutral point'. It is generally agreed that the high neutral point represents an objective finding of the negative relative accommodation, that is the amount of accommodation which can be relaxed while convergence remains fixed. The strength of the lenses at this point — that is the highest convex lenses that give neutrality of shadow — is generally stated to indicate the point of association between convergence and accommodation which brings about a comfortable adjustment between them; in actual practice the lenses will generally be found to be somewhat strong for comfort. Our knowledge of the problems raised in this way, however, is not yet quite sufficient to allow dogmatic conclusions to be drawn from the results or to assess their real use. The method is of distinct value, however, in that, just as static retinoscopy gives an objective basis for the appropriate correction for distant vision, dynamic retinoscopy provides an objective basis for the optical condition when the eye is focused for near vision, a matter which had hitherto been left entirely to subjective testing.

The determination of spectacles for near work

We have seen that the accommodation varies with age. We have also seen that if comfort is to be maintained a certain amount of accommodative power must be kept in reserve, so that special lenses are required for near work whenever the near point approaches the distance at which the work is habitually done. When the patient's symptoms indicate that such a course is necessary, the near point is determined with the distance correction still in place. He is then given the reading test types and asked to hold them at the distance at which he is accustomed to work or read. When they are not distinctly seen, appropriate convex lenses should be added to the distance correction so that the near point is brought within the working distance, and the types are easily and comfortably read.

The decision to proceed to formal measurements of the patient's power of accommodation and convergence will be taken on the basis of the symptoms. If, for example, the history appears to indicate the case to be one of simple presbyopia, then these tests are usually unnecessary and all that is required is that the patient should attempt to read the near vision test types first with the distance correction and after that with appropriate additions of convex spheres until a standard of vision is obtained allowing the patient to carry out whatever tasks he requires at his usual working distance.

Where particular reading difficulties seem to be the complaint in subjects whose accommodation might be expected to be undiminished by presbyopia, the more extensive near vision examinations should be performed. They have already been described in detail on page 186. The amplitude of accommodation is obtained by subtracting the dioptric value of the far point from that of the near point; one-third of this is

kept in reserve, and lenses are added to give the necessary amplitude.

Presbyopic spectacles should never be prescribed mechanically by ordering an approximate addition varying with the age of the patient. Each patient should be tested individually, for the individual variation is large, and those lenses should be ordered in each case which give the most serviceable and comfortable, not necessarily the clearest, vision for the particular work for which the lenses are intended. In all cases it is better to undercorrect than to overcorrect since, if the lenses tend to be too strong, difficulties will be experienced with convergence, and the range of vision will be correspondingly limited. In any case a lens which brings the near point closer than 28 cm is rarely well borne (that is, a total power of 3.5 D), and if for any reason the demands of fine work require a higher correction it is usually wise to aid the convergence with prisms as well as the accommodation with spheres.

Chalmers and Percival have pointed out that if the same spectacles are to be used by a non-presbyope for distance and near work, an error is introduced owing to the fact that in the first case the incident rays of light are parallel, while in the second they are divergent. In order that the latter may be converged to the same focus so that they fall upon the retina, a stronger correction is required than is indicated by the refraction.

The practical importance of this lies in cases of high cylindrical corrections; for in many of these, if the same lenses are used for reading as for distant vision, the result is unsatisfactory. Thus if a +5.0 D cylinder is required for distance, a +5.5 D cylinder is required for near work. To secure adequate centring, we shall see later (p. 219) that a special pair of reading spectacles is usually advisable when the astigmatic error is high, even in non-presbyopes, and the opportunity should be taken of incorporating this correction in these.

Mention has already been made of the slight amount of cyclophoric extorsion which usually occurs when the eyes are converged (see p. 121). A slight rotation of a high cylinder, particularly if it is oblique, can be made in the reading lenses in order to neutralise this, thus adding considerably to the comfort of the patient, as well as increasing his visual acuity for close work.

If near work with the reading spectacles is still giving rise to trouble which cannot obviously be explained, this is a situation in which the relative accommodation and convergence for the working distance must be estimated. It is to be remembered that the positive portion of the relative accommodation (that is, the amount in reverse) must be as large as possible, certainly larger than the negative portion. Similarly, the positive portion of the relative convergence should also be large. If the relative accommodation is deficient the spherical addition for the working spectacles should be altered; if the patient is working outside the 'area of comfort' of his convergence, orthoptic exercises should be prescribed or a prismatic correction should be ordered which brings his convergence within it.

Presbyopia is one of those conditions wherein a monocle or a lorgnette may be of real service: on the many little occasions in everyday life — when out shopping, looking at a ticket, or consulting a time-table — when taking out a pair of spectacles and putting them on for a moment become irksome, the more easily manipulated monocle may save much time and not a little annoyance. This, of course, applies to short periods only; if persisted in, the enforced uniocularity of the monocle may introduce strains of another kind.

THE DETERMINATION OF THE MUSCLE BALANCE

The next step in the examination is to test the state of the balance of the ocular muscles.

To investigate this thoroughly can be a complex and prolonged matter but for the refractionist a simplified examination will be sufficient. It usually consists of three basic examinations, the inspection of the corneal reflections; the cover test and the assessment of the ocular movements.

The *corneal reflections* are inspected as the patient looks directly at a light held by the observer immediately in front of him. The pin-point images of the light as reflected by the two corneae are compared with respect to their position in relation to the pupil and to the cornea as a whole.

The *cover test* is carried out on the basis of the corneal reflections. If the latter suggest that one eye, say the left, is deviating, the patient continues to fix a near or distant object and the right eye is covered by the hand or by a card. If the left eye is deviating and if its vision is adequate it will move to take up fixation, indicating a manifest strabismus. On removing the card, if the left eye remains fixing and the right stays in the deviated position, the squint has an alternating character. If, however, on removing the card the left eye returns to its former position and the right resumes fixation, a left (uniocular) manifest strabismus is present. If on covering either eye the other does not deviate, a manifest squint is absent. In this event the cover test should be similarly repeated but the behaviour of the covered eye is observed when the cover is removed. It may be found to have deviated while covered and to return to its fixing position on uncovering, while the other eye keeps its fixation and moves on neither covering nor uncovering. In this instance, a latent strabismus is present. If no movement of either eye occurs, any deviation that appears to exist is an apparent squint (pseudo-strabismus).

This method of performing the cover test — the method of binocular uncovering — may not always elicit a latent strabismus (heterophoria). The examiner should then proceed to the *alternate cover test* — the method of uniocular uncovering. Here each eye is covered in turn, the behaviour of each on uncovering is noted and finally both are uncovered. Attention should be paid to the speed of recovery to the binocular state. Even this may fail to break down the patient's binocular vision and it may be supplemented by making the patient follow a light in several directions with one eye, the other being covered, before proceeding to the alternate covering.

The examination of the ocular movements should be carried out in all the principal positions of the gaze and may be supplemented by the performance of the cover test in these positions. Any defective movement or complaint of diplopia should be noted. This test is crucial in differentiating concomitant from paralytic squint. In the former no defect of ocular movement is found.

Of particular importance is the examination of convergence since an absolute or relative weakness of this function can be a potent cause of the symptoms of eye-strain. The aetiology of this condition and its treatment is discussed elsewhere, but it is always to be remembered that convergence and accommodation are interconnected and weakness of one should direct attention to the other.

In very young children the last two tests may be found impossible. But even an infant will fixate a light reflexly. If the reflection occupies the centres of both corneae, it is unlikely that a squint is present. It is to be remembered, of course, that very young infants in whom binocular fixation has not yet developed exercise little or no co-ordinated control over the movements of their eyes. Before the age of 6 weeks and sometimes later, the eyes often deviate independently of each other.

We can now divide the patients into two categories — those in whom binocular fixation exists, and those in whom it does not. Those in the first class are to be subjected to finer tests to discover the presence of muscular imbalance or latent squint; those in the second should have the nature and degree of their true squint investigated, a matter outside the scope of the refractionist as such.

The investigation of heterophoria

The tests which have been suggested to investigate heterophoria are legion. They all depend upon the same principle — that of dissociating the images in the two eyes so that the stimulus for binocular vision is removed and the eyes take up the position of rest. This can be done in many ways; but the easiest, most accurate, and most generally applicable test is that of the Maddox rod.

The original Maddox rod consisted of several red cylinders of glass placed side by side in a frame. The same optical effect is produced by glass bevelled to the same general configuration, so that it acts as parallel rows of double prisms — known correctly as the Maddox groove (Fig. 22.7), but most Maddox 'rods' are of this form. When a spot of light is looked at through it, an image is formed as a focal line running perpendicular to their axes. The spot thus appears as a long red line running

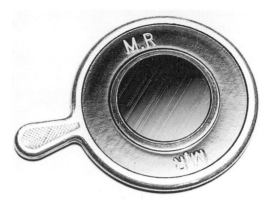

Fig. 22.7 The Maddox groove (Keeler).

perpendicularly to the direction of the cylinders. It is evident that this red line will appear completely different from a white spot of light, and so when they are seen simultaneously by both eyes there is no stimulus for fusion.

To test the muscle balance for distant vision the patient remains seated in the chair still wearing his correcting lenses, and it is essential, of course, that the centring of these be exact. A small point of light is situated 6 metres off: it is usually possible to incorporate this in the box test types. The Maddox rod is then placed in the right cell of the trial frame with the cylinders running in the horizontal direction, and the patient is asked to look at the light and say whether the red line is running through it or to one or other side.

If there is orthophoria in the horizontal direction the red line will run through the light (Fig. 22.8, B); if exophoria is present the line will be to the left of the light (Fig. 22.9, A); if esophoria, to the right (Fig. 22.9, B). The amount of deviation is then measured on a 'tangent scale' (Fig. 22.11) which registers the deviation directly; or it is estimated by placing prisms in the other cell of the trial frame with their bases in or out, until the line is made to run through the light. The Maddox rod is then rotated at right angles, when a horizontal line is seen. If this runs through the light, there is no hyperphoria (Fig. 22.8, A); if the red line appears below the light there is right hyperphoria (Fig. 22.10, A); if above, there is left hyperphoria (Fig. 22.10, B). The deviation is again measured

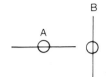

Fig. 22.8 (A) Orthophoria in the vertical direction; (B) orthophoria in the horizontal direction.

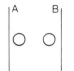

Fig. 22.9 (A) Exophoria; (B) esophoria.

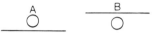

Fig. 22.10 (A) Right hyperphoria; (B) left hyperphoria.

Figs 22.8 to **22.10** The Maddox rod test for heterophoria. Relative positions of the point of light and the red line when the Maddox rod is in front of the right eye.

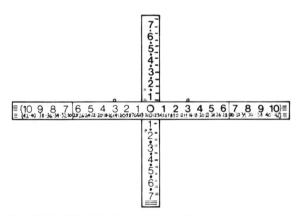

Fig. 22.11 The Maddox tangent scale.

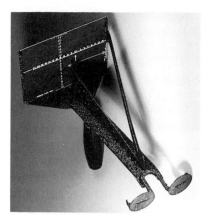

Fig. 22.12 The Maddox wing test (Keeler).

on the tangent scale or by neutralisation by prisms until the line runs through the centre of the light: in all cases, since prisms displace objects in the direction of their apices, the prism placed in front of any eye must have its apex pointing in the direction of the displacement of the red streak. If cyclophoria is present, when the Maddox rod is vertical, the red line instead of running horizontally will run obliquely; and the number of degrees through which the rod has to be tilted in order to make the line of light appear horizontal gives some indication of the amount of torsion.

The *muscle balance of near vision* must now be tested, and here again the patient wears his correcting lenses, this time, of course, with the addition for near vision. For this purpose many tests are available, but one of the best is the Maddox wing test (Fig. 22.12), which acts by separating the visual fields presented to each eye by a diaphragm and thus dissociating them. With it every type of heterophoria is investigated at a distance of one-third of a metre.

When the patient looks through the two slit-holes in the eyepieces of the instrument, the fields which are exposed to each eye are separated by a diaphragm in such a way that they glide tangentially into each other. The right eye sees a white arrow pointing vertically upwards and a red arrow pointing horizontally to the left. The left eye sees a horizontal row of figures in white and a vertical row in red; these are calibrated to read in degrees of deviation. The white arrow pointing to the horizontal row of figures and the red arrow pointing to the vertical row should both be at zero; any deviation indicates an eso- or exophoria or a hyperphoria, the amount of which can be read off on the scale.

Finally, the strength of the muscles should be estimated by forcing them to act against prisms to the limit of their power. The converging power varies very much, and with practice can be raised to the neighbourhood of 50 Δ or more; if it falls below 20 Δ, it may be taken to be definitely insufficient. The diverging power should be 4 to 5 Δ, and the normal limits of super- and subduction are from 1.5 to 2.5 Δ. Their *vergence power* (see p. 118) is thus found by placing gradually increasing prisms in front of the eye in various directions until diplopia is produced. The test should be carried out with the patient wearing his full correction. He should fix a point of light at 6 metres distance and indicate at once when it appears double.

The test is most easily done by an apparatus in which two prisms can be rotated in unison. When they are lying apex to base the combination becomes a glass plate and the prismatic effect is *nil*; when they are lying with their two bases in corresponding positions the total effect is equal to double the effect of one; and each intermediate position has an intermediate prismatic value. The deviations can be calibrated on a scale both for horizontal and vertical displacements.

Among the many other instruments which can be used for these measurements mention should be made of the Stevens phorometer. It consists of two rotating cells, each carrying a prism of 10 Δ which rotate in unison under the control of a gear-wheel, and a scale measures the strength of the refracting angle used. The whole is set on a levelling arm, and through it the patient looks at a light or a cross-line chart. When the instrument is set so that the prisms are base down before one eye and base up before the other, two images are seen on the same vertical line if there is no heterophoria; the absence of alignment indicates esophoria or exophoria, which can be measured by increasing the prismatic effect in the direction of base out for esophoria and base in for exophoria. Similarly for measuring hyperphoria the prisms are rotated so that a horizontal displacement is created by setting the prisms base in before both eyes. If one image is higher than the other the prisms are rotated until the images are made level, the pointer indicating on the scale the amount of manifest hyperphoria. The same test can, of course, be made for distant and for near vision.

The phorometer, rotary prisms, and the Maddox rods can all be combined in one instrument (Fig. 22.13); or as we have already seen, practically the entire outfit of visual testing can be condensed together in a refracting unit (p. 163), which makes these tests easier and more rapid of accomplishment. Alternatively, the deviations of muscular imbalance can be rapidly and accurately measured on the more complicated types of amblyoscope such as the orthoptoscope.

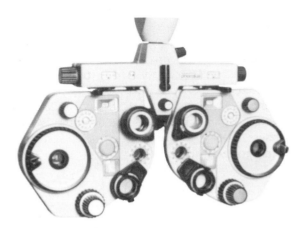

Fig. 22.13 The phorometer (Rodenstock).

By means of these tests we can thus discover the state of the muscle balance for distant vision and for near vision and at the same time we can get some information as to the nature of the deficiency. In exophoria, if the defect is greater for distant than for near vision, we refer to the deviation as the divergence excess type; if it is greater for near than for distant vision by an amount greater than the physiological exophoria (3 Δ to 5 Δ) to be expected at reading distance, it is known as the convergence deficiency type. Equivalent types are found in esophoria. The extent of the anomaly is indicated by the results of the test of the verging power.

The indications for the treatment of muscular imbalance have already been outlined (see p. 122). It may be well to repeat here that moderate hyperphoria, when giving rise to symptoms, can always be corrected in full. Greater hesitation, however, should be felt in correcting a horizontal deviation. The refraction should always be corrected and, if present, any vertical error as well; the horizontal error then frequently rights itself if the general health receives attention. In esophoria the hypermetropia is fully corrected, and the more the element of convergence excess enters into the case the greater should be the correction. In exophoria the tendency should be to undercorrect hypermetropia or fully correct myopia, and when convergence insufficiency is present the reading addition should be as weak as possible. Failure to observe this recommendation accounts for much discomfort.

Prisms, when they are ordered, should always tend to undercorrect by a half in horizontal deviations, and they should be designed to meet the case at the distance for which the glasses are to be used. In the final correction any prismatic correction is usually split between the individual correction of the two eyes so as to minimise the thickness of the lens which would result if it were all incorporated on one side.

SUMMARY OF CLINICAL METHODS

The description of clinical methods in this section may give the impression that the adequate examination and correction of the vision is a lengthy and complicated proceeding. On the contrary, it is not. Most of the tests take much longer to describe than to carry out in practice; and when practice becomes a routine, and long custom makes their execution automatic and their interpretation instantaneous, they can be performed surprisingly rapidly and at the same time accurately.

The following routine of refraction is suggested, since it saves the maximum amount of time and entails the minimum of movement. After the history has been taken, the patient should be seated in a large room which can be darkened and he need never be required to move; most patients move slowly. The following steps should then be gone through:

1. External examination in diffuse light.
2. Examination of the motility of the eyes.
3. The cover test to elicit heterophoria and squint. This is best done at this stage, before the trial frames are put on. It saves their subsequent removal and, in addition, the detection of a squint may account for a marked deficiency of vision in the deviating eye, which, if it is not recognised early in the examination, may give rise to some concern. The trial frames are then put on and centred.

4. The testing of visual acuity, uniocularly and binocularly, both with and without any correction, for near and distance.
5. The retinoscopy, and its verification with the sphero-cylindrical combination.
6. The subjective verification of the retinoscopy with the test types and then with the astigmatic fan.
7. The correction of minutiae with the cross-cylinders and the astigmatic fan, supplemented, if desired, by a 'red–blue' (duochrome) test.
8. With the full correction in place, the testing of the muscular balance for distant vision.
9. With the full correction in place, the determination of the near point of accommodation and convergence.
10. The addition of the correction for near work, and the testing of the acuity with the near types, uniocularly and binocularly.
11. With the additional correction for near work, the estimation of the muscle balance for near vision.
12. The trial frames are taken off and, if it is indicated by the symptoms complained of and the results of 8, 9, 10 and 11, the testing of the vergence power.

The position which this routine should occupy in relation to the complete general examination of the eyes is a matter of individual choice. Some prefer to refract the patient at the outset, others will wish to examine first the anterior segments and fundi.

Many will adopt a flexible routine and, indeed, the circumstances of the case may make this necessary. The precise necessity for steps 8 onwards will be determined by the patient's age and precise clinical complaint. Thus the early performance of the refraction may show that the retinoscopy reflex is poor or unobtainable pointing to an immediate examination of the clarity of the media.

23. The prescription of spectacles

The final part of the clinical routine is often to give the patient a prescription for spectacles, and the last remarks in this section are intended to round off the discussion of the indications for this.

THE PRESENTING SYMPTOMS

The prescription of spectacles should be correlated with the patient's symptoms. Where there is an obvious refractive error associated with a visual defect, the indication to order spectacles is clear; apart from such an obvious indication, however, there is a whole range of less definite complaints in which the decision may be made in the realisation that the ametropia discovered is of a degree that is unlikely to be the sole cause of the trouble. We have mentioned elsewhere the effects of spectacles as a placebo; such mild psychotherapy should, however, be cautiously undertaken lest the ocular symptomatology is merely the most obvious feature of a more profound mental or physical disturbance. Nevertheless, even in these cases the prescription of spectacles, while it may not be beneficial, does no mental or physical harm. In children, however, the prescription of spectacles for slight degrees of hypermetropia or astigmatism is to be avoided: so often a child complains of defective vision out of the desire to wear spectacles when a classmate has recently acquired them. If a minimal or non-existent refractive error is found in association with normal fundi and media, all that is required in such cases is a tactful word of explanation to the parents and a reassessment of the case in, perhaps, 3 months.

Many refractions are carried out on patients who already have spectacles but merely come for a routine check-up without symptoms and in deference to the prevailing myth that 'neglecting the eyes' or wearing wrong spectacles does harm. It must be admitted that in many cases this is unnecessary; indeed, while there may be a place for pre-symptomatic diagnosis in ocular conditions such as glaucoma, such an attitude regarding these routine assessments of optical errors is without doubt grossly inflated. Apart from the established facts concerning age changes in the refractive state, the refraction of children, adolescent myopes and hypermetropes clearly needs reviewing at intervals and it may be advisable not only to suggest re-examination in 6 months or a year but also in certain cases to indicate the likely future progression of the condition; this will forestall the frequent complaint that spectacles have 'made the eyes worse' or made the patient dependent on them.

Most subjects between the ages of 20 and 40, however, have static refractions. When a patient in this age group requires a new pair of spectacles, his present pair being in poor physical condition with the lenses scratched and the frame-joints loose or broken, it is reasonable to check that the refraction is indeed static; otherwise re-examination is likely to be superfluous at this time of life unless the optical anomaly is severe.

If a slight change in refraction is found at a routine re-examination, the examiner must be chary of invariably altering the correction, and it is good practice to make a comparison between what it is proposed to prescribe and the patient's existing spectacles. Frequently for all one's efforts the patients will notice little difference or even

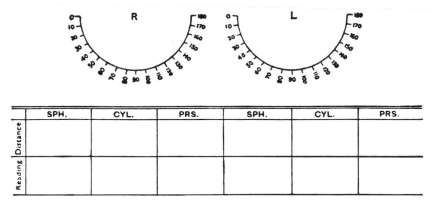

Fig. 23.1

prefer their own correction. Minor changes in refraction in the absence of symptoms can well be ignored, particularly small alterations in the axis of a cylindrical correction, or the introduction of a small cylinder where none was previously present; otherwise the result may well be the development of symptoms which were not present with the old prescription and the claim by the patient that he sees better with his old spectacles — a circumstance entailing considerable chagrin to the examiner. Even if the patient has ocular or visual complaints, the finding that his present spectacles are in some marginal degree incorrect should not always be taken as an indication to alter them, and in all cases the question should be asked whether the symptoms can reasonably be related to the change in refraction. The importance of a knowledge of the correction the patient is wearing is obvious, being of value not only in assessing the necessity for any alteration but also facilitating the examination of the refraction.

A standard type of prescription is shown in Figure 23.1. All prescriptions will indicate sphere power, cylinder power and axis and if required prism power and orientation. Some general further indication is usually necessary in relation perhaps to the type of reading addition, the form of lenses, tint, coatings, etc. As with retinoscopy results the correction for the right eye is conveniently placed on the left side of the page and vice versa.

The measurement of inter-pupillary distance, frame size, nose bridge, etc. is usually not noted by the prescriber, such features being left to the Dispenser.

Optical appliances

24. The making and fitting of spectacles

Not only is some knowledge of the processes employed in the making and fitting of spectacles of interest from the ophthalmologist's point of view, it is also of the utmost importance, for many points arise in this connection which it is necessary for him to understand. The craft of the optician is a highly skilled one, by no means without its difficulties, and the surgeon can frequently help in overcoming these. The services of both are required in the optical treatment of the patient, the one no less essential than the other, and they should have the mutual knowledge to co-operate for the comfort of the patient depends upon both.

THE MANUFACTURE OF SPECTACLES

Spectacle lenses

Spectacle lenses are now usually made of crown glass; the old-fashioned 'pebbles' of quartz, which had the advantage of being hard and scratched only with difficulty, have fallen into disuse largely because of their greater expense and their peculiar polarising properties. The glass commonly employed is a hard crown glass of refractive index 1.523, which after annealing has a high degree of transparency. Sometimes, when a glass of a higher refractive index is wanted, as in the making of bifocal or achromatic lenses, special types of crown glass or flint glass are used. (See Appendix I, Table 1.) The disadvantage of higher refractive index materials is their propensity to produce chromatism, coloured fringes to objects viewed eccentrically.

The selected glass, after annealing, is made into rough 'blanks', which are slabs of approximately the required thickness. These are subjected to grinding, a process by which the surfaces are shaped by electrically driven tools of finely grained cast iron of appropriate curvature, the necessary abrasion being effected by a hard powder such as carborundum or emery. This is completed by polishing, when a covering of cloth or wax is substituted for the powder. The product forms the uncut lens, and the spheres and cylinders and toric forms employed in ordinary use are kept in stock in quantity in this state, their further treatment being dependent upon the requirements of the individual prescription.

When the prescription is supplied, and the size and shape of the lenses have been fixed, the optical centre and the axis of the cylinder, if one is present, are determined and marked. The uncut lens is then set in a 'protractor' with the optical centre and the axis in the proper position (see Fig. 24.32), and the lens is cut to the proposed shape by a machine which engraves a deep line upon the glass. The glass is then broken off at this line by nippers, and subsequently 'edged' by a rotating carborundum wheel, which grinds it to receive the frames into which it is now fitted.

Hand glazing is now, however, only a small part of modern manufacturing practice. The whole procedure of reducing the lens blank to the required shape and size with an edge of the required design is automated to a greater or less degree. Cutting as a distinct process can be eliminated because diamond-impregnated grinding wheels remove surplus glass much more rapidly than carborundum wheels and can be used for producing a flat-edged or bevel-shaped lens of the final form from the uncut blank. By employing a 'former' or 'template', lenses of different sizes but similar shape can be produced by modern automated machines. Lastly, in the process of glazing the lenses are inserted and fitted into the frames.

A final checking completes the process. The optical centres in relation to the two visual axes (the *inter-axial* not the inter-pupillary distance) are verified and the axis of the cylinder checked. Faults or scratches on the lenses are eliminated and any strain in the glass detected by special means.

Plastic lenses

The disadvantages and the dangers of glass owing to splintering have stimulated research into the optical uses of plastics. Modern plastics possess very high optical qualities, but polymethyl-methacrylate, PMMA, (index of refraction 1.49), the original one, had the disadvantages of susceptibility to scratching and a tendency to warp when heated or put under pressure. These handicaps, however, have been largely overcome by the use of a hard thermosetting resin, allyl diglycol carbonate, CR39 which compares well with glass in resistance to scratching and is, indeed, superior to it in resisting pitting (as when used at a grinding wheel or when welding or sand-blasting) because of a difference in impact resistance. The index of refraction (1.50) is slightly higher than that of PMMA. It does not fog up so quickly as glass in changing temperatures since it warms up more rapidly. Such lenses can also be dyed to reduce their transmission of light and surface coated to reduce annoying reflections.

The making of ophthalmic plastic lenses is a relatively simple process. The plastic is cut into circular discs which are then turned on a lathe to a curvature approximating that finally required. These are heated by steam to a temperature depending upon the form and thickness of the lens. The lens blank is placed between two steel dies with surfaces accurately shaped and polished to the required optical form and pressed for several minutes while the temperature is maintained. The lens leaves the press with its surface brightly polished and may be subjected to a hardening treatment whereby a fine film of silica, a few wavelengths in thickness, is deposited on the surfaces. One of the great advantages of plastic lenses is their lightness, a property of considerable importance when high-powered lenses are required, as in aphakia.

Newer lens materials

In recent years several of these have come into wider use in response to the need for lenses which are reasonably lightweight with durable surfaces, higher refractive indices and without unacceptable increases in chromatism. One of the first was an unleaded flint glass (High-Lite) with an index of refraction of 1.70 (ordinary leaded flint glass is somewhat heavier and has an index of 1.62). There is now a glass of index 1.8 available.

Although CR39 remains the most widely used plastic material, newer resins are available now, at a price, with higher indices — 1.56 or 1.60.

Spectacle frames

The fitting of suitable spectacle frames is one of the optician's most delicate tasks, and upon his success in this much of the comfort and value of the spectacles depend. He has several interests to meet which are frequently conflicting. Most important, from the optical point of view, there are certain criteria which are essential, and it is frequently a difficult matter to combine these successfully with the requirements of an asymmetrical face (a very variable quantity) and the patient's aesthetic demands (a more variable quantity still). The essential requirements may be rapidly recapitulated.

The frames must be rigid, strong and light, and they must fit securely, yet lightly and easily causing no irritation to the points of the skin whereon they rest. They should hold both lenses firmly and constantly in a plane perpendicular to the direction of regard. Lenses for distance should therefore sit vertically, but since the eyes tend more frequently to be directed downwards than upwards, especially in tall people, they may be canted slightly downwards; an upward tilt is inadmissible for ordinary purposes. Spectacles for reading should be slightly lowered, they should converge slightly, and they should be angled downwards at an angle of from 10 to 15 degrees, depending on the wearer's habit. Moreover, the lenses should theoretically be held at a distance of 15.7 mm in front of the cornea; this corresponds to the anterior principal focus of the eye, and at this distance the images formed on the retina will be of the same size as in emmetropia. Usually this distance is not adhered to, and the lenses are placed as near to the eyes as the lashes permit, at about 12 to 14 mm distance. Finally, the lenses should be large enough to ensure a good visual field, a consideration which applies especially to children.

Conventional spectacle frames are supported by the region of the bridge of the nose and, through the side-pieces, by the ears. Apart from any cosmetic aspect, frames should be strong and durable, light in weight and capable of appropriate shape modification, usually by heat, in order to fit the lenses in them and so as to suit the individual wearer.

The materials of which they are made may be metal, tortoiseshell, plastic material or combinations of these. The metals that have been used are stainless steel, solid or rolled gold, gold plate, anodised aluminium, nickel-silver and, more recently, titanium alloy. Nickel-copper and nickel-chrome alloys are also used as well as bronze.

Tortoiseshell, derived not from the tortoise but from the back plates of the hawk's bill turtle, is available in various cosmetically attractive shades. It is durable and has the property of being bonded by heat and pressure to similar material. However it is expensive and rarely encountered these days.

Plastics such as cellulose nitrate (xylonite), cellulose acetate and propionate, and Perspex are widely used. Cellulose nitrate has the advantage over the acetate of being harder and more rigid but has the distinct disadvantage that it is inflammable, a property which has virtually excluded its use. Attractive patterns in spectacle frames can be introduced by the use of laminates of coloured acetate material. Frames can be of nylon, either pure or with embedded carbon

fibre. Copolyamide is another durable plastic in use.

Many modern spectacle frames are of all-metal or all-plastic construction, the latter sometimes being intentionally bulky in design (the 'library frame'). In others there is a combination of various types of material as, for example, where the metal is covered with plastic (the 'Windsor frame') or the metal reinforces a predominantly plastic part of the frame.

Different portions of the frame may be of differing materials. Thus the rims may be of plastic and the bridge of metal. In rimless spectacles, the lenses have no supporting rim, being connected to one another by the bridge, the side-pieces being attached either to the lenses by screws or to an extension of the bridge along the top of the lenses. A modern type of frame giving a partly rimless appearance is the 'nylon supra', in which the lower part of each lens is held to the frame by a nylon cord instead of a solid rim, or alternatively by a steel wire. In some designs the lens is either glued or screwed to the frame along its upper border.

The design of the various elements of the frame — rims, bridge, side-pieces and joints — has shown many variations. The sides, for example, usually have an angled 'hockey-end' or occasionally a 'curl-end' encircling the ear, a type particularly useful for children or sportsmen to prevent the spectacles slipping off, but sometimes the sides may be straight. The bridge in most modern frames is of the padded type having two supports for the sides of the nose, but in plastic frames a keyhole shape is a widely used design formed by the combination of a pad and the bridge itself. In some metal frames, however, the W bridge is still in use where the support is given by the bridge of the nose. Such a 'regular' bridge is occasionally found in plastic or shell frames, and further refinements of this are the 'saddle' or 'inset' varieties (Fig. 24.1). Special reversible or swivel bridges are used in reversible spectacles. Numerous ingenious devices are used in the joints of spectacle frames and many methods are used to conceal them. The introduction of sprung joints in recent years has improved the durability of the connection of front to side-piece. In very young children who wear spectacles for the treat-

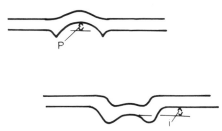

Fig. 24.1 Saddle bridge (above); inset bridge (below) p = projection. i = inset.

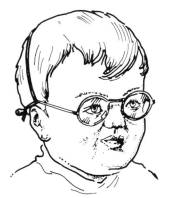

Fig. 24.2 Method of tying on spectacles in very young children.

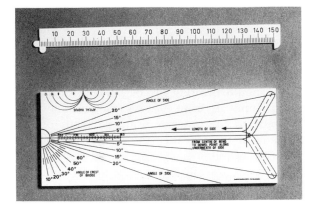

Fig. 24.3 A p.d. measure and gauge for other parameters in frame fitting (Keeler).

ment of squint, ear-pieces may be inadvisable; and if the side-pieces terminate in a metal loop, a tape arranged over the head, as in Figure 24.2, broken with a small length of elastic, provides an effective and admirable means of fixation.

Most refractive errors are corrected by lenses in spectacle frames in which the side-piece is an integral element. The spectacle frame has almost but not completely ousted *nose glasses (pince-nez)*, the sole support of which is upon the bridge of the nose. It is obvious that the former are a more adequate optical instrument than the latter and should always be preferred.

The monocle, the most difficult ornament to wear, is of little serious ophthalmological value and has been caricatured in many ways. As has already been mentioned, however, it is frequently of service to presbyopes, to whom it is useful for rapid reference. *Lorgnettes,* which are held in the hand, may serve a similar purpose. In cases of marked astigmatism, however, these are rarely

satisfactory since the adjustment of the glass is largely a matter of chance.

The fitting of spectacle frames is a highly skilled procedure. A basic measurement required for this is the inter-pupillary distance (p.d.) (Fig. 24.3). It is frequently important to measure the inter-pupillary distance not only for distant vision but also for reading and, although the centration for the latter is often calculated by rule of thumb from the former, this simple procedure may be inaccurate not only because the rule is not applicable in every case but also because the centration distance (c.d.) for near vision is not the same as the inter-pupillary distance (Fig. 24.4).

Estimates or measurements are also made of the size and shape of the bridge of the nose, the temple width, and the distance from the spectacle plane to the top of the ear. Again, there are many ingenious devices for these purposes, particularly relating to the shape of the bridge. Any significant degree of facial asymmetry may present considerable problems when fitting the frames and must be carefully studied. Thus the two halves of the inter-pupillary distance may differ, one eye may be higher than the other, the bridge of the nose may be irregular, or the ears may not have symmetrical relationships to their respective eyes. A skilful optician will be able not only to overcome the optical problems presented by such cases but, in addition, to contribute a cosmetic improvement by disguising the facial asymmetry with suitably designed frames.

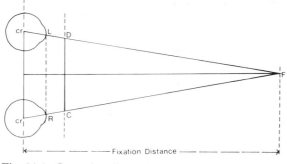

Fig. 24.4 Centration distance.

A contact dermatitis excited by the materials of which the spectacles are made is not uncommon in sensitive persons. All stages of eczematous dermatitis are met with — erythematous, papular, vesicular and even pustular — which become particularly evident where the frames contact or chafe the skin on the bridge of the nose, the temples and behind the ears. Every case of dermatitis encountered is not necessarily allergic; such a condition may be due to a traumatic irritation such as occurs when newly acquired spectacle frames bear heavily on the skin or where the surface of old spectacles has become dirty, encrusted with other material, or rough. Allergic reactions are seen particularly in the case of spectacles made of nickel or plastic.

SPECTACLE LENSES

The size and shape of lenses

There is some confusion as to the standardisation of the size and shape of spectacle lenses. The notation formerly suggested in Great Britain is not widely adhered to; this differentiated varying shapes as round, round oval, long oval, and pantoscopic (an oval with a flattened top), and indicated the sizes by the circumferential measurement. The American notation indicates the shape of the oval by a number which denotes the difference in millimetres between the long and the short axes. In practice most opticians do not adhere to these, but adopt the much more suitable procedure of varying the size and shape to conform to the requirements of the pre-

scription and the configuration of the face, as well as to the dictates of fashion.

In children especially, large glasses providing a full field are best so that the wearer is not tempted to look over them. In the case of cylindrical lenses one advantage of an oval shape is that it prevents the lenses rotating should they become loose. If round lenses are used a 'lens lock' of some form obviates the danger of a cylinder becoming misplaced in this manner in course of time.

The form of lenses

The form into which the prescription is made is a more difficult and complicated matter.

There are certain defects inherent in any system of correction of the optical anomalies of the eye by spectacle lenses. The form these lenses should take is dictated by the desire to minimise these defects, which are of two types: those due to rotation of the eye and those due to the optical aberrations of the lenses themselves.

Rotation of the eye

Difficulty may arise because the eye and the spectacle lens do not move in unison. In order to get the best optical result the eyes should remain fixed opposite the centre of the glass, and when the wearer wishes to see lateral objects clearly it is necessary for him to move his whole head in order to maintain the proper alignment, and enable him to use the lens and eye as an optically centred system. On looking eccentrically to view an object not situated straight in front, however, the pupil of the eye and the macula rotate around the centre of rotation. If a sharp image of the object is to be obtained, we have already seen that an image at the remote point must be brought to a focus on the macula. The remote point, which is conjugate with the macula, must therefore similarly move over a spherical surface, which, as is seen in Figures 24.5 and 24.6, is a *real* sphere lying in front of the eye in myopia and a *virtual* sphere lying behind the eye in hypermetropia. If the object point rotates on this sphere concentrically to the centre of rotation, it follows that in all positions

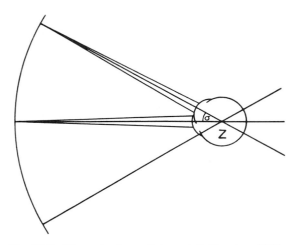

Fig. 24.5 The real sphere of sharp definition in a highly myopic eye.

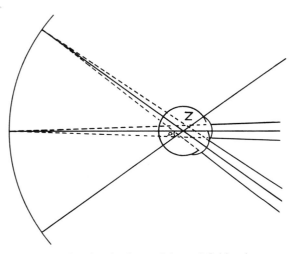

Fig. 24.6 The virtual sphere of sharp definition in a highly hypermetropic eye.

a remote sphere at the far point. In order, therefore, to make sharp images on a remote sphere concentric with the centre of rotation of the eye, the best design of spectacle lenses necessitates that the lens be bent by varying the radii of the two surfaces.

Aberrations associated with the spectacle lenses

The first of these is *spherical aberration* (p. 33), which depends on the degree of deviation of the rays of light, and is reduced to a minimum when the deviation produced at each surface of the lens is the same. A consideration of Figure 24.7 will show that this is attained when the more convex surface faces the incident rays which are more nearly parallel than the rays which leave after refraction.

The *astigmatism undergone by pencils of light falling obliquely on the lens* is a more important matter. A schematic representation of the astigmatism suffered by a pencil of parallel rays running at an obliquity, σ, to the axis of a lens is seen in Figure 24.8, exaggerated to finite

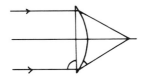

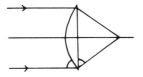

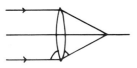

Fig. 24.7 To illustrate the best form of lens to reduce the effects of spherical aberration.

In the middle figure, when the greatest convex surface faces the incident light, the deviation produced at each surface of the lens is approximately equal.

on this sphere all the pencils of light entering the pupil will have the same convergence, and the course of the rays will be the same as if a stationary aperture (or stop) existed at Z (Figs 24.5 and 24.6). Assuming that the power of accommodation is absent, objects can be seen distinctly only if they lie on this *sphere of sharp definition*. If accommodation is present, of course, an area of sharp definition will lie between the boundary surfaces formed by two concentric spheres, a proximate sphere at the near point and

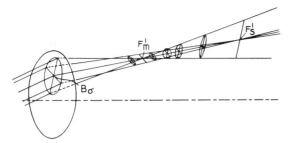

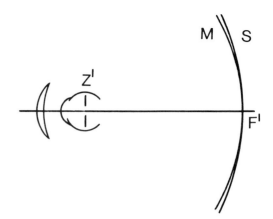

Fig. 24.8 The astigmatism of oblique pencils.

Fig. 24.10 A meniscus lens can be found with which the meridional and sagittal surfaces almost coincide.

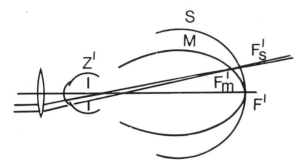

Fig. 24.9 In a symmetrical biconvex lens the meridional (M) and sagittal (S) surfaces are widely separated.

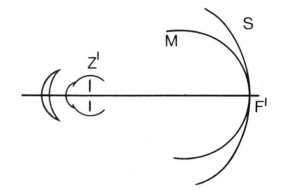

Fig. 24.11 If the bending of the lens is overdone, the meridional and sagittal surfaces again separate.

Figs 24.10 and **24.11** The astigmatic image surfaces of a convex lens.

dimensions. It is seen that two focal lines are formed, the *meridional* or *tangential focal line* (F′m) and the *sagittal* or *radial focal line* (F′s). If the obliquity of the principal ray is finite the astigmatic difference (the distance F′mF′s) is also finite and increases rapidly with the angle of obliquity. If F′m were made to coincide with F′s, no oblique astigmatism would exist. An indication of what occurs in the case of a spectacle lens is seen in Figure 24.9. By joining all the points of the meridional and sagittal foci, we will obtain two curves outlining the points at which each focal line is situated. These considerations, of course, will apply to any axial plane, and if Figure 24.9 is rotated around the optic axis of the lens the curves for the focal lines will trace out the *astigmatic image surfaces* of the lens as the loci for image formation (meridional and sagittal planes). The curve (M) represents the converging point of rays lying in the plane of the paper containing the optic axis and the principal ray (or the peripheral object point); it is therefore called the *meridional* or *tangential focal*

surface. The curve (S) represents the converging point of rays in the plane perpendicular to this and may be called the *sagittal* or *radial focal surface.* If, for example, a cross serves as the eccentric object, on the tangential surface the vertical image line is blurred, and on the sagittal surface the cross-line is blurred; and between the two surfaces will lie a third plane whereon lie the circles of least confusion. If the lens is bent into a meniscus the two planes tend to coincide (Fig. 24.10) and oblique astigmatism tends to disappear. If the bending is overdone it begins to increase again (Fig. 24.11). The other defects such as chromatic aberration, diffraction, coma, curvature and distortion of the image also exert some deleterious effect on the quality of spectacle lens imagery, and can also be taken into account to a limited extent.

Best-form lenses

The ideal lens should, of course, correct all aberrations, but this is usually impossible. The two most important are oblique astigmatism so that reasonably sharp images are obtained when looking obliquely through the lens and the approximation of the curvature of the image to the far point sphere so that continual changes of accommodation are not required when distant objects are viewed in various directions. It is found when oblique astigmatism is eliminated that the focal surface thus formed approximates closely with the remote sphere (Fig. 24.12), so that if one error is allowed for the other is automatically almost corrected. Fortunately, also, a lens of the shape required to minimise these operations also reduces the effect of spherical and other aberrations. Such a lens is termed a *best-form lens*. Huyghens (1629–95), the Dutch physicist who was responsible for the wave theory of light, first suggested that lenses should be

corrected in some such manner as this, and proposed a ratio of surface curvatures of 6:1. The English physicist, Wollaston (1804), first prepared periscopic lenses, and the best forms were worked out by Ostwalt (1898), the French oculist, and later and in more detail by Percival of Newcastle (1901). The subject is still engaging attention. Percival's recommendations for an eye the centre of rotation of which is assumed to be 27 mm behind the meniscus and useful rotation is through a solid angle of 30 degrees are given in Table 3, Appendix I.

In practice it is impossible to manufacture an indefinite number of forms, and so a limited number of standard forms is relied upon in order to reduce the number of grinding tools. The standard surface is called the *base surface*: the other surface is called the *combining surface*, and it is specially ground to suit the individual prescription. The best practical base curves are:

from +7 D to 0	−6 D next the eye
from 0 to −6 D	+6 D furthest from the eye
from −6 D to −10 D	+1.25 D furthest from the eye
from −10 D to −20 D	plane furthest from the eye

A lens with a base of 6 D is called a *deep meniscus lens*; one with a base of 1.25 is called a *periscopic*

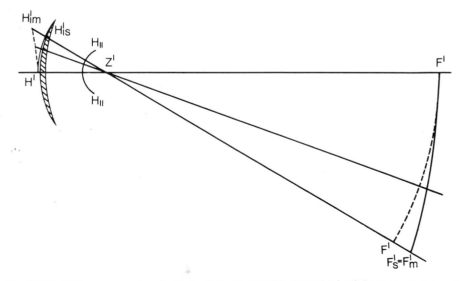

Fig. 24.12 With a convex lens in front of an eye rotating around Z', F'F' represents the remote sphere and F'F's (or F'F'm) the focal surface when the lens is corrected for oblique astigmatism. The more nearly the two curves coincide, the better form of the lens.

lens (see Fig. 24.16). For positive lenses a negative base curve is used, and for negative lenses a positive base curve; and in the fitting of the spectacles the concave surface is always placed next the eye.

The search for the ideal form of an astigmatic correction has led to the widespread use of the *toric lens*, which is a meniscus lens with a cylindrical curve ground on the spherical surface of one side. A 'torus' is a term borrowed from architecture, and is descriptive of the curvature of an Ionic column; in it the radius of curvature in one meridian is different from that of the one at right angles (Fig. 24.13). A walking stick may be exemplified as a cylinder; when it is bent it assumes a toroidal form. A bicycle tyre is another familiar example; if the tyre is 60 cm in diameter and 5 cm in thickness, the radius of curvature of the horizontal meridian is 30 cm, while that of the vertical is 2.5 cm. The base curve upon which toric lenses are constructed is almost invariably one of 6 D. A toric lens therefore consists of one spherical and one toric surface, the difference between the base curve and curvature of the principal meridian giving the cylindrical power of the lens.

It has been noted that beyond the limits of + 7 D and –20 D meniscus-shaped glasses are no longer efficient. In extreme myopia and in aphakia, therefore, no single lens with spherical surfaces will eliminate oblique astigmatism. Gullstrand suggested that the difficulty might be overcome in part by making the peripheral parts of a different curvature in the so-called *aspherical lenses*, but since in these cases peripheral vision

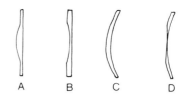

Fig. 24.14 Lenticular glasses.

(A) Plano-convex lenticular glass.
(B) Plano-concave lenticular glass.
(C) Convex-meniscus lenticular glass.
(D) Concave-meniscus lenticular glass.

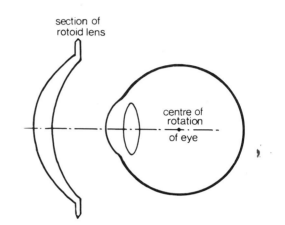

Fig. 24.15 Rotoid lens. The curve is so steep that the centres of curvature of the two surfaces approximately coincide with the centre of rotation of the eye thus allowing considerable clarity in peripheral vision in aphakia.

is at best poor the matter is as well neglected. Indeed, the greatest desideratum in such lenses is to keep down their weight and size, and for this purpose *lenticular lenses* are very useful (Fig. 24.14). In these, high-power lenses are ground only in the centre and, although the field is thus reduced, the added comfort usually compensates for the loss; they may be improved by grinding them into a meniscus shape. Nevertheless several designs of aspherical lens have been offered at various times for the aphakic patient such as Katral (Zeis), Rotoid (Fig. 24.15), Welsh four drop (the drop in power between the axial and peripheral parts of the lens). The incentive for the development of new forms for aphakia has of course declined with the advent of intra-ocular lens implantation. Nevertheless there is an active pursuit of

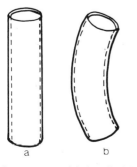

Fig. 24.13 A toric curvature. (*a*) A cylindrical and (*b*) a toric curvature.

aspherical forms quite apart from their use in aphakia. When employed in combination with the newer higher index materials advantages are said to accrue in both weight of correction and cosmetic appearance.

The modern design of lenses has been considerably influenced by the development of computers, which are a valuable aid to the involved mathematics required. Complex ray tracing is so facilitated by this means that once the criteria of the design have been agreed, a range of the best forms of lenses can be rapidly produced. A further factor influencing the design is the realisation that the centre of rotation of the eye occupies a less fixed position than had been presumed by previous workers. There appears to be a considerable variation in the distance between the lens of the spectacles and the optical 'stop' at the centre of rotation, a distance which is commonly between 27 and 33 mm (Fig. 24.14); moreover, in the same individual this distance may vary for the different positions of the gaze.

Equivalent forms and the transposition of lenses

The process of changing a lens from one form to another equivalent form is called *transposition*. This may be considered under two headings — simple and toric transposition.

Simple transposition occupies itself largely with the alteration of the form of lenses in cases of astigmatism, and with the production of periscopic or meniscus lenses or of forms which produce some of their advantages.

In the simple transposition of spheres a knowledge of the several standard forms available is essential. These are symmetrical, asymmetrical, plano, periscopic, deep meniscus, or toroidal (Fig. 24.16).

In the *symmetrical form* each side is ground similarly, and a biconvex or biconcave lens results. In an *asymmetrical lens* the two surfaces are ground differently, and in the *plano* the whole of the curvature is placed upon the one side while the other remains plane. Thus a +2 D sphere may be made up symmetrically with each curvature +1 D, or asymmetrically with +0.5 D and +1.5 D, or as a plano lens with +2 D on one

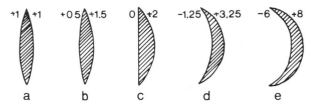

Fig. 24.16 The form of lenses.
A +2.0 D sphere made up in five different forms.

a. Symmetrical.
b. Asymmetrical.
c. Plano.
d. Periscopic (to the base −1.25).
e. Deep meniscus (to the base −6).

surface; in addition a sphere may be ground on one side and a cylinder on the other. The difference between these may not seem very material, but several considerations must be borne in mind.

The transposition of spheres into periscopic or deep meniscus forms is a question of simple algebraic addition. It is to be remembered that the given power is to be combined with a base curve of the opposite sign. Thus a +2 D sphere converted into periscopic form has curvatures of −1.25 and +3.25 D spheres. A −2 D sphere similarly converted has curvatures of +1.25 and −3.25 D spheres.

In the same way a +2 D sphere converted into a deep meniscus form has curvatures of −6 and +8 D spheres, while the corresponding concave lens will be formed by +6 and −8 D spheres.

In the transposition of cylinders two desiderata are always to be kept in view: an attempt should be made to keep the lenses as light as possible, and it is desirable to maintain the axes of the cylinders in the two eyes in approximately the same direction.

Some examples will make the matter clear.

Thus if a refraction is −0.5 D sph. −1.0 cyl. ax. 180° and it is desired to add +1.5 D sph. as a presbyopic correction, the effect is gained by transposing to a simple +1.0 D cyl. ax. 90°.

In some cases a cross-cylinder is preferable to a sphero-cylinder in that it is lighter and provides a wider field. Thus a +3.0 D sph. −4.0 D cyl. ax. 180° might well be converted into +3.0 D cyl. ax. 90° −1.0 D cyl. ax. 180°.

Again, if the refraction is given as
RE +2.0 D cyl. ax. 90° −1.0 cyl. ax. 180°,
LE −3.0 cyl. ax. 180°,
the transposition
RE −1.0 D sph. +3.0 D cyl. ax. 90°,
would be correct, but the presence of two cylinders in the two eyes at right angles would be borne with difficulty. The better transposition would therefore be
RE +2 D sph. −3 D cyl. ax. 180°.
Here, however, a thicker glass is involved, and for this reason the combination might be left in the cross-cylinder form.

Toric transposition

Toric transposition, although it appears a more complicated process, depends on the same principles and is as simple. The toric formula is written as a fraction, the numerator of which is a sphere, and the denominator comprises both the base curve and the cylinder necessary to give the required combination.

The steps in the transposition may be summarised thus:
a. Transpose the given prescription to one having a cylinder of the same sign as the base curve which is to be used.
b. The spherical surface is given by subtracting the base power from the sphere in (a). This is written as the numerator of the fraction.
c. Fix the cylindrical base curve with its axis at right angles to the cylinder in (a).
d. Add to the base curve the cylinder in (a) with its axis at right angles to that of the base curve.
These, (c) and (d), give the toric surface, and they form the denominator of the fraction of the formula.
An example will make this clear.
To transpose +3 D sph. − 1 D cyl. ax. 90° to a toric formula to the base −6;
a. is already done;
b. to get the effect of +3 D sph., the spherical surface must have a curvature of +9 D sph., i.e. the base power subtracted from the original sphere, +3 D − (−6 D);
c. the base curve required is −6 D cyl. ax. 180°;
d. the other toric power to give a resultant of −1 D cyl. ax. 90° is −7 D cyl. ax. 90°, that is −6 D added to −1 D;
this gives a combination on the one surface of −6 D cyl. ax. 180° −7 D cyl. ax. 90°, or −6 D sph. −1 D cyl. ax. 90°.
The formula is written thus:

$$\frac{+9.0 \text{ D sph.}}{-6.0 \text{ D cyl. ax. } 180°/-7.0 \text{ D cyl. ax. } 90°}$$

In the same manner the transposition of +5.0 sph. −2.0 D cyl. ax. 180° to the toric form to the base + 6 is accomplished thus.
Transposing the sign of the cylinder to correspond to that of the base, the prescription becomes:

+3.0 D sph. +2.0 D cyl. ax. 90°

A similar series of steps is now gone through, giving as a result:

$$\frac{-3.0 \text{ D sph.}}{+6.0 \text{ D cyl. ax. } 180°/+8.0 \text{ D cyl. ax. } 90°}$$

THE POSITION OF SPECTACLE LENSES IN RELATION TO THE EYE

Back vertex distance and power

We must remind ourselves that in order to correct an optical defect in the eye, a correcting lens (for distance), when placed in a suitable position, must be such that its second focal point corresponds to the remote point of the eye and the image of the remote point is brought to a focus on the retina by the dioptric system of the eye. The combination of the two will thus focus parallel rays upon the retina. It is therefore obvious that *the factor of primary importance in a spectacle lens is its posterior focal length or back vertex power*. It also follows that the shape and thickness of the lenses and their distance from the eye must be considered for these factors influence the value of the vertex power. As regards the distance from the eye we must include here a note on the *effectivity* of lenses. The prescription is determined by objective and subjective tests with a lens, or more usually a combination of lenses, in the trial frame, and the final spectacle lens must have the same optical effect if the same result is to be obtained.

How the optical effectivity of a lens varies with its position will be appreciated from the following example.

In Figure 24.17 let a thin lens placed at A correct the optical error of the eye, the far point of which is at F′. If the correcting lens were placed at B, its focal length would necessarily require to be reduced by an amount d' if it were to have the same optical effect. It follows that the two lenses to be equally effective must be of

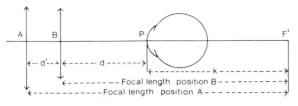

Fig. 24.17 The effectivity of lenses.

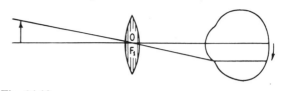

Fig. 24.18

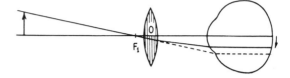

Fig. 24.19

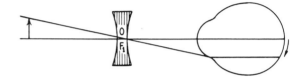

Fig. 24.20

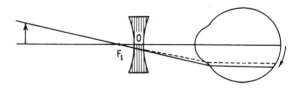

Fig. 24.21

Figs 24.18 to 24.21 To show the variation in size of the retinal image with different positions of the lens.
When the centre of the lens (O) is at the anterior principal focus (F_1) the size of the image (indicated by the arrow) is unchanged (Figs 24.18 and 24.20).
When the centre of the lens (O) is nearer to the eye than the anterior principal focus (F_1), the image in the case of a convex lens is reduced (Fig. 24.19), and that with a concave lens increased (Fig. 24.21).

different powers, the focal length of the convex lens being decreased and that of the concave lens increased, since in myopia the far point lies in front of the eye. Consequently (for parallel rays of light) the further a correcting lens is removed from the eye the weaker it must be in hypermetropia and the stronger in myopia. Conversely, the effective power of a positive lens increases as it is moved from the eye while that of a negative lens decreases.

Thus a stronger positive lens is required in the spectacle plane (say 12 mm from the cornea) than at the anterior focal point of the eye (15.7 mm from the cornea). (See Table 5, Appendix I.)

Strictly speaking we refer to the *back vertex distance* of the spectacle lens from the eye and we must therefore also concern ourselves with the back vertex power of the spectacle lens itself, a factor influenced considerably by its size, shape and form. It is most important to ensure that the combination of lenses found satisfactory in the trial frame should be ordered in a spectacle lens with a back vertex power equivalent to that of the combination. The latter may not have an optical power the same as that of a single lens ground to represent the sum of its components, particularly if these are thick — thin and thick lenses of the same surface power not being equivalent; nor are biconvex, meniscus and toric versions of a lens of the same power.

The distance at which the spectacles are worn is, as we have seen, of considerable importance in determining the effective strength of the lens; it also affects the size of the retinal image. When a correcting lens is situated at the anterior focal point of the eye, it will be seen from Figures 24.18 and 24.20 that the size of the image upon the retina is unchanged. This point, it will be remembered, is 15.7 mm in front of the cornea, and spectacles are usually worn nearer than this by about 1 or 2 mm.

If, therefore, the lens is nearer to the eye than this point, in the case of a convex lens the retinal image is diminished (Fig. 24.19), and in the case of a concave lens it is increased (Fig. 24.21). If the lens is further away, the opposite effect is produced. The difference in size, of course, varies with the strength of the lens. Consequently, when the correction of the two eyes is approximately equal, discomfort is not usually experienced, but when a marked degree of anisometropia is present, the difference between the two images may be sufficient to cause some annoyance. This effect is especially marked in unilateral cases of aphakia, for in addition to the difference in refraction between the two eyes the anterior principal focus of the aphakic eye has been altered and now lies much farther out (see p. 71).

The centring and decentring of lenses

It is extremely important that when the glasses are fitted the optical centres should correspond to the visual axes of the patient's eyes, for it is only when this condition obtains that the rays of light will travel to his eyes without suffering deviation. It will be remembered that a lens may be considered as a combination of prisms, and that when light passes through any part of a lens outside its optical centre the effect is that of a prism with its base directed towards the thickest part of the lens.

In this connection two definitions must be borne in mind. The *optical centre* is the centre of the optical system formed by the lens, and all rays passing through it are undeviated. The *geometrical centre*, on the other hand, is the point in the middle of the lens, and is merely a relation of the placement of the lens in its frame. The two need not coincide, for, depending on the shape of the orbits and the asymmetry of the face, the lens may be displaced in any direction provided the optical centre is kept in the correct position. For cosmetic reasons it is usually advisable for the geometrical centre of the lens to be opposite the centre of the pupil.

In each case, therefore, the optical centre must be determined, and the spectacles fitted accordingly. While it is usually sufficient to measure the inter-pupillary distance, this may not be adequate. Especially when the lenses are of high power, the determination must be accurate. Thus when -10 D spheres are worn, for example, an error of only a millimetre in each eye will entail a total error of convergence of 1Δ. In any case, owing to the variability of the angle α, the visual axes may not coincide with the centres of the pupils; moreover, each eye must be measured separately from the centre of the nose, for a face is rarely symmetrical. The most accurate method has already been described. It depends upon the determination of the position of the light reflex

on the cornea as the patient looks in a specified direction, and the measurement of this by means of cross-wires in a trial frame, or in a specially designed 'p.d. (pupillary distance) rule' comprised of two plano lenses with cross-lines etched upon them, one of which is moveable, carried on a calibrated bar the distance of which from the nose is marked in millimetres. The optical centres for distance lenses are thus found by asking the patient to look at a light in the distance, those for near vision by asking him to look at a light near at hand. The observer, seated opposite the patient, marks the position of the light reflex with the cross-wire in the right eye, sighting it with his own left eye, and with his own right eye similarly determines the centre in the patient's left eye.

The decentring of lenses

Lenses may be decentred in one of two ways. The optical centre and the geometrical centre may be allowed to coincide in the centre of the frame, and the frame may be displaced as a whole by lengthening or shortening the nose-piece. Or, alternatively, the lens may be displaced in its rim. Both methods give the same prismatic effect. The action of the first is seen in Figure 24.22, but for cosmetic reasons the second is usually to be preferred. In it lenses are cut eccentrically out of

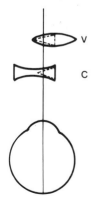

Fig. 24.22 The decentring of lenses by displacement.

If the eye figured is the right, decentring of a convex lens (*v*) outwards, or of a concave lens (*c*) inwards produces the action of a prism, base out.

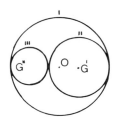

Fig. 24.23 The decentring of lenses.

I, a large lens symmetrically centred, when O the optical centre and the geometrical centre coincide. From I may be cut II and III in which the optical and geometrical centres do not coincide. They therefore act as prismospheres.

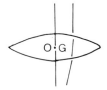

Fig. 24.24 A normally centred lens as Fig. 24.23 (I). The optical centre (O) is at the geometrical centre (G).

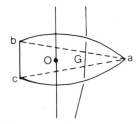

Fig. 24.25 A decentred lens, as in Fig. 24.23 (II). The optical centre (O) is placed eccentrically. A ray passing through the geometrical centre (G) will be deflected as if by a prism, *bac*.

a larger one as is seen in Figure 24.23. Here the large lens (I) is normally centred, for its optical and geometric centres coincide (OG, Fig. 24.24). The smaller lens (II), however, will have its optical centre at O and its geometrical centre at G′, and will appear as in Figure 24.25, while the smallest (III), which has its geometrical centre at G″, will have its optical centre at O, outside it altogether, assuming the form seen in Figure 24.26. In each case the optical effect will be the same as if a prism had been interpolated into the

Fig. 24.26 A decentred lens, as in Fig. 24.23 (III). The optical centre (O) is outside the lens altogether.

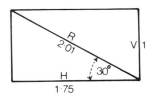

Fig. 24.27 To measure an oblique prismatic effect.

H, the horizontal component for each eye = 1.75 units.
V, the vertical component for each eye = 1 unit.
R, the resultant = 2.01 units at an angle of 30 degrees to the direction of *H*.

substance of the lens (Fig. 24.25). Such a lens becomes a *prismosphere*.

The strength of the prism will vary with the amount of decentration and with the dioptric strength of the lens: it is found that there is a prismatic effect of 1 prism dioptre per 1 D for every 1 cm of decentration which is effected. The amount of decentration in millimetres therefore equals 10 N/D, where N is the number of prism dioptres and D the strength of the lens.

Decentring a convex lens in any direction acts as if a prism were incorporated with its base towards the direction of decentration; displacement of a concave lens has the opposite effect. Thus decentring a convex lens inwards or a concave one outwards has the optical effect of a prism base in.

Where the prismatic effect required is oblique, the extent of the defect is usually calculated clinically as two components at right angles. Thus a patient may require a correction of 2 prism dioptres for a right hyperphoria, and of 3.5 for an exophoria. In such a case, as Percival pointed out, it is unsatisfactory to correct the vertical defect in one eye with a vertical prism and the latter defect in the other with a horizontal one. The two components should be resolved into one oblique deviation (Fig. 24.27), the effect being equally divided between the two eyes. Thus, in the present case, a horizontal line (*H*) of 1.75 cm is drawn, a vertical one (*V*) of 1 cm, and the parallelogram is completed: the resultant (*R*) on measurement gives the value — a prismatic effect of 2.01 prism dioptres running upwards and outwards (for the right eye) at an angle of 30 degrees. If drawing to scale is objected to, the result can be found on calculation, for it is obvious that $R = \sqrt{H^2 + V^2}$, and the angle of direction = $\tan^{-1} V/H$. In the present case, therefore, a correction of 2 prism dioptres pointing upwards and outwards at 30 degrees in the right eye and a similar correction downwards and outwards for the left eye would be prescribed. The lenses are therefore decentred in these directions by an amount in millimetres represented by 10 N/D. If the refractive error is 4 D, for example, the decentration would be 10 × 2/4 = 5 mm.

If the dioptric strengths in the two eyes are different, it follows that the amount of decentration must be different in each. If the lens is cylindrical, the amount depends upon the direction of the axis. As far as the cylinder is concerned, any decentration in the direction of its axis has no optical effect; any decentration in the direction perpendicular to its axis has the same effect as in the case of a sphere. Thus a combination of +2 D sph. +3 D cyl. ax. 90°, if decentred upwards, acts as a +2 D sphere, if decentred inwards or outwards as a +5 D sphere. If, however, the cylinders are oblique, or if an oblique decentration is required with a vertical or horizontal cylinder, the effect is more complicated.

The general optical effect of the curvature of a cylindrical surface in an oblique meridian is seen in Figure 24.28. In the plane, FAE, the surface of the cylinder is circular. In the plane of the axis MN,

the curvature is zero and in all intermediate positions it varies gradually between the two. In any intermediate position ABCD, inclined at an angle θ to the axis, the surface is an ellipse. The power of the lens in this meridian in dioptres can be shown to be represented by the expression $C \sin^2 θ$, where C is the strength of the cylinder (at right angles to its axis). This is sufficiently accurate for the small central area corresponding to the pupillary aperture. The power of a cylindrical lens, for example, of −4 D at an angle of 150 degrees, would be −4 $\sin^2$ 150° in the horizontal meridian, and −4 $\sin^2$ (θ − 90), or −4 $\cos^2$ θ, i.e. −4 $\cos^2$ 150° in the vertical meridian.

$$-4 \sin^2 150° = -4\left(\tfrac{1}{2}\right)^2 = -1 \text{ D}$$

$$\text{and } -4 \cos^2 150° = -4\left(\frac{\sqrt{3}}{2}\right)^2 = -3 \text{ D}$$

This can be simply verified: if a lens measure is placed at 30 degrees, with the plane axis of a 4 D cylinder, the reading is 1; if it is placed at 60 degrees the reading is 3. The decentration vertically or horizontally is then calculated on this basis in the manner already described.

Decentration is thus an alternative method to incorporating a prism in a lens or grinding a lens onto a prism as basis. It has the advantage of being considerably easier for the optician and considerably cheaper for the patient, since a prismatic lens has to be specially ground. The process, however, has its limits, for it necessitates a proportionate increase in weight: it is obvious, for example, that the lens of Figure 24.25 is heavier than that of Figure 24.24. In addition, a powerful prism is associated with chromatic and distortion effects. In general, therefore, decentration should be effected by displacing the entire glass as much as possible without interfering with the field of vision or with the cosmetic appearance, and the remainder should be obtained by displacing the lens in the frame. On average a decentration of much more than 4 to 6 mm will be found to be inconvenient, and it will be found better to make up the remainder (or the whole) of the prismatic effect by grinding the appropriate curvatures on a prism.

Decentring is required for three purposes:

1. To adapt a pair of spectacles to an asymmetrical face, in order to secure a cosmetic result. If one eye differs in its position from the other, it usually looks better to keep the spectacles

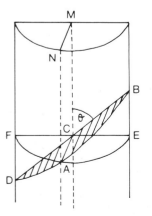

Fig. 24.28 The curvature of a cylinder in an oblique meridian.

symmetrical, and to decentre the lenses so that their optical centres are cut by the visual axes. Such a process, of course, gives no prismatic effect, and if one is desired an additional amount of decentring must be effected, the addition being made algebraically.

2. Decentring for near work. For near work the visual axes are converged and directed downwards, and the changed positions of the optical centres when the eyes are directed towards an object at any distance may be found clinically by the method already described (see p. 203). On average it will be found that the centres for reading should be about 6.5 mm below the horizontal, but the distance will depend on the habit of the individual. As a rule, when reading, the head is lowered about 20 to 30 degrees while the visual axes are further depressed by a downward rotation of the eyes through an angle of approximately 15 degrees. It is to allow for this angle that the optical centres ought to be lowered. The amount of convergence necessary will vary with the inter-pupillary distance and the distance from the eye at which the spectacles are worn: an average is 2.5 mm from the midline. It may be calculated from the following formula.

In Figure 24.29, if R denotes the centre of rotation of the eye, RS the visual axes when the eyes are directed straight forwards, and RN the distance from the visual axis of the eye to the central point of the nose, the visual axes will assume the position RO when they are directed upon a near object (O). C′ will denote the optical centre of a glass for

distance, and C″ that of one for reading, C′C″ can be calculated thus:

$$\frac{RN}{NO} = \tan RON = \tan C'RC'' = \frac{C'C''}{C'R}$$

Hence:

$$C'C'' = \frac{RN}{NO} \times C'R$$

RN is measured: suppose it is 30 mm. NO = the distance of the object from the lens + the distance of the lens from the centre of rotation of the eye, say 300 mm + 25 mm = 325 mm; and C′R is also 25 mm. Therefore:

$$C'C'' = \frac{30}{325} \times 25 = 2.4 \text{ mm}$$

If this decentration is not done, the visual axis, RO, cutting the periphery of the lens, would be subjected to a prismatic effect, and reading matter would become blurred.

In the making of bifocals the centring frequently gives rise to difficulty, and this is often the reason why these lenses may be unsatisfactory, particularly in anisometropes.

3. Lenses may also be decentred to correct a heterophoria, or to overcome a deficiency or an excess of convergence, the process being employed in place of incorporating prisms (see Chapter 17). To accomplish this the principles outlined above are applied directly.

In some cases it is an advantage that lenses should be centred in unusual ways. This is especially evident in various forms of sport. A simple way of producing the same effect for some purposes is to have spectacles provided with an adjustable degree of tilt. For instance, in golf, to be accurately centred, the lenses should be tilted downwards for putting or driving; or again, in playing a long shot in billiards they require to be tilted upwards. Similarly in target shooting, the line of vision is directed through the upper and inner quadrant of the lens, and for accuracy in aiming the optical centres, should be situated here in the lens of the sighting eye. If this is not done a considerable prismatic effect is introduced, and the object in each example (the golf ball, the billiard ball or the target) will be displaced as is illustrated in Figure 2.6, frequently with deplorable results.

Orthoscopic lenses

Orthoscopic spectacles are prismospheres which relieve exactly the same amount of accommodation

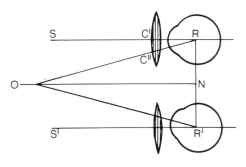

Fig. 24.29 Decentration inwards for reading.

RN is the distance of the centre of rotation of the eye from the nose. RS, the visual axes straight forwards, and O the near object looked at. The lens in front of the eye must be decentred from C′ to C″.

and convergence; thus if lenses are required of +2 D sphere for close work, prismospheres combining +2 D sphere with prisms (bases in) producing 2-metre angles of convergence would be given. The same effect is obtained if both lenses are cut from one large lens so that the two have a common optical centre. Scheffler originally proposed these lenses for presbyopes, but since the amplitude of convergence remains unimpaired while accommodation diminishes with age their use in these cases as a routine is unsound. They are frequently found useful, however, in non-presbyopic subjects who wish to increase their visual acuity for very fine work by increasing the size of the image by bringing their work close up to the eyes. If simple magnifying lenses are provided binocularly for this purpose, accommodation is relieved while convergence is not, and the strain thus thrown upon convergence becomes intolerable unless prisms are used. Such lenses are found useful in trades which demand a high degree of visual acuity, such as those working with microcircuitry, and they may well be of considerable service to the operating ophthalmic surgeon.

The verification of lenses

The verification of lenses includes the checking of the strength or, more properly, the back vertex power of the lenses, and the fitting of the frames: the importance of the first is obvious, but the amount of discomfort which may arise from the second cause is too frequently forgotten.

The surface power of a lens may be measured by special instruments, such as the Geneva lens measure, or, more exactly, by the method of neutralisation. It must be remembered, however, that these methods determine the surface or 'neutralisation' strength of the lens but do not measure its effective power — and the two may differ considerably.

The *Geneva lens measure* (Fig. 24.30) is provided with a fixed support on either side and a movable one placed centrally, so that, when placed upon a lens, the movable leg is deflected by an amount depending on the curvature of the surface. The deflection is recorded after the manner of an aneroid barometer on a scale

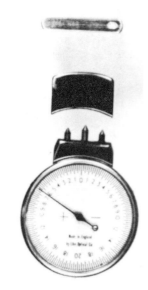

Fig. 24.30 The Geneva lens measure.

marked in dioptres, and thus the dioptric value of the lens in any meridian may be read off directly. The instrument thus gives an indication of the form (toric or otherwise) in which a lens has been made up. It is graduated for glass of a refractive index of 1.523 (ordinary crown glass), so that if any other glass is employed a correcting factor must be applied. Its accuracy should be checked periodically by standing it upon a plane surface, and adjusting it to the zero of the scale by screwing one of the stationary legs. More complicated instruments are supplied which read off the dioptric power of a lens, and record the strength of a cylinder together with the angle of its axis, but as a rule these will not be required by the practising ophthalmologist.

The *method of neutralisation* (see p. 164) is the most simple method. The examiner looks through the lens at a cross drawn on a piece of cardboard (Fig. 24.31, I). If the cross appears skewed by a scissors movement as the lens is rotated (II), it is rotated until there is no deformation of the cross-lines (III). The lens is now moved in a direction parallel to one of the lines, say up and down, when a deviation of the horizontal lines will be noticed (IV); if the curvature of this meridian is convex, the apparent movement will be in a direction opposite to that

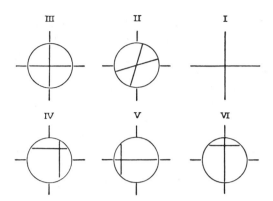

Fig. 24.31 The neutralisation of lenses.

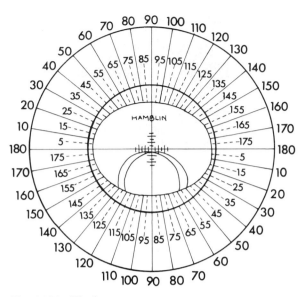

Fig. 24.32 The lens protractor.

of the lens, if concave, it will appear to be in the same direction as that of the lens. Lenses from the trial case of opposite sign and gradually increasing strength are now held up in combination with the lens under examination until this movement is exactly neutralised: this gives the dioptric value in this meridian. The lens, is then moved in the meridian at right angles: if no deviation of the line occurs, it has been neutralised in this meridian also and is a sphere; if some deviation does appear (V), it is, neutralised in exactly the same way by placing cylinders with their axes in the appropriate direction; this gives the value of the cylindrical element. It is well to mark these meridians with glass pencil; the point at which they meet is the optical centre. The lens is then laid upon a protractor (Fig. 24.32) with the horizontal diameter along the zero line and the axis of the cylinder as marked is read off. The geometrical centre can be found by measurement and any decentring immediately verified. Finally, a prism may be present. When the exact neutralising lenses are combined with the glass, the combination should ordinarily act as a glass plate, and on movement in any direction the cross should appear unaltered. If, however, a prism is present, on moving the lens there is no relative movement of the arms of the cross, but a displacement of the entire cross in one direction (VI). Prisms should now be combined with the lens until this effect is also neutralised. During the process of neutralisation the lenses should be held with their optical centres opposite each other, and they should be approximated as

closely as possible, for any degree of separation introduces an error. Where some degree of separation does exist, a condition which must obtain to a certain extent, a convex lens appears slightly stronger than it actually is, so that when strong lenses have to be employed in the process of neutralisation the convex element predominates in the combination.

If the lenses are of any considerable strength, however, their *vertex power* should be determined; in this way it is also possible to compare the vertex power of two (or more) lenses in the trial frame with the manufactured combination. This is done very simply by direct measurement with instruments known by various trade names (refractionometer, focimeter, lensometer, vertometer, ultimeter, etc., Fig. 24.33), the optical system of which is seen and explained in Figure 24.34. Electronic versions are available.

The general principle is that the image of a target, commonly a ring of illuminated dots, as seen through a telescope is focused by a standard lens; the unknown lens is then inserted into the system and its power measured by the change in the position of the target required to bring it again into focus.

If the lens is spherical, the circle of dots is refocused. An astigmatic lens splays out each dot into a linear form, these lines being made to focus

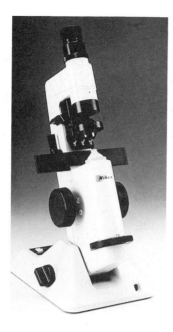

Fig. 24.33 The Focimeter.

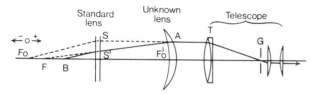

Fig. 24.34 The refractionometer.

Before the unknown lens to be tested is inserted, when the telescope is focused for parallel light, a clear image of the target (B) will be seen at the focal point of the standard lens (S) (i.e. at F_o, dotted line). At this setting the ray SAT is parallel. When the unknown convex lens is inserted at A with its back surface facing S, the light from the standard lens will no longer be parallel so that B will not be focused at G. The image of B will be formed at F, the focal point of the unknown lens. When the target is moved from F_o to F, the light emerging from A is moved from F_o to F, the light emerging from A will again be parallel, and B will again be sharply focused at G. The excursion of F_o towards F (for convex lenses) or away from it (for concave lenses) is in direct proportion to the back vertex power of the lens under test.

as sharply as possible in the two main meridia. The orientation of the line images indicates the astigmatic axis.

When the lenses are verified, their fitting should be examined. The distance of the visual axis of *each* eye from the midline is to be measured and the centring of each lens checked for distance, and for near work if necessary. Small errors here, particularly in the segments of bifocals, are productive of much discomfort; it is most marked if convex glasses are placed too far in or concave lenses too far out, so that an error of divergence is caused.

The *tilting of the lenses* should then be examined; they should lie as nearly as possible perpendicular to the visual axis so that the incident light falls upon them normally. If any tilt is introduced the spherical power is slightly increased and a cylindrical effect is added. When the lenses are of low power the change thus produced is small, but if they are of high power these effects may be considerable.

A calculation of the precise changes introduced by tilting the lens is a complicated matter, but a reasonable approximation is given from the two simple expressions derived by Martin:

$$\text{the new sphere} = D \left(1 + \frac{\sin^2\theta}{3}\right),$$

and the new cylinder $= D \tan^2\theta$

where D is the power of the sphere and θ is the angle of obliquity or tilt.

The tables printed below show the errors introduced by tilting a 1-D sphere and a 10-D sphere through various angles when the index of refraction of the glass is 1.523.

A 1.00 D spherical lens tilted

Obliquity (degrees)	Spherical value (D)	Cylindrical value (D)
10	1.0102	0.031
15	1.0228	0.073
20	1.0406	0.138
25	1.0632	0.231
30	1.0833	0.347

A 10.00 D spherical lens tilted

Obliquity (degrees)	Spherical value (D)	Cylindrical value (D)
10	10.101	0.314
15	10.228	0.734
20	10.409	1.379
25	10.648	2.315
30	10.448	3.349

This astigmatic effect produced by the refraction of a pencil of light through an inclined lens may be used to advantage by patients who require a horizontal cylinder. Thus it may be useful in aphakic patients who frequently have a cylinder in the horizontal axis, which must be decreased in strength after some weeks, a change which can be effected by merely straightening the spectacles. Another advantage of the method is that the lenses are lighter without the cylindrical addition.

If the glass is not 10 D sphere but some other value, the figures in the table are multiplied by the tenth part of the power of the lens: thus if the strength of the sphere is 9 D or 11 D, they are multiplied by 0.9 or 1.1. Hence if an effect of + 11.5 D sph. + 1.5 D cyl. ax. 180° is required, since

$$1.1 \times 10.409 = 11.5$$
$$\text{and } 1.1 \times 1.379 = 1.5$$

the effect can be obtained by prescribing +11 D sphere tilted downwards at 20 degrees.

Similarly, if a high myope of −20 D sph. −2.5 cyl. ax. 180° complains of the weight or expense of his spectacles, he can be treated in the same way. Thus:

$$1.9 \times 10.409 = 19.78$$
$$\text{and } 1.9 \times 1.379 = 2.62$$

He is therefore given −19.75 D sphere inclined at 20 degrees.

DISCOMFORT ARISING THROUGH SPECTACLES: SPECTACLE INTOLERANCE

The reasons for the inability of a patient to use with comfort the spectacles prescribed for him are varied, some of them due to the patient himself, some to the prescriber and some to the dispenser.

The patient's ocular condition may be one in which it is inherently difficult to correct the vision with spectacles. In the higher degrees of ametropia the best form of lenses does not entirely eliminate their disadvantages — optical, physical or cosmetic — as we have noted, for example, in discussing the correction of aphakia and high myopia.

One important source of trouble is the distortion of the image due to peripheral magnification. This is positive in convex and negative in concave lenses when the peripheral field is compared with the central, so that long straight lines become curved after the manner of Figure 24.35, when viewed through the spectacles. In this way objects appear to be misshapen when looked at, and since the

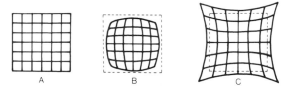

Fig. 24.35 Distortion by lenses.

(A) Object viewed through a plane glass. (B) The same object viewed through a concave lens. (C) The same object viewed through a convex lens. The dotted line in B and C indicates the real size.

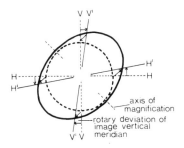

Fig. 24.36 The distortion of the image by a cylindrical lens.

VV and HH (the broken lines) represent the outline of an undistorted image; V′V′ and H′H′ (the continuous lines) represent the rotary deviation produced by a cylindrical lens the axis of magnification of which is indicated.

curvature increases as the peripheral parts of the spectacles are used they seem to move when the head is turned. They may prove extremely annoying to the wearer, but it is an unavoidable fault the effect of which can be minimised only with use or by lenticular glasses.

The distorting effects of cylinders are also important, and these vary with the relation of the direction of the axes. Where the axes are parallel and each eye is subjected to the same deviation, the effect is minimised, but when this is not so an annoying distortion occurs involving a rotary deviation in which linear objects appear to slant and flat surfaces to slope (Fig. 24.36). When any difference exists between the two eyes the lenses must be very accurately centred otherwise there will be a tendency towards distortion effects wherein rectangles appear as rhomboids; this, of course, occurs unavoidably when the periphery of the lenses is used. Where the difference in the direction of the cylinders is small (about 10 or

20 degrees), the annoyance may wear off in time; but where the difference in the direction of the cylinders is greater than this amount, the optical effect may give rise to real trouble. For this reason different spectacles may be advisable for reading and for distance and, if necessary, for work, each being accurately centred for the purpose for which they are intended. It is to be noted also that the nearer the lenses are placed to the eye, the less these distortion effects are evident.

Another important source of trouble with cylindrical corrections is an alteration in axis when re-ordering for an established spectacle wearer; even when this seems to be correct on retinoscopy and subjective testing, distortion is experienced and a reversion to the old, well tolerated axis is necessary.

Problems with peripheral magnification also apply to cases of anisometropia even when the error is spherical. On looking towards the periphery of two lenses of different power, say 1 D and 5 D, the prismatic effect is very different; if the visual axes are directed downwards 1 cm the prismatic deviation in one eye will be 1 prism dioptre and in the other 5. Here again, when the refractive error is large, the field of comfortable vision is limited to a small central area, and differently centred and tilted spectacles should be employed for near work. If prolonged work or study were attempted through the peripheral parts of the distance lenses in such a case, the difference in the prismatic effect would be intolerable, leading to disturbances of spatial orientation.

As it is, people with high errors (aphakics and high myopes) are constantly troubled on these occasions when they must look eccentrically through their lenses, as for example going downstairs. These annoyances are unavoidable and can only be diminished by custom. The corrected eye has three elements in its optical system: the spectacle lens, the cornea, and the crystalline lens. It is quite impossible to combine the three into a perfect and harmoniously working optical system, and when the refractive error is large and the lenses are strong, a certain amount of discomfort must be expected and must be tolerated.

The adaptation of an aphakic to his strong convex lenses is often a particularly trying process, apart altogether from the diplopia which may exist if the other eye retains an effective amount of vision. Fortunately many of these patients are old and sedentary and do not demand or require accurate visual perceptions. These are sometimes relatively comfortable from the start, but with those to whom accurate visual judgements are necessary and who must remain mobile, a rehabilitation problem exists which must be tackled intelligently. Initially all objects are seen larger than they appeared before (by 1/4 to 1/3, p. 71) and the distances are misjudged so that, at the least, an annoying series of accidents due to clumsiness tends to occur even in the smallest activities of life. The co-ordination of manual movements with the new visual imagery is often a difficult process which can be accomplished only by practice, preferably by repetitive exercises on such tasks as jig-saw puzzles. As a result of the spherical aberration induced by the strong convex lenses, straight lines become curves and a linear world becomes converted into parabolas which change their shape with each movement of the eyes. Thus to the newly corrected aphakic a rectilinear doorway which he approaches becomes curved inwards so as to leave a space only

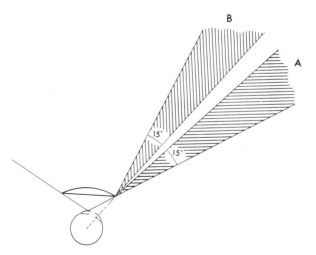

Fig. 24.37 The roving ring scotoma in corrected aphakia.

With the eye in the primary position there is a ring scotoma (A) of approximately 15 degrees. When the eye moves to the side the scotoma moves in the opposite direction (that is, towards the fixation point). It follows that if, while the eye is in the primary position, an object in the region B attracts attention and the eye is moved to fixate it, it thereupon disappears. Depending on the position of the eye, objects in this position therefore tend to appear and disappear in the most disconcerting way.

a few inches wide at the middle; it is true that if he approaches it boldly, the opening widens to admit him, but the illusion is disturbing. Only if he holds his eyes motionless and looks through the optical centre of his lens, and if he moves his head only, and not his eyes, to look at objects not straight in front of him, do these objects assume their correct shape. Once this technique of orientation has become a habit, the effects of spherical aberration disappear and cease to worry him.

Finally, as was pointed out by Welsh, the prismatic deviation necessarily occurring at the periphery of a strong lens gives rise to a ring of blindness around the central field (Fig. 24.37). For short distances (as for reading) this causes little inconvenience; for far distances beyond 6 metres (as for driving a car) the central area of clear vision is usually sufficiently large to allow adequate vision; but at intermediate distances between 1 and 3 metres the handicap presented is considerable. Thus within a room a relatively small area of clear vision is enclosed in a ring of fog. Moreover, as is seen in Figure 24.37, when the eyes move this circle of blindness moves also so that objects and persons suddenly appear and disappear after the manner of a jack-in-the-box. As the eyes move peripherally to fix an object of attention, the 'roving ring scotoma' moves in the opposite direction so that the patient suddenly does not see the person he is talking to, clumsily bumps into the furniture when he moves, stumbles on uneven ground or misses a step of the stairs with disastrous results. In time, it is true, the aphakic usually accommodates himself to these difficulties and acquires confidence, but the initial period is trying. These troubles are, of course, avoided by modern cataract surgery with lens implantation (p. 72).

Even in the lower degrees of ametropia, however, some disturbance is usual on wearing spectacles for the first time, perhaps a sensation of 'pulling' the eye and 'tightness' in the temples; this is possibly associated with the need to establish a new relationship between accommodation and convergence and is usually short-lived. The complaint of some patients that they can see reflections from their lenses can be dealt with by antireflective coating. The persistence of symptoms when wearing spectacles may simply be due to the irrelevance of the optical anomaly, although the converse is not necessarily true. It is certainly advisable in the presence of organic disease such as, for example, opacities in the ocular media, to anticipate the patient's possible dissatisfaction by giving a warning that vision will not be perfect even with the spectacles.

As far as the prescriber is concerned in the intolerance to spectacles, he may have carried out a poor refraction and ordered the wrong prescription; in another case, while the refraction itself has been impeccable in its accuracy, the spectacles ordered may have been injudicious. Thus, the sudden prescription of a high correction to a patient who has not previously worn spectacles is inadvisable, and it is wiser to advise an undercorrection which can be gradually strengthened over a period of months. Perhaps the most common fault is to prescribe too strong an addition for reading in patients with presbyopia; occasionally the opposite situation occurs and the patient returns saying he still cannot read adequately. For this no rules can be firmly laid down and few refractionists have escaped trouble from presbyopic prescriptions. It should be emphasised again that the nature of the task for which near vision is required must be carefully elucidated in each individual case, in particular the position in which a book is habitually held or the working distance and the fineness of the objects being inspected at work. Bifocal lenses frequently give rise to trouble in this respect and, in addition, complaints of dizziness on looking down while wearing them are common; in this event attention should be paid to the power, type, size and position of the segment, and where appropriate these should be adjusted, or alternatively it is frequently necessary to advise that bifocals be discontinued (see below).

Where the jump from distance portion to segment is disturbing, and especially if there is difficulty with intermediate distances, multifocals may help but these sometimes bring problems of their own.

Re-examination in cases of intolerance should always include a further assessment of the muscular balance; if it is deranged the prescription of prisms or the use of orthoptic exercises may be advisable. Finally, the prescriber may have been less than careful to eliminate organic disease during the general ophthalmic examination or, where reading difficulties seem to persist in spite of the proper optical correction, the possibility must be eliminated that the cause is not a defect of the visual field such as an unsuspected hemianopia, a small paracentral scotoma, or some alexic or dyslexic anomaly.

The dispensing of the spectacles is occasionally at fault and may be responsible for some cases of intolerance. These may relate solely to the frame or other aspect of the fitting. In practice, the form of the lenses is often left to the manufacturer, but the prescriber can and should indicate the need for any special form of lens in certain cases. The centring of the lenses and the degree of pantoscopic tilt must also be extremely accurate. A tactful suggestion to the effect that certain shapes of frames are unsuitable in the higher degrees of ametropia may prevent future trouble such as complaints of the restriction of the field. Many of these considerations apply with equal force to the changing of spectacles; a high myope, for example, may not welcome an alteration in the form of the spectacles, even if the new lenses are of the same dioptric power as those previously worn.

So far as the lenses themselves are concerned, points of importance are the occurrence of a small change in the back vertex distance in strong lenses; a change in the base curve from previous lenses; a change from flat lenses to meniscus or toric forms; and finally, a difference in the base curve in two eyes of approximately equal refraction.

SPECIAL TYPES OF SPECTACLES

Combination of lenses: bifocal spectacles

The inconvenience to the presbyope of changing his spectacles to suit the distance at which he desires to work may be overcome by the use of spectacles in which more than one lens is incorporated. The usual type is the *bifocal lens*, wherein the upper segment is adapted for distant vision and the lower one for near vision. These were first used by Benjamin Franklin in 1784, who suggested a two-piece or 'split' glass, composed of two separate segments held together

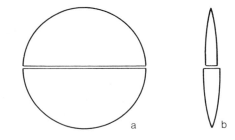

Fig. 24.38 Franklin bifocal lens. (*a*) Front view, (*b*) section.

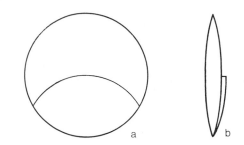

Fig. 24.39 Bifocal lens with supplementary wafer. (*a*) Front view, (*b*) section.

in a frame with a horizontal dividing line between them (Fig. 24.38).

This split bifocal is now hardly encountered, and the improvements upon it which are now used are of three types: the cemented wafer, the fused bifocal and the solid bifocal.

In the first of these a supplementary lens or 'wafer' was cemented onto the surface of the main lens (Fig. 24.39). One surface of the wafer is worked to correspond to the spherical or cylindrical lens upon which it is to lie, while the other supplies the necessary additional curvature: thus if it were proposed to add an additional correction of +3 D to a distance lens of +2 D sphere, a wafer the surfaces of which were ground to −2 D and +5 D would be necessary. The cement employed is Canada balsam, which has the same refractive index as glass, but it suffers from the disadvantage that it may dry and crystallise or may soften and allow some degree of movement. Such a lens, however, has the advantages that it is easy to make, is inexpensive, is scarcely noticeable, is easily centred, and can

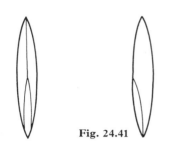

Fig. 24.40   Fig. 24.41

Figs 24.40 and **24.41** Bifocal lenses with inserted (*left*) and fused (*right*) wafers.

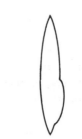

Fig. 24.42 Solid bifocal.

be removed and altered when the presbyopic error increases. An improvement in stability and in appearance was introduced by Borsch in 1899, whereby the wafer was inserted into the middle of a lens which had been split, and was cemented there (Fig. 24.40).

The split and wafer types of bifocal are, however, now virtually obsolete. Most modern bifocals are of the fused or solid variety.

Fused bifocals, introduced about 1890 by J. L. Borsch of Philadelphia, were a considerable improvement on earlier types. These 'invisible' bifocals were made by combining a lens of crown glass with a segment of flint glass of higher refractive power so that the increase in refractivity is obtained by virtue of the difference in refractive index. A depression is ground in the lens of crown glass, and a 'button' of flint glass, similarly polished and ground, is laid upon it; the two are then clipped together and heated in a furnace to 600°C until they fuse together (Fig. 24.41). The fusion is made onto the face of the lens with a spherical curve so that any cylindrical power will be the same in both portions, and the same curvature is ground all over the combined 'segment' surface. This usually means that the segment is inserted into the spherical front surface of the glass, the posterior concave surface being toric if required. The optical performance of fused bifocals is good, although with higher powered segments some chromatism is experienced because of the differing dispersions of the two types of glass.

Solid (or *one-piece*) *bifocals*, on the other hand, introduced in England in 1906, are made in one piece of glass, two distinct curves being ground upon one spherical surface, the segment side

(usually the posterior except in some high ametropias), any cylinder being ground on the other (Fig. 24.42). The production of such a combination, however, if it is to be free from optical defects, is not without technical difficulties.

In addition to the matter of their technical form, bifocals may vary very considerably in the shape, size and position of their segments, and before considering the advantages or otherwise of these many differing factors we must say something of the features which are particularly desirable from the functional standpoint. These features must take account of the optical functions and defects of bifocal spectacles as well as the purposes for which the wearer requires such a correction.

The optical function of bifocal spectacles

In the common variety the upper portion of the spectacle lens subserves distant vision and the lower, smaller segment corrects for near work. In addition to lightness and inconspicuousness, the requirements from the optical point of view are three:

1. The two portions should provide equally clear vision free from aberrations. Bending to a toric form can usually satisfy this requirement although some oblique astigmatism is inevitable because of eccentric viewing through the lower segment.

2. There should be no sudden change in the prismatic effect at the junction of the two segments so that, when the eye changes from one to the other, objects do not appear to 'jump'.

This requires that the optical centres of both distant and reading portions should be located at or near the junction of the two segments; the ideal is a *monocentric bifocal* wherein they are coincident. Alternatively, jump may be alleviated by a prism, base up, in the reading segment.

3. The centring of the two portions should be exact for their different purposes and therefore separately controllable, a matter which is far from straightforward.

In distant vision the visual axis of the eye passes through the spectacle lens at a point referred to as the *distance visual point* (DVP), which should coincide with the optical centre. On reading, each eye moves so that its visual axis now passes through the lens at a point approximately 8 mm below and 2 mm nasal to the DVP at a point known as the *near visual point* (NVP) (Fig. 24.43).

It is quite possible that there will be a prismatic effect induced at other points which may create a muscle imbalance (especially if the subject is anisometropic) or lead to displacement of objects in the near field.

As may be imagined, the elimination of all the undesirable features may be impossible, but modern bifocals are of such profuse form that an optimal correction can usually be found. In some subjects, however, this is never the case, and intolerance of bifocals is unfortunately quite common. Part of this intolerance may be due not simply to the inherent optical disadvantages but also to a failure to consider the purposes for which the bifocals are needed.

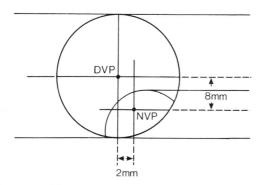

Fig. 24.43 The geometry of bifocals (see text).

Visual function with bifocal spectacles

The field of vision for near and distance viewing should be satisfactory, and here the final consideration is that the segment should not encroach too much onto the distance field. The top of the segment is usually placed 1.5 to 2 mm below the distance visual point (DVP) of the main lens but may be varied slightly for some occupational requirements, being increased to 3 to 4 mm if spectacles are continuously worn. They are often fitted with the segment top at the level of the lower lid in straight-ahead gaze.

The types of close work will influence the nature of the segment ordered. A large segment is indicated where, for example, a wide desk must be kept in view. A small one perhaps may be adequate where only casual near viewing is required such as the inspection of a theatre programme. An artist may require a predominant near portion, hence the occasional prescription of up-curve bifocals.

Particularly if the bifocals are worn constantly, some re-education is necessary in that the subject must learn to move his head appropriately for near and distance viewing, that is upwards for near and downwards for distance vision, in a fashion opposite to the way to which he has become accustomed. Some instability while walking is initially common because of the unaccustomed blur on looking downwards. To obviate this, some designs have an area for distance vision below the near segment. It should be remembered that the segment used for ordinary reading can be small, for when reading most people do not move their eyes through an arc more than 12 degrees from side to side; at the spectacle plane such a field of view is amply covered by a rectangular segment of 12.4 × 8.2 mm. A strip of only 2 to 3 mm depth will give a view of 7 or 8 inches breadth at a distance of 6 feet, which is sufficient for most purposes; at the same time it will allow a segment of 9 mm height to be used, and still leave 2 mm of segment depth in a comparatively small spectacle lens of 28 mm height.

Such a design may, however, be inadequate, and many subjects wearing bifocals of any design have difficulty in walking downstairs or stepping off a kerb. Particularly in old people, it is inadvisable to prescribe bifocals if they have not been worn previously and a considerable added correction for near vision is required; a stumble or a fall can so often have a catastrophic effect in the aged or in those with physical disabilities that cause difficulty in walking. Similarly, bifocals are best avoided by anyone prone to vertigo, whether organic or functional in origin. Moreover, some occupations, such as working at heights, also contra-indicate their use.

From the purely ophthalmological standpoint experience has shown that some conditions such as disturbances of muscle balance, especially on down gaze, and refractive anomalies such as marked anisometropia and high oblique astigmatism are particularly ill-suited for bifocal spectacles, and we should remember that the nature and strength of the subject's refractive error, as well as the required reading addition, are important factors in attaining satisfactory visual function with bifocals. The high myope with anisometropia is particularly difficult to manage with such corrections in spite of considerable ingenuity in segment design. The aphakic patient too has mixed success with bifocals, but in many subjects undue pessimism often turns out to be unjustified, and in spite of the strength of the correction it is tolerated well.

The commoner bifocal designs

The technical differences between fused and solid bifocals have been noted, and some of their functional differences are important in prescribing and dispensing them.

The fused bifocal is cosmetically very acceptable, having an impalpable break between the segments, and offers quite a range of shapes apart from the usual circular top. In the Univis designs an area of distance vision is available below the segment (Figs 24.44 and 24.45).

The disadvantages of fused bifocals include the fact that some jump is inevitable, although this may be reduced in the flat-topped shape. There is also some chromatism due to the differing refractive indices of the two glass components, and this may be troublesome in high corrections. Further, fused bifocal segments are restricted in

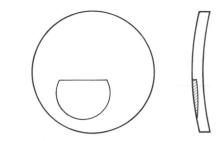

Fig. 24.44 Univis D bifocal.

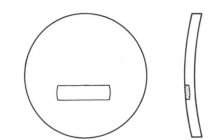

Fig. 24.45 Univis B bifocal.

size, a maximum diameter of only 25 mm being available, the usual being 22 mm. They also are unsuitable for subjects with high errors or high additions.

Solid bifocals are available with a much larger size of segment diameter, commonly 38 mm, 45 mm and sometimes 22 mm, and chromatism is slight. However, the segments are usually more visible than in the fused variety. There are visible, semivisible and invisible solid bifocals, and the degree of visibility often depends on the other optical measures required, as for example the incorporation of a prism, in order to avoid an unacceptable degree of jump. The latter results from lack of control over the optical centres in this design and is in some degree inevitable.

The break is usually palpable and the segments are not of such free shape as the fused variety. A modern flat-topped solid bifocal is the 'Executive' type in which a large reading field is available (Fig. 24.46), perhaps particularly valuable in working at a large desk. There is also a view that all round segment bifocals are best avoided if the correction is needed for VDU work.

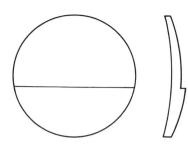

Fig. 24.46 Executive bifocal.

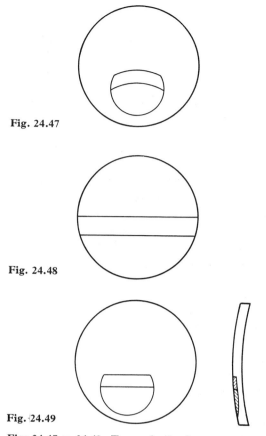

Fig. 24.47

Fig. 24.48

Fig. 24.49

Figs 24.47 to 24.49 Types of trifocals.

If a bifocal lens is so designed as to allow some selection of the sites of the optical centres, it is known as a *centre-controlled solid bifocal*. The term 'prism-controlled bifocal' is sometimes used to describe any design, not necessarily solid, in which an attempt is made to control the intrinsic prismatic effects of bifocal spectacles; it is, however, also used in a more restricted sense to describe a solid visible bifocal lens incorporating a prismatic correction solely for this purpose.

A further technical device which is frequently of considerable use is the so-called 'rising-front' bifocals. In these an adjustable step is incorporated in the nose-piece so that the spectacles can be raised or lowered. In the first position the reading segment is almost straight in front of the pupil, so that the wearer can read without having to hold the written matter below the horizontal; and in the second position the reading segment is well below the visual axis, so that the wearer is less handicapped in walking about.

As an alternative to bifocals, the additional correction for reading may be supplied as a separate pair of lenses placed in front of the distant ones ('hook-fronts'). It is more useful if these are 'pantoscopic' with 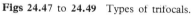 shaped lenses, so that it is easy to look over them for distant vision. To a simple presbyope lenses shaped in this way are extremely useful for reading, while the unaided eye looking over the glass is used for distance. A slight myope will frequently read most comfortably through the converse arrangement, a kidney-shaped omission, corresponding in size to an ordinary bifocal segment, being cut from the lower half of a pair of rimless distance glasses.

Trifocal lenses

Trifocal lenses were introduced in 1926 by John Isaac Hawkins of London; their designs vary

and they offer some advantages over bifocals, particularly when the amplitude of accommodation has declined to the point where intermediate distances are significantly blurred (Figs 24.47 to 24.49). In addition, the 'jump' effect of bifocals may be somewhat ameliorated. They have, however, some limitations. They are not suitable for anisometropes or when a special prism is indicated for close work; moreover, they cannot usefully be worn by those who need very small segments for occupational reasons. The strength of the intermediate addition varies in different designs but, within limits, it is usually about half the full addition required for close work.

Combination of lenses: multifocal spectacles

The modern name for these is progressive

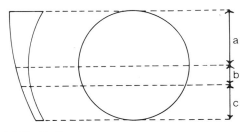

Fig. 24.50 Varilux lens.

addition lenses (abbreviated to PALs — although they are not invariably user friendly). They incorporate a near portion of the lens which has a continuously variable curve, there being a gradual accretion of power from the upper periphery to the lower reading segment where the limit of the addition ordered is attained. There are thus embodied in the one lens powers for intermediate distances from infinity to the working distance, and a sharp jump from a distance to a near focus is eliminated, incidentally conferring a cosmetic advantage. The multiple range of the lens thus counterbalances the restriction of corrections specifically for distance or for near.

One of the first types was the 'Ultifo' introduced by Gowland of Montreal in 1922. More recently the 'Varilux' lens of Maitenaz (1961–6) and the 'Omnifocal' of Volk & Weinberg (1962) were introduced. In the original Varilux lens (Fig. 24.50) the upper portion is for distance vision, below which there is a 12 mm vertical segment of increasing power until a fixed reading area is reached.

If they are tolerated, the advantages of such lenses are clearly considerable, but difficulties may arise because of restricted effective visual field and also if the corrections of the two eyes differ markedly in any respect, sphere, cylinder or axis. The lateral parts of the lenses are subject to considerable aberration on account of their non-spherical curvatures. This may lead to a sense of gross distortion on looking downwards and to the side, an effect exaggerated if there is more than a very moderate amount of astigmatism, particularly at an oblique axis. The portion of the lens which connects the distance and near

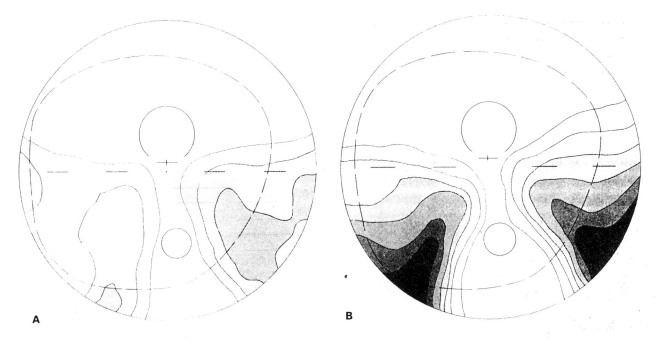

Fig. 24.51 (A) Soft and (B) hard multifocal lenses. The increasing shading indicates more oblique astigmatism and distortion.

segments, used for intermediate viewing, is distortion free in a relatively narrow corridor or channel (see Fig. 24.51B), only 2 or 3 degrees in some types.

There are now numerous designs of multifocal lens available, each attended by claims that these disadvantages are ameliorated. None eliminates them entirely, but a particular subject may be much happier with one type than another, certainly if it becomes necessary to increase the reading addition it would seem sensible to order the new multifocal correction of a form similar to that which is being worn successfully.

Generally speaking the design chosen should be such as to take into account the subject's sensitivity to distortion, the need for error-free distance correction, the width of near and intermediate fields, the precision required at these distances, and the amount of acceptable ocular depression needed for close work.

There are two extremes of design (known sometimes as 'hard' and 'soft' — terminology unfortunately easily confused with that of contact lens technology), according to the degree of unwanted astigmatism on looking downwards and nasally or downwards and laterally (Figs 24.51 A and B). This astigmatism is greater in the hard type and arises on account of the larger area of sharp definition. The opposite 'soft' design may involve some encroachment of 'add' into the upper field as well as lengthening the corridor leading down to the reading portion. Although the soft form gives smaller areas of precise definition, it is often the type preferred.

As pointed out above the choice of design is influenced by other factors, for example whether the patient is a new or established presbyope, as changing from bifocals must also be taken into account. A recent design on offer is a bifocal in which the near segment is a progressive addition lens.

Whatever is finally chosen great care must be exercised in centration of the lenses, not only in relation to the distance and near areas of the lens but also particularly in view of the relative 'waisting' of the area of intermediate vision. It has been a widespread prescribing manoeuvre to increase by 0.25 D the addition normally advised for near but this may not be necessary for some recent designs. Choice of frames with large eye sizes should be discouraged.

The verification of multifocal spectacles may be a problem. Neutralisation by lenses is complicated by the difficulty in centring over the 'maximal' add reading portion. With the focimeter some indication of the correct position is indicated by the regularity of the circle of dots, or by ensuring that the axis of cylinder is the same in the assessed reading segment as in the distance portion. Some manufacturers faintly etch the reading add on to their lenses.

OTHER TYPES OF SPECTACLES

Other types of spectacles are employed from time to time. Some examples may be quoted.

Sports spectacles may be used for specific purposes; for shooting or playing billiards the spectacles may be decentred vertically so that no prismatic effect is obtained when the eyes are rotated upwards, a device which may be supplemented by providing the side-pieces with adjustable angled joints so that the lenses can be tilted upwards for high shooting or playing long shots at billiards. In *fishing spectacles* small bifocal segments may be fitted below and to the side to allow full distant vision and provide the optical means to attach the fly. *Recumbent spectacles* are provided with prisms to allow a patient who must lie prone to read in comfort (Fig. 24.52).

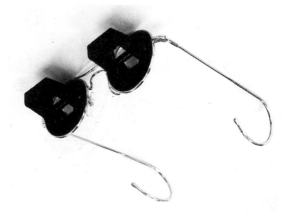

Fig. 24.52 Prismatic recumbent spectacles (Keeler).

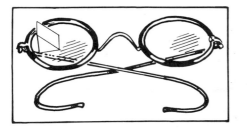

Fig. 24.53 Hemianopic spectacles.
Prismatic optical correction for hemianopia (C. A. Young).

Hemianopic spectacles are provided with a prism (8 Δ) with its base towards the blind side or a small mirror to make the wearer aware of movement in the missing part of the field, acting after the manner of the side-mirror on a car (Fig. 24.53). *Shielded* ('so lumbra') *spectacles* carry a flange which acts as a hood attached to the upper rims to eliminate glare from above, often a boon to patients with early cataract when reading. Side-shields may be similarly worn to lessen lateral glare. *Divers' spectacles* for vision under water consist of two meniscus plano lenses enclosing between them a biconcave lens of air with sufficient converging effect to compensate for the effectivity of the cornea which is abolished when immersed in water. *Crutch spectacles* are provided with a metal extension running inwards from the rim to support a drooping upper lid (*ptosis spectacles*) or evert an entropion of the lower lid.

Protective glasses

Protective lenses may be used to protect the eye from radiation by diminishing the total intensity of the light, or by cutting off a noxious portion of the spectrum, either the long heat rays (the infra-red) or the luminous (visible) rays, or the short chemically active (ultraviolet rays). Such spectacles are not necessarily used for optical purposes and therefore they will be dealt with briefly here. A very large number of various types of glass has been placed upon the market from time to time, and each has been exploited more than the other. Most of them are commercial propositions rather than scientific productions,

and few of them have anything in particular to recommend them.

They may act in one of two ways: the unwanted rays may either be *absorbed* or *reflected*. The majority belong to the first class; they are prepared by combining the glass with some chemical substance or substances with special absorbing properties, the ingredients most frequently incorporated in the glass are metals such as copper, gold, manganese, iron, cobalt, chromium and others. It can be reasonably understood that as a general rule the manufacturers are reluctant to liberate data concerning the chemical constitution of their products, but in the majority of cases the mixtures appear to be somewhat indefinite and their spectral analyses and transmission intensities often give discordant results. The prescriber will however be guided by the manufacturer's information about transmissions characteristics when deciding on the type of tinted glass appropriate to the social and occupational requirements of the patient.

Practically all these substances are coloured, and the lenses are therefore *tinted*. If they are incorporated into the glass they suffer from the disadvantage that the depth of the tint varies with the thickness of the lens; thus a convex lens will be deeply tinted in the centre while a concave one, on the other hand, will have its maximum intensity in the periphery, the central area which is really the essential part remaining more or less clear. For lenses with such '*solid*' tints, as they are known, an additional advantage is to have them as thin as possible. A considerable thickness is saved if flint glass is used instead of the usual crown glass owing to the higher refractive index of the former. A different method of procedure is to grind a plano-convex or plano-concave lens and cement a slab of a chemically tinted glass onto it or to insert such a slab into the substance of a split lens. These however suffer from the disadvantage of size and weight. Such lenses are called *isochromatic*.

The disadvantages of solid tints may be overcome by making use of the techniques of surface coating. The required tinted material is deposited on the surface of the worked lens electrolytically by the process of vacuum coating producing a fine uniform film as hard and resistant to scratching as glass is formed. This method is particularly appropriate for high myopic corrections, for certain types of bifocals and for patients with marked anisometropia where solid tints would give a different appearance of the lenses of the two eyes.

Surface coating of lenses may intentionally be varied across the surface of the lens in those particularly needed for outdoor activities, coating being denser in the upper part — so-called *gradient* lenses.

A third process is used for colouring plastic lenses, which are all surface dyed.

Alternatively instead of absorbing the unwanted rays by chemical substances, they may be *reflected* on a mirror surface as was proposed by Shreiner of America (mirrored lenses). Such surfaces are formed by layers of a metal such as gold or platinum or silver of such extreme thinness (of the order of 10 to 15 µm) that they remain to a larger extent transparent to luminous rays. The delicate lamella is then protected by incorporating it in the substance of a split lens where it is cemented or fused.

For cutting off the luminous rays and thus lessening the discomforts of glare, various forms of tinted lenses are used; they are thus of service in places where the sun is strong, or where its intensity is increased by the reflection of light from a large mirror surface such as the sea, the plains of the tropics, the desert, or a snow field. In ordinary illumination however they are quite unnecessary for the healthy eye, and the frequency with which they are employed in temperate climates depends upon fashion and erroneous ideas of the action of light upon the eye.

In addition to diminishing the intensity of light in the normal eye, tinted lenses may be of service in protecting the abnormal or diseased eye from an excess of light. They are thus useful in cases where prolonged mydriasis is necessary, in albinos, who are provided with an inadequate supply of pigment to absorb an excess of scattered light, and in cases of recent ocular surgery or anterior segment inflammation producing photophobia, such as in cases or iritis or corneal ulceration. They may also be helpful where surgical or other trauma has interfered with the contraction or integrity of the pupil. Tinted glasses may also be of considerable help in certain photosensitive diseases, for example lupus erythematosus, solar urticaria, porphyria and xeroderma pigmentosa, as well as in drug-induced photosensitivity (phenothiazines and tetracyclines are examples of such drugs).

When the eyes are healthy the ideal lens is that which cuts off as little of the light as is necessary and cuts it off throughout the spectrum uniformly so that colour schemes are interfered with as little as possible. In this way the sombre and depressing effect which all tinted glasses tend to produce is reduced to a minimum and the appearance of things is changed as little as possible. It is important to realise that the actual colour of the tinted glass, whether pink, green, brown, yellow or neutral grey, bears no definite relationship to the absorption of any particular wavelength. Having said this, however, it is usually found that for solid glass tints selective infra-red absorbers tend to be green, while those for selective ultraviolet performance tend to be brown or pink. High ultraviolet absorption is nevertheless a feature of nearly all types of optical tinted glass.

As far as ordinary *sunglasses* are concerned the most important criterion to be satisfied apart from those just mentioned is that the transmission of the invisible ultraviolet light will not be at a dangerous level. At present there are no internationally accepted standards for this particular feature. Recently, however, The British Standards Institution has adopted a system of shade numbers assigned to various transmittance classes of sunglasses which incorporate maximum permitted levels of ultraviolet transmission.

The shortest wavelength of ultraviolet (UV) radiation from the sun which reaches the earth's surface is 208 nm. Between this and the visible *wavelengths* (380 nm to 770 nm — violet to red) the ultraviolet is divided into UVA and UVB. UVA (315–380 nm), responsible for suntanning, can enter the eye but is largely absorbed by the lens. UVB (280–315 nm), which may cause blistering and sunburn, does not enter the eye significantly but is responsible for corneal epithelial disruption giving the clinical picture of photophthalmia. UVC (280–100 nm) does not reach the earth's surface, but UV light of 193 nm has some distant refractive significance in that it is the wavelength used in the Excimer laser.

Although the infra-red region region (780 nm or longer) is present in sunlight it rarely exceeds the biologically acceptable level except in particular abuse of the eyes resulting in macular burns, the condition of eclipse blindness. If specific infra-red protection for a particular subject is required it is suggested that the transmission should not exceed that of the visible wavelengths.

The actual transmission of visible light in various types of sunglasses varies enormously. Cosmetic spectacles may transmit anything from 30 to 100%, most frequently not more than 80%, of incident light. True sunglasses transmit 30% or less, but intense exposure may require even lower transmissions, down to less than 10%; in such conditions as winter sports particular attention must be paid to the ultraviolet, which is both directly and diffusely reflected from snow.

For perfectly healthy eyes transmissions below 50 to 60% are rarely required for any indoor activity. Moderate sunlight may require 30 to 50% transmission outdoors. Driving glasses for daytime use should not reduce transmission to less than 50% except in very bright conditions. Night driving should not require anything other than some antiglare formulation.

All of these conditions apply similarly to prescription tinted glasses where ordered for those cases in which an optical correction is to be incorporated.

Photochromic glass ('Photogray', 'Photobrown', 'Reactolite Rapide', 'Umbramatic', 'Heliovar', 'Colormatic') alters its colour on exposure to ultraviolet light. This property is imparted to it by incorporated submicroscopic crystals of substances such as silver halides which turn dark, absorbing white light; the more intense the ultraviolet the darker the substance goes, and photochromic materials in general are good ultraviolet absorbers. Their main function is of course to interfere with the visible rays.

Full darkening leads to the exclusion of up to 90% or more of visible light effected by a combination of absorption and reflection. The transmission figures quoted usually relate to a standard 2-mm-thick lens. The darkening and fading function does not significantly interfere with the relative perceptions of colour, and in the most modern types these functions are only slightly temperature dependent between 0 and 32°C. Absorption of ultraviolet by windscreen glass may reduce the efficiency of photochromic spectacles used for driving.

The times taken to darken and to fade differ, the latter being much more prolonged, and advanced modern glass will half-darken in 10 seconds and half-fade in 100 seconds. Photochromic glass can be used in the make-up of any prescription, whether single vision, bifocal or multifocal in type. Both laminated and high-index photochromic lenses are available. Laminated lenses are valuable for high prescriptions and in cases of anisometropia, as the photochromic property is of course independent of the final thickness of the lens. There are also photochromic plastic lens materials, but these usually take the form of a surface layer covered by a hard antireflection coating, and they are said to be not as efficient as glass photochromics.

Polaroid lenses incorporate a different principle. They consist of a film mounted between two pieces of glass as in an ordinary laminated lens, the films being a matrix of minute dichroic crystals about 10^{12} per sq. in orientated so that the whole acts as one large crystal which polarises light in one direction. In protective glasses it is used as an analyser so as to arrest horizontally polarised light. Reflected light is partially polarised in a plane parallel to the reflecting surface so that the glare from extensive smooth surfaces such as a concrete road or an expanse of water which has a significant component of horizontally polarised light is lessened. Because of this polaroid spectacles may be of value to motorists, yachtsmen and fishermen, and since they are coloured they tone down the ordinary light in addition.

Antireflective coating of spectacle lenses is said to promote the transmission of luminous rays through the glass and at the same time to hide the multiple reflective rings seen at the edge of a high myopic correction. It has also been said to be a help to those needing a correction when using a VDU, and during night driving.

Industrial protection

Apart from mechanical injury (see below)

exposure to harmful radiation may occur. Thus in metal smelting and glass blowing excessive infra-red radiation may be of such a degree as to lead to retinal damage or cataract unless appropriate protective glasses are worn.

'Arc eye', which occurs in electric arc welders exposed to too much ultraviolet light, often with a component of shorter wavelength than solar ultraviolet, produces a clinical picture similar to photophthalmia, snowblindness, which is also seen in cinema studios and in ultraviolet light clinics. It was precisely to avoid these ultraviolet and infra-red exposures that the original but now largely outdated Crookes glasses were designed (Crookes sage green glass eliminated 95% of the infra-red as well as a proportion of the luminous spectrum). Some modern tints are designed specifically for industrial purposes, especially welding ('Noviweld'). There were also multiple function glasses such as Pfunds's gold-plated, glass which consisted of a thin lamina of prepared gold reflecting the infra-red between a lens of ordinary crown glass and Crookes A which cut out the ultraviolet.

Spectacles designed as a protection against mechanical injury are usually provided with side-pieces in the form of goggles and are used in many industries. They may be supplied as flat pieces of glass, or in order to provide a greater visual field they may be blown into the shape of a globe. In the latter case however the unequal cooling of the glass often gives rise to distortion effects and they should be chosen with care. The two principal types of goggles are the cup type and the box type. Both afford excellent lateral protection, but the cup type cannot be worn over an existing spectacle correction. Simple plastic eye shields are available which can be worn as spectacles over an existing correction. Finally a spectacle correction itself may have protective side-pieces on one or both sides. This is not only of use industrially but of course also for cases where some pathological condition of the eye has increased its exposure risk, for example conditions such as corneal anaesthesia from whatever cause (see below). Other forms of ocular protection are face screens or shields, and in particular those designed for welding, where there may be a facility for interchangeable filters

which cover both gas and electric welding operations.

The possibility of mechanical damage to spectacle lenses in themselves in either industrial or other circumstances has led to measures specifically designed to avoid the danger of splintering.

Triplex or one of the more modern forms of non-splintering glass may be used in spectacles. They are especially useful for car drivers and pilots or for children or those who play games wearing spectacles. A Triplex lens consists of two segments of glass, between which is a plate of cellulose acetate, the three being cemented together in a manner sufficiently adhesive that if the whole is shattered it cracks into fragments but does not splinter and fly while at the same time it remains airtight and watertight. It can be ground into any lens form in the ordinary way. In the more recently produced types of glass the interpolated material is itself adhesive; consequently no sealing is required at the edges and the lens is considerably thinner. Plastic materials such as Perspex and CR39 do not splinter and thus have a considerable safety factor.

A further method of avoiding splintering is the use of a case-hardened (or toughened) lens of glass which is prepared in the ordinary manner so that there is a minimum central thickness of 3 mm. The lens is then heated to 1330°F in an oven and rapidly cooled by an air draft or oil immersion. This temperature is just insufficient to distort the glass yet adequate to anneal it so that when it is rapidly cooled the outer shell hardens more quickly than the inner mass. The resulting compression generated within the lens makes the outer layer crumble on impact without the lens fracturing or breaking into pieces. Finally, mention must be made of a very common process applied to spectacle lenses these days, which is to coat them with some material which makes them scratch resistant.

Though all sports involve a risk of ocular injury squash seems to be a particularly dangerous one, racquet and ball being the offending articles. This is now so well recognised that special squash protection spectacles are available and should always be used. Ocular protection is also advisable if the eye itself has some anomaly making it susceptible to what a healthy eye would withstand. Protective side-pieces are often fitted in cases of potential exposure problems whether due to pathology leading to corneal anaesthesia, treatment for trigeminal neuralgia or other involvement of the trigeminal nerve or to lagophthalmos as in a prolonged Bell's palsy.

25. Contact lenses

INTRODUCTION

An optical correction worn in apposition with the cornea has several advantages over spectacles. The first of course is cosmetic, and indeed most contact lenses worn today are prescribed for this reason. There are however many ways in which a contact lens may be optically superior to spectacles. For example it moves very largely with the eye, and vision through it is therefore much less liable to the peripheral distortion which occurs on eccentric viewing through a powerful spectacle lens. Furthermore, the size of the retinal image may be more physiological, thus facilitating binocularity in anisometropia or uniocular aphakia. Being bathed in tears, contact lenses are not subject to 'misting up' as are spectacle lenses in humid or other climatic conditions.

BASIC CONTACT LENS TECHNOLOGY

Modern contact lenses are classified as rigid or non-rigid according to the type of material of which they are made (Fig. 25.1). The term *rigid* contact lenses covers both types of what are known as *hard* lenses. The material is either 'Perspex' (polymethylmethacrylate, PMMA), the common plastic from which most contact lenses were made until the late 1970s, or one of the large number of new substances characterised by their permeability to gases, particularly oxygen. Most rigid lenses prescribed today are of this *gas-permeable* type.

Non-rigid lenses, usually referred to as *soft*, may also be made from any of a different group of newer plastic materials.

A further distinction between rigid and

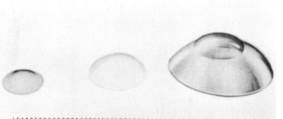

Fig. 25.1 The various types of contact lens. Hard, corneal, soft and scleral from left to right. A mm scale is shown.

non-rigid lenses is the degree to which they cover the eye. Rigid lenses, whether PMMA or gas permeable, are essentially corneal lenses, their overall size being less than that of the cornea. Non-rigid soft lenses extend 1.5 to 2 mm beyond the limbus to cover the most anterior part of the conjunctiva and sclera (Fig. 25.1).

In physical dimension, they are a reduced version of the now largely out-moded *scleral lenses*. These were the original form of contact lenses, initially of glass and later of PMMA or gas-permeable material which had a large portion (the haptic — hence the alternative name for scleral lenses — *haptic lenses*) resting on the sclera. We shall make brief reference to these below.

THE PRACTICAL PROBLEMS OF CONTACT LENS FITTING

The decision to fit a patient with modern contact lenses involves making choices based on the experience of the practitioner. Here are some of the factors to be taken into account:

1. *To fit or not to fit?* Clinical suitability, psychological, physiological and physical, for contact lenses at all; conditions for which the lenses are indicated; the reason they are desirable, be it cosmetic, or visual or both.
2. *What type of lens?* Is the lens to be rigid or non-rigid, for daily wear, extended wear or disposable?
3. *What parameters should the lens have?*

Clinical indications and contra-indications

The type of optical error

In *myopia* the corneal contact lens finds its most widespread clinical application. In lower degrees the main advantage is cosmetic; spectacles are avoided and the appearance of a small eye produced by myopic spectacle lenses is also abolished, a large attractive globe being seen instead. To this are added the optical advantages of increased size of the retinal image obtained with contact lenses, and effectively wider field of vision, and the elimination of the distortion experienced when looking through an eccentric portion of a spectacle lens. A counterbalancing fact to these advantages is the relatively greater effort of accommodation and convergence required in the myope when wearing contact lenses; this may be of no consequence in young subjects but is important in presbyopic patients in whom difficulties in near vision may be precipitated.

A variety of fitting techniques and designs is available, the choice of which depends on the personal fancy and experience of the individual practitioner. In the higher degrees the optical advantages of contact lenses are correspondingly increased but problems arise in their fitting. Such lenses are relatively heavy and every effort is made to reduce them to be as thin as possible.

In the *hypermetrope* the incentive to wear contact lenses is on the whole much less, for most young hypermetropes do not need a constant optical correction and older patients are not so concerned with cosmetic considerations. In any event the optical advantages of contact lenses in preference to spectacles are marginal. There may

be a reduced requirement for accommodation and convergence resulting from the approximation of the optical correction to the eye, as well as the avoidance of the prismatic effect of strong convex spectacle lenses. The size of the retinal image is smaller in hypermetropia with a contact lens than with spectacles.

In *aphakia* the patient corrected with a high convex spectacle lens experiences several untoward effects which we have already discussed; when a spectacle correction is worn the size of the image is 1/4 to 1/3 larger than in the phakic eye (involving an intolerable aniseikonia in uniocular aphakia), peripheral vision is accompanied by distortion due to oblique astigmatic effects and other aberrations, and the prismatic effect of the edge of the lens leads to a roving ring scotoma in the field of vision which in any event is restricted. Many of these unpleasant optical effects can be eliminated by wearing contact lenses, of either the hard or soft variety, a mode of correction employed for binocular as well as uniocular aphakia, and in those cataract-operated patients in whom intra-ocular lens implantation was impossible or considered undesirable.

In *anisometropia* contact lenses are of value because they abolish the prismatic effects obtained with spectacles when the eyes look through parts of the lenses other than their optical centres. Moreover, the size of the retinal image when contact lenses are worn differs from that obtained with spectacle lenses so that they may diminish the aniseikonia. There is some dispute as to whether this applies to all types of anisometropia. Theoretically, the advantages of contact lenses over spectacles should be most marked in refractive rather than axial anisometropia, and in the reverse condition spectacle lenses should be preferable. In view of the complex inter-relationships of the components of the refraction, however, it is not possible to determine clinically whether the eyes of a subject with anisometropia have refractive or axial anomalies, and it is likely that many subjects have a combination of both. It thus follows that a trial of contact lenses is clinically justified in any type of anisometropia, certainly if a correction by spectacles is not acceptable.

In other optical conditions contact lenses may

be advantageous; these include a moderate (not excessive) degree of astigmatism, presbyopia and keratoconus. As these give rise to special problems relating to the type of lens required, they will be discussed in more detail below.

The ophthalmological findings

Only general guidance can be given about how particular ocular conditions affect the likelihood of successful contact lens wear. There are no absolutely hard and fast rules.

Active ocular disorders are usually definite contra-indications; these include inflammatory diseases of the lids, conjunctiva, cornea or anterior uveal tract. Lid conditions such as squamous or rosaceal blepharitis, styes and chalazia, or any condition where excessive sebaceous or Meibomian secretion is formed, are unfavourable to contact lens wear. Redness of the bulbar conjunctiva and the presence of follicles or papillae on the inner tarsal surface, whether allergic or infective in origin, may also indicate an unsuitable subject. Lacrimal anomalies must also be considered, e.g. defective secretion of tears associated with keratoconjunctivitis sicca, rapid break-up time of the tear film or corneal dry spots on fluorescein staining. Small pinguecula need not be a contra-indication but a pterygium is. Trachomatous corneal scarring does not preclude wear if the corneal vascularisation is light, nor does old interstitial keratitis. Corneal anaesthesia from whatever cause strongly contra-indicates the wearing of contact lenses.

Glaucoma, either simple or closed angle, need not necessarily be considered a contra-indication; special techniques may be adopted if a drainage bleb is present. A history of retinal detachment or a tendency to it raises some problems, particularly in high myopes. There is no evidence that the wearing of any type of contact lens increases the likelihood of this complication, but it is obvious that a patient who is apt to be clumsy in manipulating the lens into and out of the eye is unsuitable.

Corneal surgery, as for example after trauma or grafting procedures, is no contra-indication to wearing a contact lens, and may in fact be a positive indication. The ophthalmological examination as a whole is of course highly relevant to the non-optical use of contact lenses for either prosthetic or therapeutic purposes, and some reference to these will be made later.

General findings

These may also have a bearing on the ability to tolerate contact lenses. Allergic diseases of the upper respiratory tract such as asthma, hay fever or vasomotor rhinitis are often reflected in sufficient conjunctival hyperaemia and irritability to make wearing lenses difficult. Similarly a history of contact dermatitis should be regarded with suspicion in view of the possibility of allergy to plastic material. Fitting is also inadvisable during pregnancy, and this is believed to be associated with changes in the corneal shape, possibly due to oedematous swelling. The taking of oral contraceptives has been blamed for poor tolerance of contact lenses.

The manual dexterity of the patient must of course be taken into account as, apart from the patient himself, the conditions in which the lenses are to be worn must also be considered. Hot dusty atmospheres are unsuitable, and those engaged in dirty occupations or exposed to chemical or conjunctival irritation will probably be unable to tolerate the lenses. Similarly high altitudes as in flying may give rise to discomfort owing to changes in the atmospheric pressure.

Psychological factors always need consideration. Many subjects are highly motivated to proceed to contact lenses either from cosmetic considerations or because of promised visual advantages especially if there is a need to wear contact lenses during the subject's occupation. Nevertheless some patients are appalled at the idea of any physical object approaching or 'in' their eyes and cannot even consider embarking on a trial. Sometimes this factor emerges only after starting the fitting procedure. In other instances an impression of personal untidiness may suggest an increased risk of corneal infection if a less than scrupulous regime is likely to be followed in the insertion, cleaning and storage of the contact lenses.

It will be appreciated that a full ocular history and examination as well as a review of the patient's general health are essential before a decision can be made as to whether to attempt to fit corneal lenses, but summarising the positive factors the ideal contact lens patient will be highly motivated, with good manual dexterity and scrupulous personal hygiene; ocular examination including slit-lamp inspection will show no abnormality of the lids, lashes and lacrimal apparatus, cornea or conjunctiva with a good blink rate and normal closure. Age itself is, within limits, immaterial; although most wearers are young adults, both children and the old can learn to wear lenses successfully.

The choice of the type of lens

Two questions have to be answered. First, is the lens to be the hard or soft type? Secondly, having decided that, what material is the lens to be made of?

Hard or soft?

With regard to the choice of hard or soft lens, the initial consideration is always that a soft lens is likely to be more comfortable but problems arise with respect to visual performance, especially in cases where there is a significant degree of corneal astigmatism. In the optical system of an eye wearing a hard lens any astigmatic effect of the cornea is abolished because the corneal substance and tears have almost the same refractive index as the material of the contact lens and the front spherical surface of this lens becomes effectively the front surface of a uniform ocular system. The majority of soft lenses are spherical in design and being pliable simply conform themselves to an astigmatic corneal surface, thereby losing the optical advantage of the hard lens. If therefore one is prescribing for a patient with a refraction having less than 1 dioptre of corneal astigmatism a soft lens will usually be first choice. With astigmatism of greater than 1 D, the alternatives lie between choosing a hard lens and trying a soft lens of special design. Between 1 and 2 D of astigmatism, a spherical soft lens may be satisfactory if the patient is prepared to accept less than perfect corrected vision.

Similarly for a patient with other corneal irregularities such as keratoconus, again a soft lens is likely to be optically poorer than a hard lens, in fact the optical performance of hard lenses is always likely to be better than that of soft ones and, even though toric soft lenses are now widely available, a hard lens of purely spherical dimensions may still be the first choice if only on grounds of simplicity of the fitting procedure and economy, particularly if absolute clarity of vision is felt by the patient to take precedence over comfort.

Nevertheless, patients thought to be particularly sensitive to the 'feel' of contact lenses should be advised to try soft lenses even though most types are more expensive.

Any occupation or leisure activity such as sport which may be embarrassed by the lens displacing itself perhaps indicates soft rather than hard lenses, the latter being more prone to get out of position.

An important environmental or occupational factor militating against soft lens wear is the possibility of absorption into the lens material of atmospheric toxic substances, or of regularly used eyedrops. For a similar reason, patients with marginally adequate tear secretion will do better with hard non-absorbent lens materials.

A patient's own ideas about which are desirable are important. The prospect that little handling of the lens would be required in an extended-wear regime may be welcome and usually indicates soft lenses, and gas-permeable lenses should not be worn this way except on a very limited basis (2 days).

Other factors to be weighed in the choice between hard and soft lenses include the relatively simple care regime for the former as well as their durability. Soft lens wear brings with it a greater possibility of infective and allergic reactions.

The need for a bifocal correction must also be taken into account — does the patient want to avoid the use of spectacles altogether?

At the time of writing, it looks as if all our criteria may have to be re-examined with the forthcoming increase in availability of disposable soft lenses which will offer a different kind of reduction in handling and wearing problems.

There is a whole group of contact lens wearers

for whom a change in contact lens type is indicated; this may be hard to soft for comfort or hard to gas-permeable if optical conditions are appropriate. It should, however, be stated that change for the sake of change without an optical or ophthalmological reason is undesirable. This particularly applies to long-standing and happy users of PMMA lenses who are persuaded on dubious grounds to embark on gas-permeable or soft lenses, often adding to or creating problems of storage or disinfection.

Lens material

The question of the *lens material* is in theory extremely complex, but out of the numerous choices available each practitioner will select from a personally restricted range known to be clinically satisfactory for the hard or soft lens to be prescribed. Because of their better tolerance, gas-permeable lenses are now most often prescribed if hard lenses are indicated. The classical PMMA has really become somewhat dismissed for a new contact lens wearer.

The basis of the practitioner's original selection lies in the diverse characteristics of the material. These include chemical composition, stability and inertness. Physical properties such as transparency, refractive index, good thermal conductivity, resistance to excessive heat and mechanical deformation, lightness in weight and factors influencing tolerance by the eye such as oxygen transmission, water content, wettability and, when made up into lenses, the method of manufacture, the durability and reproducibility of the finished article. Add to this considerations of cost and an element of commercial secrecy about the exact chemical make-up and it will be appreciated that an individual practitioner's choice of lens may have to be a compromise in face of the fact that an ideal contact lens material does not yet exist.

There are now so many materials marketed that some classification is needed which gives the practitioner an overall idea of the properties of the materials he is dealing with. In order not to interrupt the practical emphasis of this work, some basic information has been gathered in Tables 1, 2 and 3, Appendix II.

Three parameters are however always to the fore in considering contact lens materials, gas transmission, water content (strictly speaking saline content) and wettability, all of which are important for patient satisfaction. Patient satisfaction depends on comfort and good vision while wearing the contact lens, which in turn relate primarily to continued health of the cornea.

The cornea gets its oxygen supply from the tears, and in the contact lens wearer, oxygenation of the tears under the lens is maintained both by constant renewal of the tears under it and by oxygen transmission to the tears through the lens itself.

Tear renewal depends on slight movement of the contact lens over the cornea, especially in response to blinking. Oxygen transmission depends on the nature of the contact lens material and the thickness of the lens, hence the objective of making the lens as thin as possible compatible with physical stability. We characterise the intrinsic gas permeability (its oxygen transmission) by the Dk value.*

Gas permeability is also a correlate of water (or saline) content of soft lens materials — for example, a 20% increase in water content doubles oxygen permeability.

Gas-permeable soft lenses are largely of hydrophobic material and are therefore poorly wettable. Most soft lens materials are hydrophilic and their good wettability is an important factor in patient comfort.

Hard lens materials. Polymethylmethacrylate ('Perspex' 'Plexiglas' 'Lucite'), PMMA, is one of the enormous family of chemicals, the polymers. These essentially are chains of repeating units, the individual units being known as monomers.

The chains may in some instances consist of

---

* The Dk value is defined as the volume of oxygen in ml passing in one second through a piece of the material polymer 1 cm thick over an area 1 cm^2 for every 1 mm Hg partial pressure difference across the specimen at a defined temperature, (the European Standard is 35°C). The actual performance of a lens in transmitting oxygen is defined as Dk/L where L is the central thickness. For most contact lens materials, the Dk value is quoted as a number between 0 and 100. This multiplied by 10^{-11} gives the oxygen passage as just defined.

over 100 000 monomers. Although many polymers are naturally occurring, PMMA is a synthetic product, the monomer of which it is made up being methylmethacrylate.

The gas-permeable materials belong to one of several groups. The first is a modified polysaccharide, cellulose acetate butyrate (CAB). The most widely available of the new materials are co-polymers of siloxane and methylmethacrylate, and these have largely superseded CAB. The important qualities for contact lens consideration vary between these types of hard lens material. PMMA is a durable optically clear material, easily machined but with poor wettability and very poor oxygen transmissibility so oxygenation of the tears under the lens depends very largely on renewal by blinking.

CAB has the advantage of good oxygen transmissibility but it is also poorly wettable and can become warped if water is absorbed.

Siloxanyl methacrylate co-polymers are the basic formulation of many of the hard gas-permeable lenses in use today. As the generic name suggests, the material is characterised by good gas transmission imparted by the siloxanyl element. Nevertheless the hardness and rigidity and optical properties compare favourably with that of PMMA. Most of these gas-permeable materials are poorly wettable and cannot be heat sterilised. Recently a new group of gas-permeable materials containing fluorocarbons has been introduced. These are claimed to have the greatest oxygen transmissibility as well as significantly improved resistance to deposits and wettability. In spite of this wetting solutions are advisable when using most forms of rigid corneal lens (see Table 1, Appendix II).

Soft lens materials. A large and ever-increasing number of these materials exists, but historically soft lens materials originated by the Czech chemist Otto Wichterle. In the late 1950s and early 1960s, he introduced the first optically useful hydrogel. A hydrogel is in essence a gel which is a cross-linked polymer that swells by imbibition of water. The characteristic chemical feature is the introduction of hydrophilic groups into the monomer unit of which the polymer is made. In Wichterle's original polymer, the monomer was hydroxyethylmethacrylate (HEMA).

The property of water imbibition confers on lenses made of such material the softness and high oxygen transmissibility. Since the original polymer of Wichterle, a tremendous number of new ones has been introduced, and some of the chemical characteristics of these can be obtained from Table 2, Appendix II, indicating that soft lenses are commonly of HEMA-containing material, either alone or co-polymerised with other monomers, such as N-vinyl pyrrolidone, which are introduced to enhance some particular feature such as water imbibition or mechanical stability.

The second group of soft lens materials have no HEMA in them but contain similar substances.

Thirdly, there is a much smaller group of silicone rubber lenses; these elastomers, as they are known, are soft materials but differ fundamentally from other soft lens materials in being extremely hydrophobic, although with very good oxygen transmissibility.

Generally speaking, hydrogel soft lens materials are of either moderate (35–50%) or high (50–80%) water content, and very roughly the former are designed for daily wear and the latter for extended wear. Perhaps the commonest moderate water content material is still one of the original hydrogels based on poly-HEMA, known in the US as Polymacon or in British terminology Filcon 1a (38) (see Table 2, Appendix II).

Why the extreme diversity in the continued search for new materials? The answer to this is that the hydrophilic property and good oxygen transmission may be counterbalanced by other factors. These include mechanical qualities such as fragility (which also limits how thin the lens can be made), susceptibility to chemical insult, problems of manufacture, etc.

Some HEMA lenses contain ionisable material, and this leads to a pH-determined swelling of the lens material by water imbibition in a relatively less acid environment. Although such material may help to stabilise the water content, any pH change may have other disadvantages (see p. 256). Other chemical factors include the degree of cross-linkage of the polymer chains of which the material is made up; the more cross-linkages there are, the better the physical stability of the material.

Determining parameters of the lens

We begin this section with a description of the essential measurements in contact lens wear, the curvature and size of the cornea and dimensions of the lenses themselves.

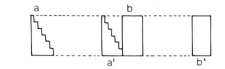

Fig. 25.2 See text.

Measuring the eye

In most reliable techniques for contact lens fitting, *keratometry* is essential. Keratometry, measurement of the curvature of the anterior corneal surface, makes use of the first Purkinje image. The corneal surface acts as a convex mirror so that the size of the image produced varies with the curvature — the greater the curvature of the mirror the smaller the image. A luminous body is therefore held up before the cornea and the image as seen therein is measured; hence, knowing the size of the object and its distance from the eye, the radius of curvature of the cornea can be deduced.

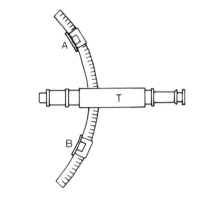

Fig. 25.3 See text.

The accurate measurement of such an image however raises a problem since it is impossible to immobilise the living eye completely while the image is under observation. This has been overcome by devices using the *principle of visible doubling*. In one type of instrument the image is doubled by refraction through two rotating glass plates, which are then adjusted so that the lower edge of one image coincides with the upper edge of the other; if the eye moves during the process, both images move together, and therefore difficulties in adjustment are avoided. From the amount of rotation of the glass plate necessary just to double the image its size can be calculated. A modern version of this is the Bausch & Lomb instrument in which the movement of prisms changes the degree of doubling.

In other types of keratometer the amount of doubling produced by a Woolaston prism is fixed, but the size of the external object can be varied. This consists of a plate of two rectangular quartz prisms cut in opposite axes, cemented together.

The classical Javal–Schiotz instrument is of this type: the objects reflected on the cornea are situated in a circular arc rotated round the axis of the instrument. The objects themselves, known as mires, are shaped as a and b in Figure 25.2

Fig. 25.4 See text.

and are considered as the end of a linear object, AB (Fig. 25.3) which appears on the cornea in duplicate as ab and a'b'. A and B are adjusted on the arc so that the two images of a' and b touch each other as in Figure 25.2. The arc is now rotated through 90 degrees and a similar reading taken. If the curvature in this meridian is the same, the mires will again approximate, but if the second meridian has a greater curvature the sizes of ab and a'b' will diminish and the mires will overlap (Fig. 25.4). One mire (A) is so constructed that each step of the image 'a' corresponds to a dioptre of difference of refractive power, so that the difference in refractive power between the two meridians is readily read off by counting the degree of overlap. In the Haag-Streit keratometer (Fig. 25.5) based on the Javal–Schiotz design the mires are red and green

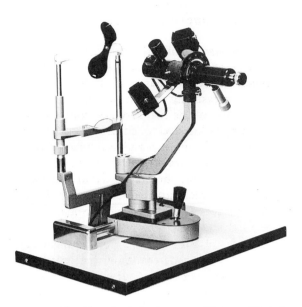

Fig. 25.5 The Haag-Streit keratometer (Clement Clarke).

objects and are internally illuminated. A third form of keratometer, the autokeratometer (Fig. 21.47) makes use of three infra-red light beams and measures the corneal curvature on each of three points of fixation.

Certain additional features particularly important in contact lens wear need noting. First, it is generally accepted that only the central 3 to 4 mm of the cornea, the optical cap or apical zone, is actually reliably measured by this technique, and in fact it is only this part of the cornea which can be regarded as having a surface of almost true optical regularity, either spherical or astigmatic.

Even if this zone is accurately measured by the correct keratometry technique, the observer must pay attention to the calibration of the particular instrument used, especially relating to the conversion of dioptric power to radii of curvature. Keratometers are usually but not always calibrated so as to read directly the radius of curvature of the cornea as well as the dioptric power. The latter figure is usually calculated on the basis of a deliberately chosen low value for the refractive index of the corneal substance, thus taking into account the slight refractive effect to

its posterior surface; the reading is therefore a net dioptric value for the central part of the cornea as a whole. For contact lens work it is of course the actual radius of curvature (not the dioptric power) which is important.

In any event, the range of some keratometers may be inadequate for the extremes of corneal curvature occasionally encountered. Provision for this is made in the Bausch & Lomb instrument, in which by interposing a +1.25 D or −1.00 D lens a range of 36 to 52 D (6.5 to 9.38 mm radii of curvature) can be extended to one of 30 to 61 D (5.6 to 10.9 mm)*. Keratometry, of course, only measures cord length between two mire images. In certain cases, the cornea between these points may have an unsuspected irregularity or distortion (see Keratoconus).

Further out than the optical zone, the peripheral cornea flattens and it remains a subject of controversy as to how much the routine fitting of contact lenses should concern itself with attempts to depict, measure and record this flattening. Most techniques take the flattening into account pragmatically but include no formal method of measurement even though a large number of methods are, in fact, available. These include simple techniques such as eccentric keratometry to determine where precisely the cornea starts to flatten. The Topogometer for example, consists of a fixation line which can be moved to various positions, at each of which keratometry is performed. When the Topogometer indicates flattening, this marks the limit of the optical cap, and the size of the apical zone is a parameter some consider helpful in contact lens fitting.

There are more advanced photographic methods such as photokeratoscopy based on reflections from the cornea of concentric black and white rings such as originally used on the placido disc. Arbitrary boundaries are defined between intermediate and peripheral zones, and it is fair to say that these methods have no application to simple contact lens fitting although

---

$$*D = \frac{337.5}{r(mn)}$$

they may have a place in cases of complex corneal topography.

Corneal diameter can usually be assessed well enough by simple inspection, but specially designed rulers are available. An assessment of *palpebral aperture width* as well as of *pupil size* in dim and bright illumination may also be clinically valuable.

Measuring and inspecting contact lenses

Lens power is assessed by one or other type of focimeter. Modern focimeters (Fig. 24.33), either optical or electronic, measure the back vertex power. Because of the much steeper curvature of the posterior surface of a contact lens as distinct from spectacle lenses, an error of measurement may occur if a contact lens is simply applied to the stop of the focimeter and a specially designed accessory stop or choke is best fitted. This is of standard design with a measuring area between 4 and 5 mm in diameter. Test lenses of known power are used to provide a calibration curve for the particular instrument. The lens to be measured is placed with its back surface on the stop and the back vertex power measured is then used to obtain the true back vertex power from the calibration curve.

Soft lenses should be dried by lint or by paper tissue and given perhaps 10 seconds before being placed on the focimeter.

Other lens parameters include the several dimensions: overall diameter, diameter of its various zones both posterior and anterior and the radii of curvature of these as well as lens thickness.

Overall diameter is simply estimated by ruler or by simple band-measuring device (see Fig. 25.6).

Although a band-measuring device may be useful for measuring the diameter of clearly delimited zones of the two surfaces, sophisticated methods may be needed to identify the diameters of the optical and more peripheral zones if there is blending between one zone and the next. These methods depend on the regularity or otherwise of light (in one technique, fluorescent) reflected from the surface. These may be informative not only as to the actual dimensions of the various zones but also about the quality of the blend, an important feature in determining lens comfort.

Radius of curvature can be measured in various ways. The radiuscope (Fig. 25.7) is simply a low-power microscope which makes use of the Drysdale principle. A convex lens is situated between a point source and a reflecting surface that is being measured so that it focuses an image at the surface itself. Keeping the distance between lens and source fixed, both are approached to the reflecting surface so that at one position the reflected image is focused at the same place as the source. The distance both lens and source have had to move equals the radius of curvature of the surface. This method applies particularly to hard lenses.

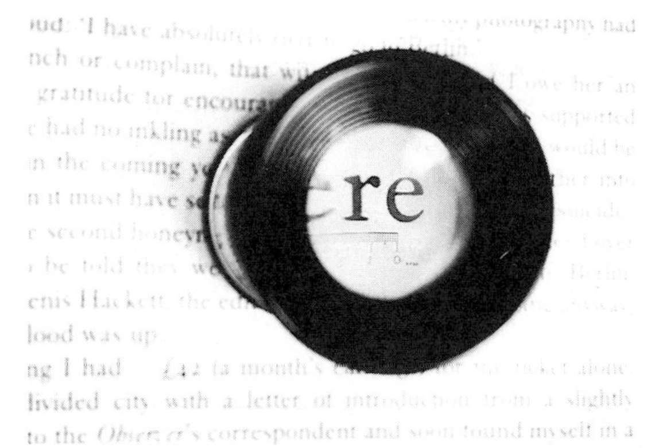

Fig. 25.6 Band-measuring device.

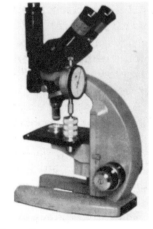

Fig. 25.7 The radiuscope.

An alternative curvature-measuring technique for either type of lens is to use a keratometer with an attachment that incorporates a 45-degree mirror (the Conta-check). This simply reflects the image of the mires on to the horizontally placed contact lens.

Other methods for soft lenses involve estimation by simple mechanical or by ultrasonic apparatus of the sagittal depth. Laser interferometry is also used.

Some method for *lens thickness* measurement is essential and it is estimated by one of the many gauges available. Other features of importance are best carried out by simple estimation by the naked eye or by loupe or slit-lamp magnification. These include optic and surface quality as well as the very important features of edge design, ideally rounded and being neither too sharp nor too blunt.

HARD LENS FITTING

The design and parameters of hard corneal lenses

An essential feature in the design of a hard corneal lens is that the posterior surface must conform to a greater or lesser degree with the shape of the cornea; any significant disparity in this respect will lead to a lack of adhesion between the lens and the eye or in some cases to the precise opposite. The parts of a hard corneal lens are shown in Figure 25.8. It will be remembered that the cornea has an axial region of varying size of largely spherical curvature, peripheral to which there is a band of progressively decreasing curvature. The central portion of the posterior surface of a corneal lens is therefore the most steeply curved, the curvature usually being spherical and occupying a proportion varying from one case to another.

In British terminology, the back optic zone thus has a spherical curvature measured as the *back optic zone radius* and an extent known as the back optic zone diameter. The expression 'back optic' is often used for the back central optic surface. In America, the back optic zone is frequently referred to as the optical zone and the back optic zone radius is described as the central

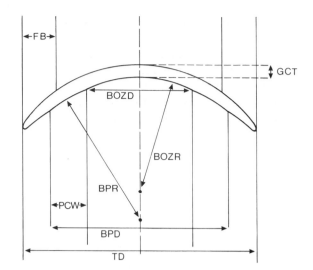

Fig. 25.8 The parts of a hard corneal lens.

BOZR: Back optic zone radius
BOZD: Back optic zone diameter
BPR: Back peripheral radius
BPD: Back peripheral diameter
GCT: Geometrical centre thickness
TD: Total diameter
PCW: Peripheral curve width
FB: Front bevel.

If there is more than one peripheral curve, these are referred to numerically, i.e. first back peripheral radius, second back peripheral radius, etc.

posterior curve, the optic zone radius or the base curve radius, and the back central zone diameter is known as the optical zone diameter.

The peripheral part of the posterior surface of a corneal lens again follows the corneal property, being less curved than the axial region, but designs show great variety. In its simplest form, there is a single peripheral curvature, the radius of which is greater than that of the optic zone; such a lens is known as a bicurve. In more complex designs, there may be two or more peripheral curves, tricurve or multicurve lenses. In all these, the central curvature of the peripheral curve lies on the axis of symmetry of the whole lens. The curvatures of the peripheral zones or bands progressively decrease; the width is a matter of great variation, the most peripheral usually being narrow and forming part of the edge. The inevitable discontinuities at the junctions of the zones of different curvatures can be eliminated to some extent by the process of blending or by arranging that any two different curvatures have a common tangent at the point of interception. Such offset lenses are usually bicurve in design and the peripheral curvature may be conic, e.g. paraboloidal. Other forms include continuous-curve lenses which flatten in non-spherical fashion from the axis outwards. The design of the edge of the lens is also very important; too sharp an edge may dig into the corneal or limbal tissues; too thick an edge may irritate the lids. Furthermore, the form of the edge influences the centration and stability of the lens.

The extent to which the curvature of the most peripheral band differs from that of the back central optic radius is a measure of what is known as 'edge lift', also sometimes known as the Z factor. In PMMA lenses the edge lift needs to be slightly more than for gas-permeable lenses because of the greater need to ensure tear renewal. If edge lift is excessive however, the adherence of the lens to the eye may be compromised.

The form of the anterior surface is entirely or largely spherical. Its parameters are given by the ametropia to be corrected, which determines the curvature of the axial region of that surface. A small peripheral zone may be present, sometimes referred to as a front bevel. Such a very distinct zone is present on the anterior surface of *lenticular* lenses, a design that is sometimes necessary in order to reduce the thickness of the edge in a highly myopic correction or to diminish the weight in high hypermetropia or aphakia.

Although custom-design lenses are available, many practitioners restrict themselves to the designs available from a limited range of products. This means that the choice of trial lenses and of the lenses finally ordered for the patient is to a degree dictated by what is offered by a particular manufacturer, but this is of course itself determined by what is most frequently required.

Thus the total diameters of modern hard lenses are usually between 8 and 9.5 mm; microlenses, a term used to describe small-diameter lenses (less than 8.5 mm, and even as small as 6 mm), are less commonly found today because

gas-permeable materials allow larger diameter lenses to be worn successfully. Indeed such larger lenses may be necessary for stability or optical reasons.

Within one particular design of lens back optic zone radii may be available in a range commonly from 7 to 8.5 mm in 0.05-mm intervals. A choice of back optic zone diameter is much more limited and is often fixed for one particular design, usually somewhere between 7.4 and 8.4 mm. Central thickness is often fixed for one particular style and varies between manufacturers from 0.1 to 0.2 mm. A wide range of optical powers up to ± 25 D is commonly available.

The fitting procedure

The practitioner will usually carry out keratometry and fit from a trial set made up of lenses of a standard favourite design. The same trial set is usually appropriate both for PMMA and for gas-permeable lenses. Although it is possible to order contact lenses based on trial lenses alone or on keratometry alone the combined method is preferable.

In selecting from the trial set, a total diameter of 9 mm is appropriate for the fitting of gas-permeable lenses in a new contact lens wearer with an average corneal diameter, and palpebral aperture. If these are small an overall diameter perhaps 0.5 mm less may be selected, conversely for large cornea and wide aperture.

The next consideration is the back optic zone radius of the trial lens to be selected and this should be derived from keratometry. Usually one starts with a base curve that is either the mean of the two keratometry readings or nearer the flatter one. However this practice varies between different fitters, and some use nomograms perhaps related to the particular lens type to indicate which radius to try first. In the type of fitting known as On-K, the back central optic radius of the lens is made the same as that of the flattest meridian of the apical zone of the cornea. In other cases a spherical cornea may require the curvature of the optic zone to be slightly flatter than K in order to encourage the free flow of tears.

The eye is topically anaesthetised with two

drops of Benoxinate 0.4% and a trial lens is inserted of the indicated overall diameter and base curve and with a power as close to the patient's refraction as is available in the trial set. For this purpose we take the patient's spectacle refraction in negative cylinder form and use the sphere only as the power of the trial lens, perhaps corrected for back vertex distance in subjects with high ametropia.

After an interval of perhaps 30 minutes to 1 hour to allow lacrimation and discomfort to subside, the lens position and its movement are noted. Ideally the lens should be well centred on the cornea and its optic axis should coincide with that of the eye. From the practical point of view this means that the position of the corneal lens should be such that its geometrical, which is usually its optical, centre is opposite the midpoint of the pupil. Whenever a lens is significantly decentred its optical function suffers to a degree. This impairment is small in low degrees of ametropia, and if some parts of the optical quarter of the lens remain opposite the visual access the degree of oblique astigmatism is negligible. If the decentration is gross however the optical function through the edge of the lens may be poor.

Nevertheless an eccentrically located lens which remains on the cornea may be optically acceptable but, if the eccentricity is such that the lens permanently positions itself over the limbus at one point, discomfort may arise whatever the optical state. A dropping lens is usually less comfortable than one which is well centred or rides high. Even so, many such lenses continue to be worn without ill-effect, though there is no doubt that in fitting the lens accurate centration should be attempted.

A corneal lens of large diameter, 9 mm or more, often lies with its upper edge covered by the upper lid for 2 to 3 mm; this exerts some backward pressure, keeping the lens in place. In this connection, there is a tendency for corneal lenses incorporating myopic corrections to ride high because of the increase of thickness towards the periphery while the lids combine with gravity to act in the opposite sense in a case of high hypermetropic corrections wherein the lens often tends to ride downwards. The lower lid usually exerts no supporting influence on a lens except when in contact with its lower margin. Though undesirable this may have no untoward consequences, but a situation where the lower lid actually covers the lower margin of the lens is usually thought to be unacceptable since it causes pooling of tears between the lens and the lower part of the cornea.

Some degree of mobility of a corneal lens is to be expected; rotation of the lens without actual translation is common and may not cause any optical disability or lead to any discomfort. Also, with temporal movement of the eye, the lens approaches the nasal limbus; the precise degree of such movement — the 'excursion' lag — that is acceptable is difficult to define, but in horizontal movement should not be greater than 2 mm for lenses of total diameter of 9 to 9.5 mm. Anything more than a slight overlap of the limbus on ocular movements is usually not well tolerated.

More important are the movements which occur on blinking. A properly fitted lens moves downwards relative to the cornea with the descent of the upper lid and is rapidly taken upwards to a level above its static position as the upper lid ascends and finally settles down again more slowly to its initial position. Any undue delay in this may give rise to a temporary blurring of vision. This mobility during blinking is believed to be of importance for the continued health of the cornea, giving temporary relief to the part of this tissue which physically supports the lens in its central position and allowing the tear flow under the lens to be renewed. Any theoretical optical advantages that might arise from the lens remaining fixed in the centre of the cornea are considerably outweighed by the damage that would occur as a result of immobility and the stagnation of tears.

The overall picture of the mobility of a corneal lens is sometimes characterised by the terms 'tight' or 'loose-fitting' based on the criteria we have just discussed. A tight lens moves little on blinking and ocular movements and may even resist movement if pushed externally and may be so tight as to leave an imprint of its edge on the cornea. Loose-fitting lenses, besides having optical disadvantages, lead to excessive awareness of their presence because of their free mobility; this may be to such a degree that gross displacement of the lens may occur on to the conjunctiva, into one or other fornix or even off the eye altogether.

The way the lens is co-apted to the corneal surface, the bearing relationship, is then gauged by using fluorescein. A small drop of 1% solution is applied to the upper limbus with a glass rod, or with a prepared strip. Naked eye inspection with light filtered through cobalt blue glass or ultraviolet black light (Fig. 25.9) will indicate the proximity of the cornea to the lens at various sites as shown by the degree of fluorescence. Slit-lamp microscopy of the lens/cornea interspace with a narrow beam may provide additional information. The fluorescein pattern is not static, since the tear film in the interspace alters with every movement of the lens; it is examined initially with the lens centred and the lids retracted and will indicate that the central portion of the posterior surface of the trial lens matches the corneal apex, an alignment fit, or is clear of it, an apex clear fit, or lies too closely upon it, flat fit. These terms do not necessarily correspond with the fitting system based on keratometry (on K, steeper than K, flatter than K). Astigmatic factors may also be shown by the fluorescein appearances.

The relationship generally favoured is that of minimum apical clearance (Plates 3, 4, 5). In this case a uniform film of tears intervenes between the optical zone of the lens and the optical zone of the cornea, thinning somewhat so that the green pattern becomes darker in the intermediate zone where most support is given to the lens. At the extreme periphery the green colour again becomes more intense; this indicates greater clearance of the cornea, allowing free access of tears to the interspace and counteracting stagnation, although if this is excessive it indicates too much 'edge lift'. A progressive dilution of the fluorescein in the lens/corneal interspace should be seen to occur, indicating that tears from under the lens are being constantly renewed.

Much experience is required in the interpretation of the fluorescein patterns, which vary with the technique of examination and the parameters of the lens, but the pattern just described indicates that in the mid-periphery there is an annular area which has the greatest load-bearing function. However peripherally this area is situated, its breadth will vary with the design of the lens; in some it will be at the periphery of the back central optic zone, in others it will be an intermediate area of flatter curvature. Again, the part of the lens receiving the maximum support will depend on the degree to which its back central optic zone and the apical zone of the cornea are matched, intentionally or otherwise, in curvature and diameter. Astigmatic corneas tend to show a typically dumb-bell shaped area of either fluorescence or touch.

These various patterns, taken in combination with centration and lens movement, will indicate that the trial lens is or is not satisfactory according to the above fitting criteria. If the fit of the trial lens is unsatisfactory, it should be replaced by one with slightly different parameters and re-assessed according to the criteria of movement, centration and fluorescein pattern. It should be noted that changes of fitting pattern can be altered just as well by changing the diameter of the back optical zone as by altering its radius of curvature. A larger back optic zone diameter will give a tighter fit.

Once a lens of satisfactory fit has been found it may be advisable to carry out an overrefraction. This is particularly so if the trial lens is very different from the patient's refraction, as may occur in the higher dioptric ranges and in such

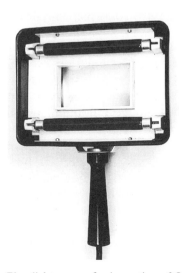

Fig. 25.9 Blue light source for inspection of fluorescein patterns.

cases effectivity considerations enter (see Table 5, Appendix I). Just ordering from the patient's refraction may also be undesirable if the type of fit found to be adequate is not close to the alignment type.

If for any reason the back optic zone radius of the lens to be ordered differs from that of the trial lens (or indeed that of the one that the patient may already be wearing) the power ordered should be changed by 0.25 D for every 0.05 mm change in radius, more minus being needed as the radius is steepened.

Ordering hard lenses

This may simply be from a manufacturer's known style specifying back optic zone radius and power and any other parameter such as total diameter, variation of which is offered within the range (see Table 3, Appendix I). Otherwise it is a matter of ordering a more custom-designed lens when greater detail will obviously be necessary. This will include the material of which the lens is to be made, the form of the anterior and posterior surfaces, the total diameter, the parameters of both curvature and diameter of the posterior surface zones both optical and peripheral, the centre thickness, and of course, the power corrected for effectivity at the cornea (see Table 5, Appendix I). A typical prescription might be:

7.50 : 7.00/8.30 : 8.50/9.00: 9.50

power — 4 D.

Here the back optic zone radius is 7.50 mm in back optical zone of 7.00 mm diameter. The first back peripheral zone extends out to 8.50 mm and is of 8.3 mm radius and the lens is of overall diameter 9.5 mm with second peripheral zone radius of 9 mm.

This is the formulation of a tricurve lens and it also allows one to quantify the 'edge lift'* (see above) the difference between the optical and peripheral zone radii, here 9.00 mm minus 7.50 mm i.e. 1.5 mm. Edge lift of less than 1 mm may be acceptable for a gas-permeable lens but would be inadequate for a PMMA lens.

---

* There are other more precise definitions of edge lift; these are more complex and too technical for inclusion here.

THE PATIENT'S MANAGEMENT OF THE HARD LENS

Education

This involves teaching the patient the technique of insertion and removal (Figs 25.10, 25.11 and 25.12) hygiene, and a regime of building up tolerance starting with 2 or 3 hours twice a day and then progressively extending to all-day wear. Although some forms of gas-permeable lenses are being recommended for extended wear, this is far from generally acceptable to either patients or practitioners. In some individuals it may be helpful to teach them how to blink naturally.

Hygiene

Hard lenses are usually cleaned by and stored in solutions containing preservatives with varying degrees of antibacterial activity. Nearly all of them contain benzalkonium chloride (approximately 0.02%) and disodium edetate (approximately 0.1%). Some contain chlorhexidine, and there are still some available that incorporate mercury-containing preservatives, in particular Thiomersal (the American anagram is Thimerosal). We should note here that benzalkonium chloride is not included in soft lens solutions and the continued use of Thiomersal in any solution for any type of lens is highly inadvisable (see below).

The materials of which hard lenses are made are thermoplastic; heat would damage them and as a consequence heat disinfection is not practised for such lenses. They are kept as infection free as possible by cleaning them after removal and then storing them in a recommended soaking solution. Prior to insertion some advise further cleaning, but solutions are available which putatively carry out all the functions, cleaning, soaking and wetting. In any event a wetting solution (usually containing polyvinyl alcohol) should be massaged into the lens prior to insertion; this again contains preservatives together with a wetting agent such as polyvinyl alcohol and perhaps some other constituent to increase bulk and viscosity, such as methyl cellulose.

Simple daily cleaning may be inadequate to remove certain debris on the lenses and the

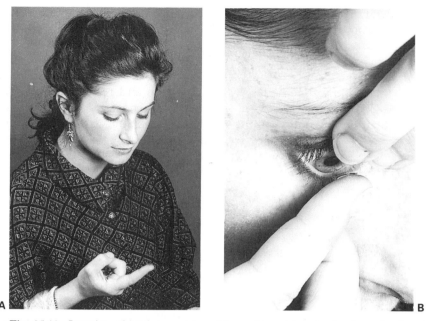

Fig. 25.10 Insertion of hard corneal lens. The moistened lens is placed on the tip of the right index finger (A) and brought to the eye (B) while the lids are retracted and the eye gazes steadily at the approaching lens until it is applied to the cornea. When the lens is in position the upper lid is released first and then the lower.

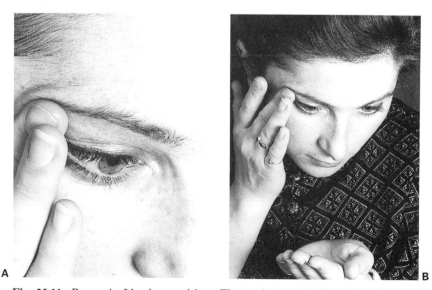

Fig. 25.11 Removal of hard corneal lens. The eye is opened wide so that the lid margins are beyond the lens edge. A finger is placed at the outer canthus (A), possibly touching the sclera, and, with firm pressure backwards, stretches the skin and therewith the lids laterally, expelling the lens on to the lashes or a waiting hand (B).

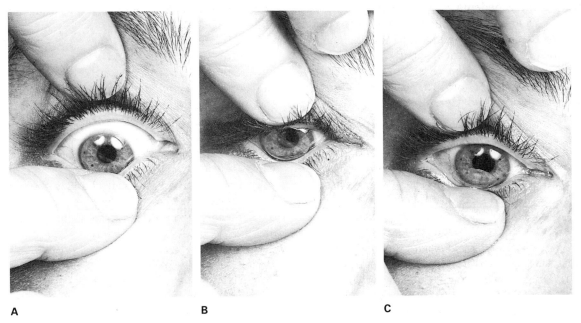

A   **B**   **C**

Fig. 25.12 Removal of hard corneal lens by practitioner. The practitioner steadies the lower edge of the lens by light pressure through the lower lid (A) and the subject then looks down (B). The upper lid is then gently pushed down and slightly rearwards to tease the upper edge of the lens forward off the globe (C). It can then be retrieved from the lashes or elsewhere.

intermittent perhaps weekly use of an enzymatic cleaner can be helpful. Many of these contain papain, a protease; others include enzymes attacking starch and lipids.

It goes without saying that scrupulous personal hygiene must be observed in the handling of all types of contact lenses. Hands must be washed thoroughly and nails brushed.

Storage cases for all contact lenses have less attention paid to their hygiene than is desirable. They should be periodically inspected, thoroughly cleansed, disinfected and if appropriate renewed.

HARD LENS FOLLOW-UP AND PROBLEMS

The patient should be followed up frequently in the few weeks after the initial fitting and then at progressively decreasing intervals. Provided there is no trouble, all that is necessary may be an annual check-up, but even this is something that many longstanding hard lens wearers forego provided their eyes are comfortable, they are seeing well and the lenses are not obviously deteriorated.

For a routine follow-up visit it is important to see the patient at the end of the wearing period, and enquiries should be made about any visual or non-visual symptoms experienced. While the lenses are still in position, the visual acuity is checked and an assessment is made of lens centration and mobility as well as of the state of the lenses themselves (scratches, deposits, etc.).

General inspection reveals whether the eye looks quiet; both the conjunctivae and the lids should be noted, the former for injection and any sign of follicles or papillae, the lids for any Meibomian gland anomalies, cysts or excessive secretions.

Slit-lamp examination is then carried out, first with the lenses in situ and then after they have been removed.

Signs without symptoms

Corneal abnormalities are particularly important,

and of these oedema is a frequent pathological sign. This arises in a variety of circumstances but the factors in its genesis include mechanical trauma to the cornea, negative hydrostatic pressure under the lens, hypoxia of the epithelium and anomalies of the tear film, particularly its lipid layer, as well as the effects of drying.

Generalised oedema to a degree sufficient to produce the effect on vision known as veiling is uncommon, but localised oedema, seen by retro-illumination with the slit lamp, is often present and may be associated with corneal fluorescein staining. Minor degrees of oedema are made evident by the technique of sclerotic scatter in which only the limbal region of the sclera is illuminated; sclerotic scatter oedema is the commonest and earliest change in the cornea and with it there may be no associated staining.

Areas of punctate corneal fluorescein stain are frequently seen; whether because of an actual loss of epithelial cells or because of some alteration in the cells themselves, disappearance of the stains is often remarkably rapid after removal of the lens, so rapid indeed that it has been suggested it is caused merely by the destruction of the normal lipid cellular relationship. On the other hand, some simple stains may take days to disappear, especially those developing after oedema. Microcystic change may be evident in the epithelium.

'Dimple veiling' a form of corneal staining associated with the trapping of small bubbles of air under the lens may occur centrally or peripherally. Since it is very transient it is of no pathological significance.

Mechanical trauma often presents as punctate stains where undue pressure is exerted by the lens on some area of the cornea. This will clearly be aggravated by spasm of the lids. Imperfect blending between two of the curves on the posterior surface of the lens or poor polishing may lead to an arcuate area of stain. A similar pattern may occur as an abrasion caused by insertion, and the upper part of the cornea may be traumatised due to the edge of the lens either riding high or being of poor shape. Staining will of course occur if a foreign body gets under the lens leading to an abrasion. The symptomatology

may however be minimal and a linear track stain may be the only evidence.

Staining at 3 and 9 o'clock may be traumatic in nature or it may be related to drying of the cornea when the lens prevents contact between the lids and the globe (see Plate 6). This is a serious type of pathological change following the wearing of corneal lenses and is associated with oedema and anomalous blinking as well as other factors including grease on the lenses and lenses which ride low on the cornea.

Quite apart from corneal changes there may be abnormalities of blinking, either frequent or deficient, corresponding to a spasm of the orbicularis or levator respectively, and arising from a desire to reduce the discomfort. Excessive blinking may be accompanied by an abnormal tilt of the head so as to minimise the sensation arising from the movements of the lens. On the other hand the failure to blink resulting in a staring appearance may lead to the stagnation of tears under an immobile lens; such patients should be taught to exercise their blinking, as also should those who close their lids incompletely in this reflex. An incorrect movement of the lens when the patient blinks normally may indicate a deficient fit. If the lens is relatively fixed it may be too steeply curved or too large; the opposite holds for a too mobile lens when irritation of the lens may occur, and occasionally the lens may be completely displaced. It is possible to modify a lens to correct some of these defects either by altering the overall size or the curvature of the optical zone or occasionally by adding further intermediate posterior curves.

Lens intolerance and discomfort

As far as non-visual symptoms are concerned in the initial stages of wear there is an inevitable awareness of the presence of the lens lasting for a few minutes. This is accompanied by the symptoms and signs met with at the first insertion every time the lens is inserted. As the wearer becomes adapted the time taken for this to disappear shortens to a few seconds.

Awareness of the presence of the lens developing at a variable period after its insertion, associated with increasing discomfort and perhaps watering and photophobia, may be caused by a poorly fitted lens either because the design is bad or the edge poorly polished or because it is rough, chipped or scratched perhaps with dried debris adherent to it. In such cases as the discomfort increases there is associated blinking and spasm of the lids and this may also result from a conscious effort to clear the vision, which is often blurred. As has been noted the basis of these symptoms may be hypoxia of the cornea if it is not mechanical trauma. In any event in any serious case of discomfort the patient will of course be too distressed to keep the lens in for any appreciable period.

Photophobia by itself is not infrequent and is thought to be associated with some definite change in the cornea such as punctate staining or oedema. Tinted contact lenses may be prescribed.

The management of these complaints consists of reviewing the lens fit, cleaning and polishing the lenses and either modifying or replacing them where appropriate. As we have already remarked, the substitution of gas-permeable lenses for the older PMMA variety offers one possible solution to those problems related to corneal hypoxia. Such lenses may be ordered with larger overall diameter if indicated. Even gas-permeable lenses may be insufficient and recourse is still occasionally had to the manoeuvre of fenestration, even for the gas-permeable type, in those subjects particularly prone to oedema; one or more tiny holes about 0.3 mm in diameter is drilled in the lens either centrally or peripherally. A simple alternative is to switch to soft lenses where appropriate.

Acutely painful episodes may occur if the cornea is abraded by the lens or fingernail on insertion or if a foreign body has got underneath it. Another important clinical appearance is that sometimes known as the 'over wearing' syndrome. Here, following epithelial oedema, symptoms of epithelial loss may not come on until some time after removing the lens when the patient experiences intense blepharospasm, pain, watering and foreign body sensation. Less acute but often recurrently painful eyes may occur from the breakdown of cysts in a microcystic epithelium.

In all such cases withdrawal of lens wear is of course the first therapeutic measure, and whatever else is needed to encourage the re-epithelialisation of the cornea is then started: padding the eye, perhaps mydriatic drops and antibiotics if there is any suggestion of an infective element to the epithelial loss.

Whether and when lens wear may be resumed is a matter of judgment in each individual case. Chronic microcystic disease for example may lead to slow healing and the necessity to withhold lens wear for a prolonged period; the over wearing syndrome on the other hand may require the lens to be left out only long enough to ensure that the new epithelium is stable and properly grounded and that the lens and its fit are satisfactory.

Poor vision

This may be due either to incorrect optics in the lens eye relationship or some abnormality of the cornea developing on wearing the lens.

In the first place the patient's refractive error may simply not be corrected properly by the contact lens; if the spherical correction incorporated is inadequate small modifications are usually possible such as a correction of −0.75 D. The correction of residual astigmatism, although much less of a problem than with soft lenses, may be dealt with by such expedients as the incorporation of toric surfaces (see below). The altered accommodative requirement compared with spectacles may give rise to visual difficulties with close work. This applies particularly to a high myope whose distance vision is much better with contact lenses than with spectacles but who reads comfortably when the latter are removed. Other visual symptoms may arise from the effects of the peripheral curves, the edge of the lens or from the tear meniscus at this site if and when they obtrude over the pupil, perhaps especially when this is large in a dim environment. This 'flare' or 'ghost images' may be described as double vision or multiple images. The lens as a whole or its back optic zone diameter may be too small and its mobility may be excessive. The lens may centre poorly or the size of the pupil may be larger than had been estimated. The substitution of a larger gas-permeable lens may be helpful.

Progressive blurring of vision which worsens the longer the lenses are worn may occur from increasing corneal oedema if the lens fit is poor. If the oedema becomes sufficiently severe the phenomenon of veiling which we have noted above may occur with haloes around lights. The remedy again here is to change the lens design or material.

Visual impairment may also result from the accumulation of debris or sebaceous secretion in the lens–cornea interspace or on the anterior lens surface. Other causes of visual problems may be warping of the shape of the lens, to which some modern gas permeables are particularly prone, putting the lens into the wrong eye and displacement of the lens off the cornea sometimes into the upper fornix where it may become implanted subconjunctivally, even to the extent of it being regarded as lost. The management of these problems is usually evident once the precise cause is identified.

The influence of a rigid corneal lens on the shape of the cornea is important. An extremely common phenomenon amongst wearers of rigid lenses is that of *spectacle blur*, an indistinctness of vision experienced when using the spectacle correction after removing the lenses.

This is due to two factors: in addition to the element of oedema, there may be some degree of warping or distortion of the cornea to allow it to conform to the shape of the posterior surface of the lens, particularly if that is steeply fitted and sometimes if there is an increase in the thickness of the cornea. In association with these changes, the visual disturbance may or may not be correctable by optical means. The oedema often clears rapidly after removal of the lens with the warping effect of the cornea persisting for long periods. It may change the patient's refractive error, usually myopic, considerably — even to the point of giving good unaided vision. Unfortunately, this state of affairs is temporary if contact lenses are abandoned.

Intentional flattening of the corneal apex by the use of rigid lenses was the basis of the practice of 'orthokeratology' and may have been part of the explanation for the presumed 'arrest of myopia' said to have been a benefit of rigid contact lens wear in some subjects.

Another aspect relates to optical corrections when contact lenses are discontinued temporarily or permanently. Here any spectacle correction may be exasperatingly temporary and short-lived in value — a significant alteration in the correction required occurring even in the interval between the examination of the refraction and the receipt of the spectacles.

If a patient who has been wearing rigid contact lenses comfortably for some time wants to have spectacles for occasional use, it may be inadequate to allow merely an interval of, say, 7 days after removal before carrying out refraction. The actual interval varies widely between practitioners, some arguing that refraction immediately after lens removal may be of more practical use. It might be suggested that one criterion of an ideal rigid contact lens is the ability of the wearer to see clearly with spectacles when the lens is not used. In fact many wearers of such lenses no longer possess spectacles, but this is undesirable as it may lead to difficulties when for any reason the lenses have to be discontinued temporarily or permanently.

Finally it should be added that the warping effect of hard lenses is not so marked with the modern gas-permeable type as it was with those of PMMA.

SOFT LENS FITTING

The design and parameters of soft lenses

As with hard lenses and perhaps even more so a wide variety of soft lenses is available particularly in relation to material, lens thickness, and other factors such as the precise geometrical design of front and back surfaces. The front surface may be spherical or bicurve in form and is often lenticulated to reduce weight. The back surface may be spherical — monocurve, bicurve or continuous curve — or aspherical in form. No one manufacturer produces lenses of all these designs. The practitioner usually bases his work on an association with a strictly limited number of products.

Another matter influencing product choice is

the technique used for manufacturing lenses; lathe-cut lenses offer the widest range of curvatures and diameters. However, whilst this variety may not be extensively shared by lenses produced using the other two manufacturing techniques, moulding or spin casting, these latter have other advantages. Both avoid the susceptibility to surface scratches of the lathe-cut type. Moulded lenses can be faithfully reproduced; spun cast lenses are largely a product of one manufacturer, Bausch & Lomb, and these have intentionally aspherical posterior surfaces, again with easy reproducibility, and of surface and edge features which are said to promote comfort.

There are two approaches to the lenses used for fitting trials. In one a relatively small number of diagnostic lenses with a limited range of dimensions and a few powers is present.

In the second type of approach a considerably larger and therefore much more expensive range of lenses is employed. From this a lens is likely to be available for trial virtually the same as that required so that it can be supplied on the spot.

The fitting procedure

Selection of the lens to be tried is based on several factors. These are the K readings, the corneal diameter, sometimes referred to as the horizontal iris diameter or horizontal visible iris diameter (HVID), the shape of the limbal sulcus and the type of soft lens material, whether high or low water content.

The overall lens diameter is usually taken as 1.5 mm greater than the horizontal iris diameter, but this figure is not absolute and may be greater if the limbal sulcus is not very pronounced.

The base curve of the lens is chosen flatter than the flattest K reading, and how much flatter is determined by the overall lens diameter. The smaller the latter, the steeper the lens to be tried. For a patient with a cornea of 12 mm diameter and K readings of 42 D and 43 D, a 13.5-mm-diameter lens will be selected. The base curve to be used would be 0.6 mm flatter than the flattest K. A K reading of 42 D represents a radius of 8.036 mm, and the ideal base curve would be 8.63 mm in ideal terms, in practical terms 8.5 mm. Generally speaking one might take a base curve 0.3 mm flatter than the flattest K for a 13.0-mm-

diameter lens increasing by 0.3 mm of flattening for every 0.5-mm increase in lens diameter.

Two other factors have to be borne in mind. First high water content lenses such as might be used for extended wear, particularly in aphakia, need slightly steeper fitting than lower water content lenses, as the former are relatively somewhat more flexible; thus, whereas a low water content lens of overall diameter of 14.5 mm might indicate a base curve 1.2 mm flatter than the flattest K, 1 mm or less of flattening might be adequate for a high water content lens.

Finally a pronounced limbal sulcus might indicate that the lens should not be so large in overall diameter and the base curves should be selected a little less flat.

Having decided on the overall diameter and base curve, lenses are selected for trial with power similar to what is indicated by the patient's spectacle refraction.

After insertion the fit is evaluated after giving time for hydration of the lens to settle in the tear environment; it is best to wait 20 minutes for a low water content lens and 5–10 minutes longer for one of high water content.

A properly fitted lens will centre well and its edge will not dig into the conjunctiva. Particular attention should be paid to movement of the lens on upgaze and on blinking. On looking up a soft lens should not lag more than 0.5 to 1.5 mm, and on blinking in the open position the lens should be carried up about 1 mm before it recentres. Excursions smaller or greater than this indicate tight or loose fittings respectively.

Another indication of an unsatisfactory fit is the effect of blinking on the vision. With a tight lens usually vision will be clearer after a blink. The reverse is true of a loose-fitting lens.

A regular retinoscopy reflex through the trial lens and undistorted keratometry mires are taken by some practitioners as indications of a good physical lens fit. It should be mentioned that fluorescein is not used in soft lens fitting evaluation.

The result of the retinoscopy carried out with a trial lens of optimal fit in place is used as the basis for subjective tests to assess the required power of the lenses to be ordered.

No hard and fast rules can be given as to the change to be made if one trial lens is unsatisfactory but the following are guidelines. Better centration may be achieved by increasing the overall diameter. Edge compression may be diminished by flattening the base curve. A tight lens as indicated by its lack of mobility should be replaced by one with a smaller overall diameter or flatter base curve or both, conversely for a loose lens. These however are general indications, they may not be absolutely correct for every style of lens and every cornea. This is because the bearing relationship of soft lenses is complex, involving ideally touch of the lens not only to the apical cornea but also to the upper and lower limbal conjunctivae. In addition the flexibility of movement of such lenses also leads to contact with the peripheral cornea and other areas of the limbus.

Ordering soft lenses

Where the practitioner does not supply lenses from his own stock at the time of trial, these are ordered from a particular manufacturer's product list guided by the overall diameter, the base curve, the power and the desired lens material.

A typical example might be as follows:

Menicon Soft M, 8.00/13.50 (8.00 mm base curve, radius 13.50 mm overall diameter) and of the required optical power.

The fitting process may of course reveal that a particular cornea has features which would best be served by a lens that is not standard in the manufacturer's list and here as with hard lenses it is perfectly possible to order a custom-designed lens specifying overall diameter, base curve, back optic zone diameter for the commonly prescribed bicurve posterior surface, and central thickness, which in some modern lenses may be down to almost one-third of a millimetre, particularly for some extended-wear lenses.

THE PATIENT'S MANAGEMENT OF THE SOFT LENS

Education

Insertion and removal of the lens is taught (see Figs 25.13 and 25.14) and the patient is shown how to recognise when soft lenses have become

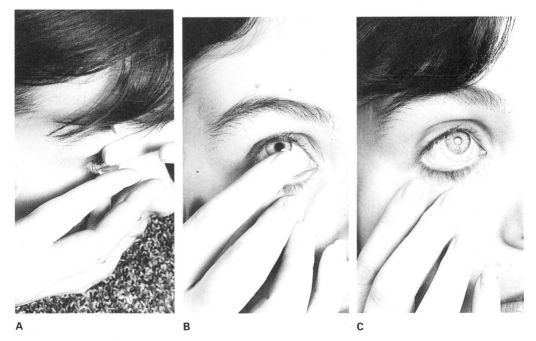

A **B** **C**

Fig. 25.13 Insertion of soft lens. This may be as for a hard lens (A) or the lens may be placed initially on the sclera (B) and eased across on to the cornea (C).

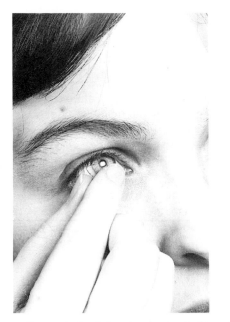

Fig. 25.14 Removal of soft lens by simply pinching the lens out (this method can be used by a practitioner).

inverted. A build-up of wearing time to all-day wear is arranged and this regime can usually be more rapid than with hard lenses.

Soft lens hygiene

All daily-wear soft lenses should be disinfected at every removal either thermally or chemically, and whichever method is used the lens should be cleaned beforehand (see below).

Thermal disinfection is usually carried out in specially designed apparatus with the case containing the lenses immersed in saline solution, exposed to dry heat (90°C approx. for 10 minutes). The method is somewhat cumbersome, may cause lens deposits to become even more adherent and is not completely bactericidal although probably more efficient in this regard than chemical or 'cold' disinfection. All heating methods probably shorten the useful life of soft lenses. Various types of saline solution have been promoted at one time or another. Saline, possibly buffered but without preservatives, is preferred.

Cold disinfection is by one of a number of chemical solutions. Hydrogen peroxide 3% is popular at present but must be neutralised before the lens is inserted in the eye; this neutralisation is carried out in one of several ways, chemically with sodium pyruvate, sodium bicarbonate or sodium thiosulphate, enzymatically, or by a platinum-coated disc.

It is believed that the relatively short periods of soaking in hydrogen peroxide may be ineffective in dealing with the organism acanthamoeba, and if overnight disinfection with hydrogen peroxide is not carried out the lenses should be left at least 4 hours in the disinfecting solution.

Other methods of cold disinfection include solutions releasing sodium hypochlorite and numerous 'preservative' solutions which are now waning in popularity. Many of these contain chlorhexidine 0.002 to 0.003%, thiomersal 0.001 to 0.004% or disodium edetate 0.01%. Thiomersal particularly is now known to give rise to unfavourable reactions (see below). One particular preservative, benzalkonium chloride, should never be present in any preparation used by soft lens wearers.

Hydrogen peroxide has come under criticism recently on the grounds that even after it has been neutralised some of it may remain in the substance of soft lenses. The latest proposed disinfecting solution, 'polyquat', is said to have no deleterious effect at all on the corneal epithelium and to penetrate soft lenses poorly if at all.

After disinfection, soft lenses should be stored in a sterile, preservative-free normal saline solution. Reinsertion when required can then be carried out simply by retrieving the lens from the storage case. Rinsing of the lens with normal saline solution may be advisable, before reinsertion, if the hygiene regime involves a storage fluid other than saline.

Daily cleaning of soft lenses is usually by solutions containing non-ionic, surfactant chemicals, oxidants or fat solvents (e.g. isopropyl alcohol). Enzymatic cleaning is also advisable weekly in order to reduce protein deposition and the protease, papain, is popular for the purpose. Other enzymatic preparations contain amylase and a lipase as well. An additional type of cleanser incorporates minute polymeric beads and acts mechanically to debride the lenses.

DAILY SOFT LENS WEAR: FOLLOW-UP AND PROBLEMS

Signs without symptoms

These may affect all contact lens wearers so supervision is essential to detect problems that are arising but may not yet have caused any complaint. The appropriate management of these will perhaps prevent their developing to the point where symptoms are actually present.

Follow-up should always be timed towards the end of the wearing period. A search is made during routine follow-up for abnormal signs in the eye itself, particularly in the cornea and conjunctiva, both bulbar and tarsal, as well as in the contact lens itself.

Corneal anomalies include punctate epitheliopathy (staining spots, erosions, microcysts), infiltrates with or without fluorescein staining, limbal vascularisation and, finally, oedema, perhaps with folds in Descemet's membrane.

The conjunctiva may be engorged and the everted upper lid may show a folliculosis or papillae over the tarsal plate. The contact lens may be obviously damaged, chipped or torn or scratched. It may also show deposits of various foreign substances on its surfaces.

It goes almost without saying that at each follow-up visit vision, and if appropriate refraction, should be checked with the lenses in place. If spectacles are worn at other times, the clarity of vision with the spectacles should be enquired about.

What should be done about any abnormal findings discovered at a routine examination is not a matter for dogmatic pronouncement. Experienced practitioners may decide that the degree to which these abnormalities are present does not justify any particular course of action. If, however, any treatment is necessary it will follow the lines of what is now to be discussed when these signs are found in a contact lens wearer with actual symptoms.

Acute complications of soft lens wear

The painful red eye may be due to a variety of causes. Perhaps during but often typically a few hours after the lens has been worn, a build-up of oedema in the corneal epithelium which becomes necrotic leads to ulceration and erosion of its surface. Altering and blurred vision are other features of this 'overwearing syndrome' as with the same event in a hard lens wearer. It is managed by keeping the lens out for a few days allowing it to heal over by conventional methods of treating corneal ulcers — padding the eye and antibiotic ointment and, if necessary, a mydriatic.

Once the episode is over, an assessment of the appropriateness of the lens itself, e.g. its water content, its fit etc., is required. Measures to be considered are reduction in wearing time, a change to a higher water content lens or a looser fit, all of which would increase the oxygenation of the epithelium, thereby reducing the likelihood of oedema.

Similar symptoms may be given by a corneal abrasion, possibly caused by clumsy lens insertion or removal, or associated with a foreign body under the lens. Here a sharply delineated fluorescein staining area is formed. After routine treatment has allowed restoration of epithelial continuity, resumption of lens wear may be considered.

If there is discharge from the eye, a particularly serious view must be taken in view of the possibility of an infective keratitis. Recent surveys show that up to 40% of all types of infective keratitis are associated with contact lens wear, especially soft lenses. The cornea shows ulceration and infiltration and culture or scrapings or both for microbiological investigation should be taken immediately. Culture of the lens itself and lens case may also yield relevant information. There seems to be a particular predisposition to infection with *Pseudomonas pyocanea* and antibiotic therapy, typically gentamicin locally and perhaps systemically but based on organism sensitivity, is urgently required in such cases. Lens wear should, of course, be discontinued immediately.

Microbial keratitis is a particular feature of extended lens wear and it has now begun to be recognised that overnight wear itself is a crucial factor in this; the occasional soft lens wearer who leaves the lens in overnight is at increased risk of infective keratitis.

Fortunately as yet not very common, but nevertheless of considerable importance, is corneal ulceration due to the organism *Acanthamoeba histolytica* although neomycin and bacitracin may have some effect. This may not present acutely but is characterised by an indolent central ulcer, sometimes in a ring shape and preceded by a dendritiform figure, (Plate 7) attended by marked pain which is disproportionate to the appearance of apparent epithelial involvement. There is evidence that the use of home-made salines may be responsible for some cases; tap water may contain the organism.

Treatment is problematical as the organism is little sensitive to conventional chemotherapy. Curiously enough, the time-honoured remedy of propamidine has been found to have some effect in this situation. The antifungal clomitrazole has also been successfully used.

Small areas of superficial corneal infiltration may be infective or non-infective (Plate 8A, B), and experience seems to show that such infiltrates 1 mm or less in diameter in the corneal periphery should not be taken too seriously if cultures are negative. Many resolve spontaneously if lens wear is stopped; some believe that local steroids help their resolution. Thiomersal sensitivity may be responsible in some cases.

Poor vision

If vision is poor at the outset in a soft contact lens wearer who is comfortable and has no other symptoms or signs, the first investigation must be optical. Over-refraction should be carried out, and this may indicate inadequate correction by the lens either in its spherical element (an under-correction of increasing myopia for example) or because of astigmatism; the latter may be of a degree that is giving unacceptably poor vision. A change to a hard lens or to a different more complex type of soft (toric) lens may be indicated.

It should be noted that the most elementary cause of poor vision on lens insertion is putting the lenses (hard or soft) in the wrong eye.

Blurring of vision that develops as the lens is worn may be due to corneal oedema, either epithelial or stromal. This again may be a phenomenon of the early stages of wear and the problem may decrease with time, perhaps if wearing time is reduced initially to be built up again progressively. If the problem persists, a lens with a looser fit or a higher water content should be considered.

Another important condition blurring vision is excessive mucus production. Amongst its many causes may be the condition called 'giant papillary conjunctivitis' (GPC — see below) or lipid which greases the lens. The latter is Meibomian secretion overproduced by a mechanically induced chronic meibomitis.

Lens spoilage

Any deposit on a lens may interfere with vision. There are many such substances, mostly arising, like mucin, from the tears. Mucin deposits appear as low humps on the lens. Lipid deposits produce sharply reflective patches, sometimes with fingerprint impression where the lens has been handled. Calcium deposits appear as white plaques. If surfactant cleaners do not dislodge them, the lenses should be replaced.

Lens spoilage due to protein deposits is particularly prone to affect high water content lenses and those made of highly ionic materials. Enzymatic removal of protein is important, and it is better to avoid heat disinfection of lenses prone to them as they may be baked on, making removal virtually impossible.

Pigment, either melanin or a type originating externally such as nicotine or eyelid cosmetics, may also be responsible for spoilage.

Finally, the lens may have its quality deteriorated by contamination with infective organisms, both bacterial and fungal. Each may form a film over the lens surface, and fungal deposits can appear in a wide variety of colours. This biofilm may form very rapidly and may be resistant to conventional cleaning methods. The bacteria within it produce a polysaccharide onto which tear proteins deposit. Significant biofilm formation is much commoner with soft than with rigid lenses.

Chronic inflammation and discomfort

The first inspection should be concerned with the fit of the lens; is its mobility correct, is blinking adequate, are the lens parameters ideal, are the lenses in the correct eyes? Even if one specific condition is not obvious lens hygiene should be gone into with the wearer and the physical state of the lenses inspected for damage and deposits. Anomalies in either or both of these departments may be the simplest explanation for what has become known rather vaguely as the 'contact lens red eye'.

Turning now to more specific causes, a very common finding is punctate fluorescein staining of the cornea which will disappear once the lens is removed, only to reappear when wear is resumed. Oedema may be the basis of this and refitting should be considered.

Apart from chronic infections unrelated to contact lens wear, either bacterial, chlamydial or viral, we have to consider four important causes of persistently uncomfortable eyes in soft contact lens wearers:

1. *Giant papillary conjunctivitis* (GPC) (Plates 9, 10, 11). Although this condition occurs with hard lenses very occasionally, it is far away most frequently seen in the soft lens wearer. Characterised by a burning sensation, excessive mucus production interfering with vision and the presence of very marked papillary change on the upper tarsal surface, the appearance resembles that seen in spring catarrh. It eventually will lead to total non-tolerance of contact lens wear. Its exact cause is unknown — an allergic aetiology is likely, perhaps hypersensitivity to protein deposits on the lens. Mechanical factors may play a part and total duration of wear of the lenses is perhaps also important. It improves sometimes slowly without treatment soon after lens wear is discontinued, although itching and mucus production may continue for a while. Some believe that steroids hasten resolution, but this is not proven. Sodium cromoglycate may also be helpful. Enzymatic cleaning of the lens may help to get rid of protein deposits. In some other patients, the condition may resolve with a completely different soft lens, perhaps of a new material or modified design, or a disposable type.

2. *Thiomersal keratoconjunctivitis*. It is now recognised that the inclusion of Thiomersal as preservative in contact lens solutions, whether used for cleaning, rinsing or for heat disinfection, can give rise to particular clinical problems in soft contact lens wearers. Whether it is directly toxic or allergic is not certain. The clinical picture is of irritation and discomfort, even photophobia, at a variable but progressively decreasing period after lens insertion with upper conjunctival injection and superficial vascularised keratopathy in the upper part of the cornea (Plates 12 and 13). There may be some papillae on the tarsal plate, and some believe that the sterile small infiltrates in the cornea are also produced by Thiomersal toxicity.

The vascularisation resembles the condition of superior limbic keratitis of Theodore. It is, of course, not characteristic only of Thiomersal toxicity but occurs even asymptomatically in many soft lens wearers: usually it is superficial but stromal new vessels must be taken much more seriously.

Treatment is to recognise the cause and withdraw all solutions containing Thiomersal. The Thiomersal should be removed from the lenses themselves by repeated soaking in preservative-free saline. Clearing of the condition is sometimes slow.

Although Thiomersal is a common and recognised offender, other preservatives such as chlorhexidine and benzalkonium chloride can also produce toxic keratopathy. The latter has now largely disappeared from modern soft lens solutions, but a soft lens wearer may occasionally develop a quite severe acute toxic reaction from it if some solution intended for hard lens wearers is mistakenly used.

In an attempt to identify the individual factor, often the remedy is to change the solutions used and hopefully this lens fluid-related toxic keratoconjunctivitis can be avoided. As with Thiomersal, the fluids concerned may be those used for cleaning, rinsing, disinfecting, soaking or wetting.

3. *Microcystic epitheliopathy*. This is more a common feature found in hard lens wearers but it also does occur in soft lens wearers. The minute epithelial cysts may rupture causing pain and discomfort when the lens is worn. Owing to

defective oxygenation, it is best managed initially by lens withdrawal and then by a change to a lens regime using different material which allows more corneal oxygenation.

4. *Chronic Meibomitis* will also lead to a form of keratoconjunctivitis. Here the important features are punctate epithelial changes in the cornea with excessive lipid production, the patient complaining of a persistent discharge. This, as we have noted, may be deposited on the lens and interfere with vision. Another result may be the development of Meibomian cysts which are a relatively common occurrence in contact lens wearers.

Finally, it has to be admitted that in some cases, we cannot fathom precisely what has caused an intolerance, and this is particularly so when the patient complains of one eye only. There is often no obvious clinical explanation although unsubstantiated explanations, such as 'the eyes are dry', are often offered. An empirical approach may be adopted, changing fluids, changing lens materials or, if there is an unacceptable mechanical touch, refitting with a lens of different parameters, but it is hardly surprising that there is a multitude of placebo drops ('in-eye' comfort preparations) for use in such cases.

Extended-wear lenses

Some years ago, it seemed that there was a real possibility of contact lens wear which could be described as 'fit it and forget it', and it is certainly true that in selected cases soft lens wear with the lens in place for extended periods, weeks or months, is practised and safe.

Any of the common conditions for which the wearing of soft lenses is thought appropriate may be suitable for trial of extended (or as it is now sometimes referred to, prolonged) wear. Special problems do arise on such a regime however, and extended wear has not attained the universal applicability at one time hoped for. Nevertheless, it is worth considering in several clinical situations, particularly where there is difficulty or perceived inconvenience in daily handling. This applies to some clinically inept subjects, to others who are too frightened to get themselves into a routine of insertion and removal and especially to the elderly aphakic subjects. On the other hand, those with deficient tear production or chronic lid disease should be discouraged from even attempting to wear soft lenses on an extended basis.

The type of lens which is appropriate is usually a high water content hydrogel with minimal central thickness. The classical material was Permalens Perfilcon A of 71% water content. Sauflon PW is another popular material, as is Lidofilcon B, which has 79% water content. One lower water content lens (the 'CSI') can be manufactured so thin that this compensates for what would otherwise be its low oxygen transmissibility.

A silicone rubber, Silsoft, has also had some success but is less popular now.

Hydrogels are fitted as for other soft lenses but with a tendency to slightly more loose fit. Base curves of 8 to 9 mm and overall diameters of 13.5 to 14.5 mm are common.

Follow up of extended-wear cases

It is usually advisable to see a patient embarking on extended wear within the first 24 to 48 hours, and if no untoward signs have developed it is then most important that the practitioner establish a revisit schedule, perhaps every 2 or 3 months, when the lenses can be inspected in situ and either replaced or removed for cleaning and reinsertion. It is quite common practice if the lens is seen to be in good condition in situ, with a symptomless patient having no abnormal corneal or conjunctival signs, simply to leave well alone and not even to remove the lens. Indeed some patients in this category approach continuous wear but should still be re-examined every 3 to 4 months. In others, the inspection may show some abnormalities of the lens or cornea even in the absence of symptoms, but it is vital for the patient to report immediately if anything untoward is occurring between routine visits — pain, persistent discomfort, redness or disturbed vision — and it is important as well to try to teach the patient to remove the lens at the first sign of trouble.

Complications of extended wear

Any complications known to occur with soft lens wear in any regime may occur. There are, however, particular complications associated with extended wear.

The *tight lens syndrome* is a painful red eye developing acutely, commonly on waking and characterised by an immobile lens which is partially dehydrated. It seems to be gripping a cornea oedematous on account of poor oxygenation. Not only may the cornea show abnormal signs — epithelial loss and stromal oedema — but there may also be chemosis and anterior chamber reaction with cells and flare. If neglected, there is a risk of secondary infection.

Treatment is to remove the lens for a week or so; the cornea usually returns to normal without particular medication such as cycloplegics or antibiotics. A change to a looser fitting lens should be considered, either by reducing the overall diameter or fitting flatter.

Other complications to which extended wear lens are particularly prone are the accumulation of deposits (see below), especially protein and mucus, a susceptibility to infective keratitis (see below) and corneal vascularisation seen especially in aphakics, particularly across the upper limbus at the site of the surgical section. Both superficial and deep vessels may grow into the cornea and deep vessels may be further complicated by lipoid deposits which can reduce vision. An added problem in aphakics is the possible presence of significant astigmatism requiring a spectacle overcorrection to be worn, or indicating an attempt at toric lens fitting.

SPECIAL FITTING PROBLEMS

Astigmatism

If total astigmatism of the eye were entirely due to the anterior surface of the cornea and if the refractive indices of the contact lens material, the tear fluid and the corneal substance were identical, a properly centred lens of appropriate power with spherical surfaces would fully correct the ametropia. The optical effect of the astigmatic cornea would be eliminated by the absence of refraction at its surface. As these refractive indices are not absolutely identical, and as some astigmatism is not corneal in origin, this theoretical situation is rarely seen. As the result, the optical system of an eye corrected by a spherical corneal lens almost invariably shows some astigmatism.

Residual astigmatism is the term used in this respect to describe the astigmatic error found when refracting a patient wearing any type of hard contact lens, particularly a spherical lens from a trial set. It is made up of two elements: a true residual astigmatism of the eye itself, largely lenticular in origin, and factors caused by the contact lens. These include the astigmatic effect caused by the difference of refractive indices mentioned above, the tilt, eccentricity or warping of the corneal lens and intended or accidental toroidicity of its surfaces.

These factors cannot easily be assessed, and it is therefore impossible to estimate the residual astigmatism from a keratometric reading or from the patient's refraction. Fortunately, it is usually small (about 0.5 D against the rule) and has so little effect on the visual acuity that it can be ignored. In higher degrees however spherical corneal lenses may not give adequate vision.

The physical fit of a rigid spherical lens with spherical back surfaces on an astigmatic cornea is a further important consideration. We have already seen that in the fitting of such lenses, the selection of the curvature of the back central optic zone is usually made in close relation to the mean curvature of the corneal meridian. When the astigmatism is small, the moderate lack of co-aptation between the lens and corneal surfaces is of physiological value in encouraging the flow of tears through the interspace, but in high degrees difficulties may arise; thus discomfort may occur if the lens rocks or becomes decentred and the corneal periphery, in the flatter meridian, may be unduly traumatised. Moreover, 'flare' may interfere with the vision and spectacle blur may be a problem.

In spite of the possible disadvantages, in lower or moderate degrees of astigmatism rigid spherical lenses fitted on K or slightly steeper are often adequate. A small total diameter, 8.5 mm or less, may be suitable incorporating a small back optic zone diameter. Lenses of gas-permeable materials can be ordered slightly thicker than PMMA lenses, thereby reducing the likelihood of warpage or flexibility to which some types are susceptible. Both of these distortions may compromise vision.

In larger degrees, toric designs are necessary — back toric or bitoric. A conflict exists between the physical fit and the optical performance of a back toric hard lens. This arises because the exact physical approximation of such a lens to the back surface of the cornea produces an induced astigmatism on account of the greater refractive index of plastic material as compared with tears, thus introducing an extra optical factor, the *lacrimal lens*. In order to avoid this, close approximation to toroical cornea is avoided, and often this partial approximation will give adequate centration and rotational stability. A typical compromise might be to match the flattest back surface of the toric lens to the flattest meridian of the cornea but to make the steepest meridian of the lens one-third flatter than the steepest corneal meridian. If a compromise of this type does not give adequate positioning of the lens, a more exact fit is looked for and any induced astigmatism is corrected by incorporating a front toric surface as well — a bitoric lens. Such a design may also be required if there is a significant degree of both corneal and residual (lenticular) astigmatism.

If residual astigmatism without corneal astigmatism is a problem, front toric lenses are helpful and a lens that does not rotate, or does so minimally, is called for. For this purpose, many ingenious devices exist to prevent rotation (Fig. 25.15). These include prism ballast, usually of 2 prism dioptres power, or truncation, which is frequently combined with prism ballast. Such devices are usually not necessary for back toric lenses, which often stabilise without needing them. Indeed, in some cases, a toric periphery alone may be enough to allow the lens to settle in the appropriate orientation without the necessity for a full toric back surface.

The fitting technique for all toric hard lenses is usually based on spherical trial lenses with keratometry, fluorescein patterns and over refraction forming the basis of the often complex calculations to be made before ordering. Each practitioner has his own method of relating these to the manufacturer's products. When discomfort has caused rigid contact lens wear to be abandoned, soft lenses are considered. These are perforce of toric design, either front or back, and all require some feature to maintain rotational stability such as was noted with hard lenses. These include truncation of the lower edge, prism ballast and chamfering (thinning) of the upper lower edges — one form of so-called dynamic stabilisation. Simple back surface toric design, which is effective in preventing rotation in some types of hard lenses, is not enough by itself for soft lens correction of astigmatism but a special trial set of soft prism ballast truncated lenses is available. Each lens has reference marks or lines on it to indicate how it is orientating itself on the eye. Over-refraction is carried out, and from this and the parameters of the satisfactorily fitting lens together with the information about its orientation in relation to the reference marks a lens can be ordered empirically. This is often from tables supplied by manufacturers of a particular style of lens.

The process is not simple; none of the devices for stabilising lenses is completely reliable and a lens ordered may not perform visually as it should either because the lens still rotates during blinking, giving variable vision, or is relatively stable but at an incorrect axis. The often frequent necessity for a change of lens for these reasons or on account of the added discomfort because of the

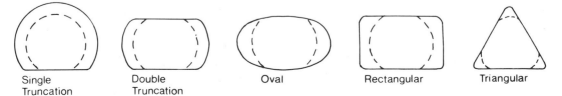

Single Truncation   Double Truncation   Oval   Rectangular   Triangular

Fig. 25.15 Devices for prevention of rotation.

greater contact with the lower lid as compared with spherical lens fitting makes the whole procedure both time-consuming and expensive. Even with the most assiduous attention, the success rate of toric soft lenses leaves something to be desired. If these are not successful, other techniques are on offer. Classical scleral lenses have a small part to play if modern toric corneal lenses cannot be satisfactorily fitted to give good vision.

Other designs of corneal lens are also available, such as the Saturn lens, which has a hard centre and a soft edge; a more recent version of this type is the softperm, in which a gas-permeable rigid centre is blended into a 25% water content soft 'skirt' periphery. Another ingenious design is the piggy-back lens, which essentially is a soft contact lens over the centre of which a hard lens is fitted. This is particularly suitable for irregular astigmatism but may also find a place in high degrees of regular astigmatism where other methods of fitting a corneal lens have proved inadequate.

Irregular astigmatism

Whether primary or as a result of corneal pathology this may be helpfully served by contact lens wear. Irregularities of surface may be optically eliminated because, although the refractive index of the tears, cornea and lens material differ, as we pointed out above the differences are not sufficient to affect the improvement given by a corneal lens with simple spherical front and back surfaces.

Presbyopia

Contact lenses are only exceptionally the primary optical correction for presbyopia in the emmetrope; on the other hand, several choices are available for a patient wearing contact lenses for ametropia who has become presbyopic. The simplest expedient is to use a spectacle correction for near work in addition to the lens. Alternatively, both contact lenses may be made with slightly more plus power in early presbyopia or dissimilar contact lenses can be used, one for distance and

one for close work, often with surprisingly little disturbance of binocularity; if necessary, a spectacle distance correction may be worn at times to correct the eye that has the presbyopic lens. Such a correction may be advisable, for example, when driving. A further possibility is a bifocal contact lens, but the number of designs of these now available is unfortunately some indication that, as yet, none is entirely satisfactory. It follows from considerations of effectivity that the power of the near addition needs to be slightly greater in a bifocal contact lens than in bifocal spectacles.

The types of bifocal contact lenses

Two principles are to be considered; these are, first, simultaneous or bivision and, secondly, alternating vision. In bifocal designs using the simultaneous or bivision principle, the retina receives optical images of both distance and near vision and it is up to the patient to take notice of the one that is of interest and to ignore the other one mentally. Those types using the alternating principle have different portions of the lens to subserve different functions. It must be stated at the outset that many bifocal lenses currently available do not operate exclusively on one principle or the other; the three main designs are annular (or concentric), segment and diffractive.

Annular bifocals. Here the central portion of the lens is of one optical power, usually for distance, and is surrounded by a corrective zone for near vision. In some designs, the zone functions are reversed. Simultaneous vision is present but some alternation is possible if the outer portion is for near because on looking down the lower lid pushes the lens up, bringing the periphery opposite the pupil. There are also multifocal designs where the distance and near portions blend into each other, or the lens surfaces are intentionally aspherical.

In *segment* bifocals, the lens is constructed so that a portion, usually crescentic in shape, has the near correction, and this is orientated downwards by prism ballast and truncation. Again the lower lid is central to the intended function of alternating vision. Here, of course, the degree to which distance and near vision are separated depends on how much the segment obtrudes over the pupil in distance vision and whether any of the remainder of the lens is over the pupil in near vision. Some simultaneous vision with this type of lens is unavoidable, but the best subjects for avoiding this are those with small pupils and relatively highly positioned lower lids, i.e. above or level with the limbus. When these conditions do not obtain, simultaneous vision may be more successful.

The latest type of bifocal contact lens, the *diffractive* lens, works on this principle. Etched on to the posterior surface of the lenses is a series of concentric rings which, acting by diffraction, give a presbyopic power up to +3D. This last type has been hailed as a great advance, but as with all simultaneous vision lenses success depends on ignoring the unwanted image. Furthermore, the compromise of clarity for both near and distance fractions may mean that one or other is unacceptably blurred — a level of 30% blur is quoted, though what that equates to in terms of visual acuity is uncertain, and near vision may be relatively poorer in dim illumination.

All these types of lens are available in both hard and soft lens materials, although hard lens materials are most commonly used for annular bifocals. The diffractive type has until recently been fashioned only in gas-permeable materials but a diffractive soft lens bifocal is now available, the hydron echelon lens. As with many sophistications of contact lens design, bifocal and multifocal lenses require a longer fitting regime and are more expensive than single-vision lenses; they are also significantly less successfully worn. Those subjects most likely to do well will be highly motivated and in public view, where they feel that their image or occupation would be damaged by having to wear spectacles. This would embrace stage and television performers, politicians and musicians.

Keratoconus

The contact lens has a valuable part to play in the treatment of this condition, but the fitting techniques are diverse, complex and specialised. Nevertheless contact lenses should always be considered, even though in milder cases of the condition spectacle corrections may suffice; here an astigmatic correction based more upon subjective testing than on an often uninterpretable retinoscopy may produce a surprisingly satisfactory corrected visual acuity. When spectacle lenses are inadequate because of the extreme irregularity of the astigmatism present, rigid corneal contact lenses, usually gas permeable, are indicated. Many styles are on offer, but fitting with standard lenses, albeit of higher posterior curvatures, is feasible.

The approach to fitting varies considerably. Small diameters (8.5 mm or less) are widely favoured in the United States, particularly if the cornea is not too eccentric. Larger lenses are needed if the cone is not central, often being displaced downwards and inwards. Some believe that these larger lenses encourage corneal scarring.

The fitting procedure begins with keratometry, but this will be merely indicative of the curvature needed in an acceptable lens because the mires are very often considerably distorted. Particular features to be sought are good centration and a fluorescein pattern showing apical light touch and two zones of mid-peripheral contact (the 'three-point touch') with an adequate degree of edge lift. The last factor is particularly important in keratoconus fitting where the lens, of necessity of steep posterior curvature, may dig into the periphery of the cornea.

Numerous specialised lens forms have been tried. The Soper lens (8.5 mm total diameter) has an especially steep central portion to its back optical zone which vaults the corneal apex. Soft lenses are rarely of value except perhaps in kerataconus occurring in Down's syndrome. The Saturn lens with a CAB central area set in a hydrophilic surround has had some limited success. Scleral lenses used to have wide application and still have some place if other types failed.

Finally it will be noted that progression of keratoconus is uninfluenced by contact lens wear; there is neither aggravation nor amelioration; nor is kerataconus produced by wearing contact lenses in those not previously suffering from it.

Aphakia

Although cataract surgery with intra-ocular lens implantation has considerably reduced the indication for contact lens wear in aphakia, there remains however a rump of aphakics who have had cataract surgery for which lens implantation was considered unsuitable, as for example in children, or was found impracticable.

Several features of the aphakic eye are pertinent to contact lens wear. After cataract surgery, a corneal hypoaesthesia is frequently present. Although it allows relatively early fitting without discomfort, it is an indication for close supervision thereafter. The fitting of hard corneal lenses in such patients poses special problems; if the whole of the anterior surface is of uniform curvature, the lens will be of excessive central thickness and heavy, a so-called *single-cut lens*, and it will tend to ride downwards. Not only will this interfere with vision, it may also create an unwanted prismatic effect. Lenses of small diameter overall, although recommended by some practitioners, may also not centre well so that special designs are often employed for the anterior surface of larger lenses, for example greater than 9 mm in overall diameter.

A *lenticular* form is the popular design alternative to the single-cut lens. The carrier periphery is designed to be of minus power ('negative carrier') and the relative concavity of this part of the lens allows the edge to tuck in and be held by the upper lid. The lenticular design has therefore two immediate and related advantages — less weight and better centration.

In deciding between the two designs, a single-cut lens may be preferred in the lower aphakic powers and in subjects with narrow palpebral apertures, but on the whole lenticular designs are more widely used. The total diameter of the lens may be anything from 8 to 10 mm, the outer 1 mm of the posterior surface being devoted to peripheral curves, giving a large optical zone.

In fact, the average pupil size is an important determinate of lens size in that the larger the pupil, either naturally or on account of surgery, the greater the back optical zone diameter should be in order to avoid flare from the edge of the lens and to keep optimal visual performance. A small total diameter may be quite suitable for a cornea with steep curvature and also in subjects with a narrow palpebral aperture.

Centre thickness is obviously less with the lenticular design (best about 0.4 mm) than with the obviously heavier single-cut lens where the minimum thickness cannot usually be less than 0.5 mm.

The posterior surface of the lens is usually designed with the back optic zone radius on K or steeper than K according to the amount of corneal astigmatism. This may be not inconsiderable and against the rule or oblique, adding to fitting problems, particularly with centration. It is important with a lenticular design to keep the diameter of the back optic zone smaller than that of the lenticular zone on the front surface.

The procedure of fitting is best carried out with a trial set of lenses closely similar in design and power to that which it is proposed to order, an over-refraction being carried out to find the appropriate power for the lens. Here, as with all high-power lenses, attention must be paid to the back vertex power of the correction as in the trial frame, to the thickness and to the design of the contact lens. All these factors affect the power of the contact lens to be ordered. In a subject with no particular feature of pupil size, upper lid tightness or palpebral aperture and average aphakic power, a lenticular design lens of large diameter should be tried first. If this does not centre reasonably well with the carrier under the upper lid, a single-cut lens with a smaller diameter should be tried. Further more specialised devices include the prescription of lenses with toric back surfaces if the astigmatism is appropriately severe.

The above refers to hard lens fitting but soft lenses of both lenticular and single-cut form are widely used, especially in extended wear (see above).

It should perhaps be noted finally that aphakic contact lenses retain one clear advantage over intra-ocular lenses — their power can easily be changed if it is incorrect.

DISPOSABLE CONTACT LENSES

The recognition that some of the problems of soft lens wear could be attributed to lens spoilage, that the complex regimes of disinfection, cleaning and storage are inconvenient, expensive and not necessarily effective and that, in any event, the useful life of such lenses is limited prompted the search for a product that is both disposable and economically acceptable.

The first of these to be marketed, Accuvue a 58% water content soft lens, can apparently be mass manufactured by a new technique of modified soft cast moulding and the lenses are available in the limited range of plus 6 D to minus 6 D. There are already at least five other varieties of disposables now marketed, but it is as yet too early to say how far this type of contact lens will come to be accepted as the normal, ousting traditional lens wear regimes.

Some advantages are already appreciated by patients, notably convenience of care systems and economy in solution purchase, though in regard to the latter the lenses themselves are expensive. It seems likely that there will be a significant reduction in the incidence of preservative-related keratitis and probably also in giant papillary conjunctivitis.

In fact a change to disposables has allowed some GPC sufferers to continue contact lens wear which might otherwise have had to cease; furthermore they may have a special place in some subjects such as atopics who have found conventional soft lens wear regimes unsatisfactory.

A typical protocol is to dispose of the lens every week or fortnight and to use the lenses on a daily wear basis with hydrogen peroxide disinfection overnight. The necessity for supplementary solutions is totally eliminated. Others are using them in a modified extended-wear fashion keeping them in for 7–14 days before replacement. A balanced view is perhaps not to extend to more than two nights of continuous wear.

The concept of 'one day' disposables has been mooted but is regarded as a manufacturer's nightmare at present.

THERAPEUTIC USES OF CONTACT LENSES

Although this work is primarily concerned with the optical problems to which contact lens wear relates it would be a glaring omission to make no reference to those clinical conditions where the devices have a non-optical or only partly optical role in treatment.

Occlusive lenses are used in albinism or aniridia in order to reduce light exposure. In occasional cases of strabismus either in the management of amblyopia, where the good eye is fitted, or in intractable diplopia a contact lens with a pupillary area occluded has some part to play.

Tinted lenses are available in numerous formulations. In the common types a moderate to high water content soft lens is made of homogeneously tinted material. Such lenses are used for photophobic subjects, for purely cosmetic eye-colour-changing wear and for hiding obvious ocular anomalies such as white pupils from cataract, corneal scars, heretochromia and obvious iris anomalies such as colobomata. A black pupil can be painted on the front if necessary. Heat disinfection is unsuitable, hydrogen peroxide being best.

Lenses made of homogeneous materials are not fully occlusive. For the latter purposes completely opaque lenses are used perhaps such as in cases of albinism with a clear pupillary area. The remainder of the front surface is white and onto it is painted the appropriate colour with or without iris pattern. Like the homogeneous variety these are soft lenses of high water content and can also be worn on an extended-wear basis. A further variety is an opaque filling within a poly-HEMA sandwich.

Hand-painted and laminated rigid lenses are also available, and these are usually best for disguising an unsightly blind eye or masking a marked strabismus. Custom-fitted painted scleral shells are also used for these purposes. Colour matching with the normal eye should be performed in daylight and a woman should be wearing her normal make-up.

In the complex optics that may arise after corneal transplantation the contact lens is of great value in bringing up visual acuity if a satisfactory fit can be achieved, although this may not be easy. The cornea, which may be thicker than normal and anaesthetic, often has a distorted anterior surface, the graft being tilted or eccentric, or simply bulging. Even if the astigmatism found present is regular, it may be of very high degree.

Rigid lenses with steep back optic curves bridging the graft, perhaps fenestrated, are one approach to the problem and as with keratoconus (see below) lenses of the Saturn type may be helpful.

A *bandage* soft lens is the type used for corneal conditions marked by chronic severe oedema with repeated painful epithelial droplet rupture — bullous keratopathy. Typical of these is aphakic dystrophy following cataract surgery whether without, or more commonly with, pseudophakic implantation. Other cases of bullous keratopathy may arise from chronic intractable glaucoma, typically rubeotic, following central vein thrombosis, from Fuchs' dystrophy of the cornea, or from patients who have had multiple intra-ocular surgical interventions.

Extended wear with its attendant advantages and complications employing a thin, high water contact lens is customary. Lenses are removed and replaced or reinserted at 3 to 6-monthly intervals. There may be a place for continuous prophylactic topical antibiotic therapy in these subjects because these are usually sick eyes, and as with all extended wear there is a significantly increased risk of suppurative keratitis.

The severity of the ocular pathology which has led to bullous keratopathy precludes any very great improvement in vision by bandage lens wear. The objective of this type of management is simply patient comfort.

Soft contact lenses have a minor place in the care of some patients with corneal epithelial pathologies, particularly those characterised by failure of the epithelium to regrow over denuded areas, either because it does not properly adhere, as in recurrent erosion, or because a chronic ulcerative process destroys it as may occur in some corneal dystrophies.

Bandage lenses have been tried at least as a temporary measure in a few cases of corneal perforation, whether ulcerative or traumatic in origin.

There have been cautious trials of soft lens wear in dry eye conditions. However, as has already been pointed out, such subjects are often unsuitable for routine contact lens wear and the hydrophilic nature of the hydrogel may be disadvantageous for therapeutic use; hydrophobic silicone rubber lenses have been tried. Soft lenses

soaked in some medication have been used as a slow-release method for delivery of a drug.

All types of lens have at various times been used to play a part in ocular protection; lagophthalmos of any degree may be suitably managed, whether traumatic or paralytic in origin. In these cases however contact lenses should be regarded very much as a second line of treatment to other surgical measures such as tarsorrhaphy or conjunctival flaps.

The therapeutic use of scleral lenses, as with their general application, is declining, but they still have some part to play in conjunctival cicatrisation such as may result from the Stevens–Johnson syndrome, trichiasis, and in atopics or those with dry eyes. A scleral lens has also been used as a method of supporting a ptosed upper lid.

SCLERAL LENSES

Scleral lens fitting has declined considerably in modern contact lens practice, and the following account is included partly for historical reasons but also to indicate the routines of practice where this is still continuing.

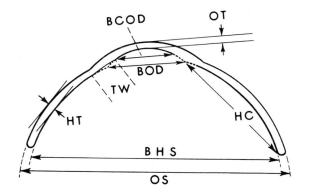

Fig. 25.16 The parts of a scleral lens.

HT: Haptic thickness
OT: Optic thickness
BOD: Back optic diameter
BCOD: Back central optic diameter
TW: Transition width
HC: Haptic curve
BHS: Back haptic size
OS: Overall size.

Types of scleral lens

Many modern scleral lenses are of the moulded variety, although pre-formed lenses based upon geometrical concepts or upon differing established ocular shapes are still extant (see Figs 25.1 and 25.16).

Moulded scleral lenses are based on casting taken from the individual patient's eye. These are carried out by introducing into the palpebral aperture a readily impressionable material in a melted form which sets rapidly and firmly to form a negative cast — such a substance as ophthalmic Moldite (made of gypsum, light magnesium carbonate, dental plaster, trisodium phosphate and sodium alginate) or a newer material, Panasil. The chief advantages of such materials are that they can be inserted cold and set rapidly. Special plastic shells are employed to apply the material to the eye (Fig. 25.17). From the impression a model of the anterior segment of the globe is made in a dental plaster; a shell is now fashioned by pressing a sheet of heated plastic onto the mould.

If the scleral lens is for optical purposes its back surface is usually cut or ground so as to give the lens minimal apical clearance from the cornea, the back surface of the optical portion being made slightly flatter than that of the subject's cornea.

Although some sealed (non-ventilated) lenses are still in use, most are ventilated by either fenestration or channelling (see Fig. 25.18) and,

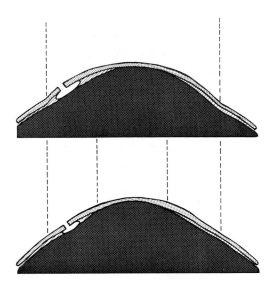

Fig. 25.18 Ventilation of a scleral lens.

in order to avoid pressure on the limbal circulation, a transition is usually ground between the optic and haptic portions of the posterior surface.

In a lens intended for therapeutic use however, the flush-fitting shell, the posterior surface of the lens closely follows the anterior surface of the cornea.

Most scleral lenses are made of PMMA but some gas-permeable materials have also been tried although there are manufacturing problems as they do not exist in sheet form.

The fitting of scleral lenses

A properly fitting scleral contact lens for optical use has the following features. The haptic (scleral portion) lies in even contact with the globe to within 2 or 3 mm of the limbus with no very tight or loose areas, its temporal and superior regions being as large as possible and the nasal flange fitting moderately loosely to encourage through flow of tears and the outflow of debris.

The limbal region is cleared and there is no sharp transition between the haptic and optic portions, the optic is well centred on the cornea and except in the flush-fitting variety clears the apical region, perhaps in its axial two-thirds, by

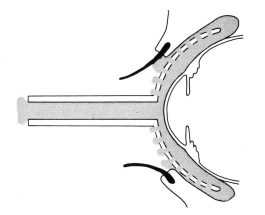

Fig. 25.17 Shell for moulded scleral lenses.

0.1 mm. Although a minimal clearance is the theoretical ideal it is likely that light central touch is present even in the primary position of gaze. In the peripheral zone of the cornea clearance becomes progressively greater until the limbal region is reached where it is at its maximum (see Fig. 25.18).

There must be no excessive lag of the lens on ocular movements, nor must it sag under its own weight; some relative movement however is inevitable and probably desirable in order to encourage the exchange of fluid under the lens. Because of the progressive clearance towards the periphery of the cornea a concave meniscus of fluid exists between the lens and the eye, and when ventilated the fenestration or channel (groove) must communicate with this perilimbal meniscus (see Fig. 25.19).

A fenestration is placed in the palpebral aperture, usually the temporal border of the optic and slightly below the midpoint of the pupil. A bubble of air forms here beneath the lens. In a well-fitted scleral lens the bubble is bean shaped, about a quarter of an inch by an eighth of an inch wide in the primary position, and with movements of the eye it moves round the limbus. It may alter in size as the air is sucked in or forced out; the increase in the size on extreme ocular movements should never be so great that on return to the normal position there is undue delay in the refilling of the chamber between the lens and the eye. The bubble should remain confined to the limbal region and preferably

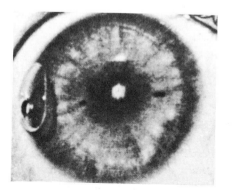

Fig. 25.19 Bubble beneath scleral lens.

temporal portion; in the inferonasal region it may interfere with vision.

The above criteria of a well-fitting scleral lens are what should be aimed at in the clinical assessment of a patient as to suitability for scleral lens wear.

The procedure adopted varies with different practitioners. The fit may be inspected after inserting the lens dry, but more commonly it is inserted with fluid to which a drop of fluorescein has been added. The lens is marked to indicate the horizontal diameter before it is inserted (by comparison with the mould) or when it is in situ.

The factors to be considered after insertion are the overall size and shape of the lens, its movement with the eye, the haptic bearing relationship, the transitional zone between the haptic and optic portions and the clearance and centring of the optic. If the lens is too small it may be cosmetically unacceptable because the edges of the haptic are visible. Conversely too large a lens can be reduced to the appropriate size. If the lens rotates, fitting is grossly wrong, and it may be necessary to carry out a fresh moulding if that is the technique used. Some modification to the tight areas of the haptic seen by the blanching of the underlying conjunctival vessels, or to its edge if this is loose, may also be necessary. Once the overall size and stability are established any fenestration or channelling is carried out and then the fit of the lens is re-examined.

Examination of the fluorescein pattern is important. Ideally, about the limbal region there should be a ring of fluorescence some 2 to 3 mm in width if the clearance there is adequate. It is important to assess the fluorescein pattern not only in the primary position but also on movement of the eyes. Digital pressure on the lens may give some indication of the freedom or otherwise if the fluid can enter and leave the space behind it.

Areas requiring modification are marked and the lens is removed. Precisely how these procedures are carried out is not within the scope of this book, but in principle tight areas are ground out and polished and the region surrounding a loose zone similarly treated. Heavy apical touch of the cornea requires increased clearance, which can be obtained by grinding the posterior surface of the optic. A final haptic thickness of about 0.6 mm is aimed at.

Once the physical fit is satisfactory a refraction is carried out and the centre of the pupil is marked with the eye in the primary position. Objective and subjective refraction are performed with the contact lens in place. The appropriate optical power is then worked on the front surface of the lens.

In the majority of cases the refraction of a subject wearing a contact lens with a spherical anterior surface will show a simple spherical correction since the optical effect of the corneal astigmatism is eliminated; in some instances however a significant degree of residual astigmatism is found. This can be corrected by modifying the front surface of the optical part of the lens to a toroidal form. In ordering the incorporation of an optical correction it is usual to undercorrect myopia or overcorrect hypermetropia, since in subsequent modifications it is easier to make the correction more myopic or less hypermetropic than the reverse.

Complications of scleral lens wear

During the process of adaptation — initial symptoms caused by the presence of a large foreign body and many of the reflex responses to it — become much less marked. Thus pain, lacrimation, blepharospasm and conjunctival injection may be present in the early stages but later disappear together with the sensation of a foreign body and a burning feeling and a sensation of stretched eyelids. This may partly be because the fit of a scleral lens alters with the passage of time in a process sometimes referred to as settling; to some extent this may be a moulding of the ocular tissues in association with the development of local oedema or a herniation forward of the corneal apex.

However, residual symptoms or discomfort remain in many subjects which limit tolerance and finally wearing time and may finally cause the lens to be abandoned.

The most important complication is the development of corneal oedema producing blurring of vision and 'veiling' (Sattlers' veil) at a variable interval after lens insertion. As we have noted fenestration, channelling and transition width are all important to allow renewal of the tear flow under the lens, adequate oxygenation of the tears being required to prevent this veiling. In very longstanding wearers corneal vascularisation may occur.

The time, expense and results of scleral lens fitting were all factors prompting the development of the corneal lens, and their routine prescription for simple optical defects has been largely abandoned. Therapeutic flush-fitting shells continue to have an important place in ophthalmology, and there is perhaps a very limited indication for scleral lens wear in sports activities, particularly swimming, where it is the only type of contact lens not liable to be lost, and in other sports where repeated loss of a corneal lens, rigid or non-rigid, has occurred. The other specialised uses of scleral lenses have been mentioned throughout the text. They may be valuable in light exclusion in albinism and aniridia. They have some part to play in the management of high astigmatism, particularly residual astigmatism or where it is markedly irregular, perhaps with consequent failure of a corneal contact lens to centre properly. The particular variety of astigmatism where it has been most applied is of course in the management of kerataconus, but even here, as with all these other indications just mentioned, scleral lens trial has now become a last resort after all other types of contact lens have proved unsuccessful.

CONTACT LENSES AND THE GENERALIST

What has gone before has been intended as a concise overview of contact lens practice, acquainting those outside the field with its methods and the rationale behind it and introducing an approach to the subject which will allow the reader to embark upon lens fitting if so desired. There are however many eye-care professionals, some ophthalmologists, optometrists, medical personnel or those in other ancillary occupations such as orthoptists or nurses, whose clinical exposure to the contact lens patient is minimal but when it occurs relates only to complications of wear of one sort or another. What follows is therefore directed to their recognition and handling of such problems and related issues. Some of these have already been detailed in the formal account above but this section is for the non-specialist.

Perhaps the first thing to emphasise is that any 'anterior segment' complaint or visual disturbance in a contact lens wearer must be attributed to that cause before considering any other aetiologies.

It is astonishing to have to state this but it often happens that contact lens wearers are reluctant to admit to someone from whom they seek advice either that they wear or have in the recent past worn lenses or that their trouble could possibly be related to them. They are often so anxious not to be told to leave them out, the latter being the first obvious therapeutic measure for their problem, indeed the beneficial effect of so doing may already be known to them.

This situation occurs especially when the complaint is neither of vision nor of pain and discomfort and is typically found when the symptom is simply a red eye or a slight discharge.

In fact when in the general ophthalmological clinic a patient describes symptoms of external eye disease an important direct question should always be 'do you or have you ever worn contact lenses?'

When the answer is 'Yes' a routine of other questions should follow: 'Hard or soft?', 'How long?', 'When last worn?', 'What relation of symptoms to periods of contact lens wear?', 'What wearing regime?', 'What solutions are being worn for storage, soaking, cleaning, wetting, etc.?', 'When were lenses last cleaned professionally?', 'How old are the current pair and what is the age of the storage case?', 'Has the lens type been changed?', 'Why were the lenses changed?', 'What methods were used to insert the lenses?', 'What is the hygiene regime and how good is compliance to it?', 'What advice was given by the fitter about the presenting problem?', 'What kind of follow-up regime was there after the lenses were fitted?', 'Does the wearer carry any identification of the type of lens worn?'

Although the generalist will not have the complex instrumentation of the full-time contact lens practitioner it will usually be possible to inspect the lenses for the presence of deposits or scratches and indeed for their intactness. This inspection may be done either in situ or with the lenses removed. Simple neutralisation will allow one to gauge the power of the lens. Their optical efficiency is assessed by visual acuity, by retinoscopy and by overrefraction with lenses and a pin-hole. A myope for example may be discovered to be undercorrected in spherical power or, in the case of soft lenses, an uncorrected astigmatic error may show up. With the lenses in place a check should be made of centration, mobility and whether the patient appears to be blinking adequately.

The precise nature of the complaint will prompt a search for particular physical signs. All acute painful episodes are likely to show some degree of conjunctival or circumcorneal injection, an area of corneal staining in a subject with a watering half-closed photophobic eye being a very common finding in these circumstances. Corneal infiltrates should always raise the spectre of infective keratitis, although as we have seen in some soft lens wearers small peripheral infiltrates are often quite sterile.

Oedema of the cornea, epithelial or stromal, may be associated with any kind of insult whether overwearing or a fitting problem, a purely mechanical effect or an infection. Recurrent non-acute problems of poor tolerance may occur with corneal microcystic disease, or with 3 and 9 o'clock staining.

Limbal vascularisation may be found in daily or extended soft lens wearers, in aphakics and in some cases of Thiomersal toxicity.

Excessive grease on the lens or in the conjunctival sac should raise a suspicion of giant papillary conjunctivitis in the soft lens wearer and it is mandatory in every contact lens follow-up to evert the upper lids to look for this condition.

A final question is what to do about these problems. Should a generalist handle the situation or should there be a referral back or on to a more specialised professional — ophthalmologist or optometrist. There is no definitive answer to this problem but perhaps the guideline should be to act on the identifiable problem up to the point where it is felt that the only remaining step is to refer for refitting.

The first measure is obviously to stop lens wear for a period of time. This is always the case with acute episodes, particularly of course if the subject has been unable to remove the lens himself. Doing this may not be easy in an eye with marked blepharospasm and pain and local anaesthesia should be used without hesitation.

What is more difficult to decide is when to allow resumption of lens wear. Here one must be guided by the way the cornea returns to normal and by assurance that all other factors — lens cleanliness, sterility and handling, case sanitation and the appropriateness of fluids used — are satisfactory. When lens wear is resumed frequent follow-ups may be advisable again.

The regime to be followed after particular complications has been detailed in previous chapters, but it would certainly be perfectly appropriate for the 'general' professional, in referring back to the contact lens specialist, to comment on what was felt to be the cause of the problem, specifically this could indicate the need for more corneal oxygen, i.e. for thinner or higher water content soft lenses or for a fit which would be preferable, either tighter or looser, or for a change of lens type from gas permeable to soft or the reverse.

Changes of fluid should be advised if there is the slightest question of preservative toxicity or sensitivity. Most countries' handbooks of contact lenses now list types of available contact lens fluids with their compositions. It is a good idea for the generalist to have such a reference source available. The possibility of reducing dependence on contact lens fluids is now somewhat more in prospect following the introduction of disposable lenses. However the regimes for using these in some cases still seem to include a number of pharmaceuticals.

Two related topics which the generalist should be aware of are lens compatibility with ophthalmic medication and in women (most often) with eye cosmetics.

As far as medication is concerned there is no great problem with hard PMMA or gas-permeable lenses. For soft lens wearers these may in fact potentiate the action of some habitually used anti-glaucoma drops such as Timoptol; adrenaline may cause pigmentation of lenses so some caution is needed and lens renewal may be required more frequently. Antibiotics and steroids in drop form are well tolerated. As a matter of practice the drops should be placed in the lower fornix. Something to watch out for in the chronic drop user is a possibility of preservative-induced keratopathy, the possible offenders being Thiomersal or, particularly in soft lens wearers, benzalkonium chloride.

With regard to *cosmetics* the situation appears to be that only a minority of contact lens wearers run into trouble from this source. The simplest problem arises from lenses that become dirty or stained or contaminated with cosmetic products, often mascara, and here as with cream eye shadows their containers may act as a source of repeated reinfection of the eye. Certainly mascara particles are frequently found subtarsally and in the fornices whether contact lenses are worn or not. It is believed that fibrous, waterproof varieties are the more abrasive; the particles of pearlised crayons and eye shadow may act similarly.

Oil-based products which are widely used as make-up removers may intermingle with the pre-corneal film and deposit on the lens. Finally, the possibility of true cosmetic allergy should be considered, especially if there is an obvious blepharitic element.

The likelihood of cosmetics problems in the contact lens wearer will of course be significantly reduced by scrupulous hygiene in relation not only to the products and implements used for applying and removing them but also in lens and lens case hygiene itself.

Finally the generalist may be faced with a patient wearing contact lenses to which the problem complained of is perhaps totally unrelated. Here it may incidentally be observed that some symptomless anomaly is present such as a minor degree of 3 and 9 o'clock staining, a poorly centring lens, or minimal limbal vascularisation. In most cases such findings should be noted for further reviews at suitable intervals (or earlier if relevant symptoms develop) and no further action should be taken.

26. Visual aids

Failure of the visual acuity to correct to a normal level with standard optical techniques is characteristic of many important ophthalmic diseases, but in a significant proportion of such cases some improvement in vision can be obtained by the use of special optical devices known as visual aids or low-vision aids. The vast majority of these are for magnification of the image, and how helpful they are depends on many factors. The patient's pathology and temperament, the purpose for which they are required and the enthusiasm and sympathy of the prescriber all play a part in what is always a clinically difficult situation, overshadowed as it is by the knowledge that the patient's basic eye disease is one for which the ophthalmologist has nothing further to offer.

What type of patients might benefit?

Most patients coming to a visual aid assessment have macular problems, either age related or due to high myopia, but a trial of these devices is also worth while for those with many other conditions such as advanced glaucoma, diabetic retinopathy, optic atrophy or even strabismic amblyopia.

There is no absolute standard of vision above which visual aids will be useful and below which they will not. Much will depend on the nature of the visual loss. Is it a central scotomatous effect? Is it a general lowering or homonymous defect of the visual field? Is the field severely contracted? Nevertheless, there are suggestive features. An acuity of no better than hand movement from whatever cause is unlikely to be helped; someone with a macular pathology but who has good navigable vision, perhaps with some retained ability to recognise large coloured objects, may be educated to make further use of eccentric viewing and of magnification devices.

What usual activities is the patient interested in attempting to improve?

Many of the patients are old and frequently relatively immobile so that the retention of some ability to read is of vital importance to their happiness. Both in them and at younger ages other leisure activities involving near work are important and the necessity for some useful near vision in the subject's occupation is a powerful stimulus to attempting to use these devices.

Visual aids are also available to help distance viewing, but they are less practical than those for near. In addition however there are many other specific activities which may need to be considered. Signing cheques, recognising paper money and coinage, playing cards, cooking and consuming food are examples of these.

Clinical assessment

As full a refraction as possible should be attempted, and a subjective test should be performed with special test types, of which there are many. Three-metre charts for distance and low-vision near charts (Keeler, Sloan) are those commonly used.

As far as the distance correction goes this need not be refined to more than perhaps + or −1 dioptre of sphere if the best acuity is less than 6/60. Cylinders in the final correction can often be ignored unless of very high power. A trial frame and lenses should always be used, not a large refracting unit, which may interfere with the patient's use of eccentric viewing. Encouragement to poorly responding subjects will sometimes be given by putting a special telescope (2.2 × magnification, Keeler) into the trial frame to demonstrate that some useful distance sight is available.

With regard to near vision, the various special charts will indicate the reading vision and the magnification or addition required to attain a particular level. The charts should be employed at the recommended distance, the Sloan M charts at 40 cm, the Keeler chart at 25 cm. The patient should wear a distance correction with a spherical addition appropriate to these distances (+2.5 D for the Sloan and +4.00 D for the Keeler) so as to eliminate any accommodative requirement.

In the Sloan system a series of M cards is available numbered 10 to 1. M1 corresponds to newsprint (J5) or a distance acuity equivalence of 6/12 or slightly better. These are presented in decreasing print size and the smallest seen is identified; this will have an M number, say 5, the reading add required is 5 × 2.50 = 15 D (2.50 D is the dioptric value of 40 cm, the test distance).

In the Keeler system, at 25 cm test distance

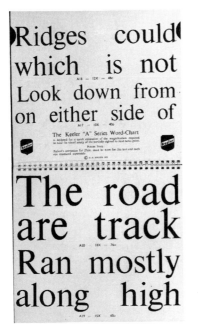

Fig. 26.1 The Keeler low-vision reading chart.

the magnification required can be assessed from the test card (Fig. 26.1 and Table 26.1) and the appropriate add is obtained by multiplying the magnification by 4 (dioptric value of 25 cm).

A useful rule of thumb for the near addition may be calculated from the distance Snellen acuity. The reciprocal of this acuity gives an approximate guide to the near lens power for attempting to read newsprint (J5 or N6–8, printers' 8 point type). The lens power should be the reciprocal plus the patient's own refraction, and where indicated with 1 or 2 dioptres more added. Stronger lenses are needed for telephone directories (J3 or N5), and if an attempt is to be made at the smallest print (Bible type J1 or N4.5).

THE MANAGEMENT OF LOW VISION

General factors

Whatever size of retinal image is considered appropriate, its distinctness and its contrast should be optimal, and this means that accurate refraction and appropriate illumination should be ensured. The targeted object should not have any undesirable features that can be avoided, such as glossy printed material.

Magnification

This is the basis of most techniques used in the low-vision clinic. There are three methods of enlarging the retinal image: approximating the object, magnification of the retinal image, and increasing the size of the object to be viewed.

1. *Bring the object nearer*

   This leads to an increase in the visual angle subtended at the eye by the object. The retinal image is made optically as clear as possible by the use of convex lenses to supplement or replace whatever accommodative power the eye has; such power may be quite high in a young subject, and in the high myope a lens may be unnecessary as the far point will be very close to the eye anyway, no accommodation being required.

   Where a lens is necessary in a subject of an age in whom accommodation has vanished, a

Table 26.1   Keeler system

Actual visual acuity (ametropia corrected) (at 25 cm)						Magnification needed to read			
Snellen fractions		%	Jaeger	Times New Roman	Keeler 'A' series	N12 (J10)	N10 (J8)	N8 (J6)	N6 (J4)
English	American								
6/18	20/60	33	J4	N6	A6				
6/24	20/80	26	J6	N8	A7				1.3
		21	J8	N10	A8			1.3	1.6
6/36	20/120	17	J10	N12	A9		1.3	1.6	2.0
		13	J12	N14	A10	1.3	1.6	2.0	2.5
6/60	20/200	11	J14	N16	A11	1.6	2.0	2.5	3
		8.6			A12	2.0	2.5	3	4
		6.9			A13	2.5	3	4	5
3/60		5.5			A14	3	4	5	6
		4.4			A15	4	5	6	8
		3.5			A16	5	6	8	10
		2.8			A17	6	8	10	12
		2.3			A18	8	10	12	15
1/60	3/200 (approx.)	1.8			A19	10	12	15	18
		1.4			A20	12	15	18	23

Newspapers ⟶ (N8)

Telephone directory ⟶ (N6)

The level of visual acuity in many visually impaired patients is commonly 6/12 (20/40) or worse. Standard optometric test types have insufficient ranges with irregular intervals which make estimating the magnification requirement of patients more difficult. In order to overcome these disadvantages, Keeler use a system of grading acuities was developed based on a logarithmic scale. Each grade or 'A' number represents a constant fraction of 80% of the size of the preceding number. Snellen 6/6 (20/20) is designated A1. Therefore 80% of the size 6/6 will be A2, and so on. In turn A20 represents 1.4% approximately of 6/6. Near vision letter (see Fig. 26.1) and word charts are available too, and allow estimates of magnification required to be made for reading, based on similar principles of size scaling.

simple high addition to a presbyopic correction may be helpful. This type of optical manoeuvre inter-relates with a group of devices known as spectacle-borne aids (see below). This method of approximating the object is of course of particular value only if the task is one relating to close work. Truly distant objects, road signs for example, or bus numbers, have to be managed in a different way.

Psychologically it is very difficult to persuade many patients to bring objects close to their eyes, and certainly at very close distances binocularity will be impossible. However education should persist in attempting to persuade the patient that no harm comes to the vision from viewing objects at a very close distance, and in particular they should be advised to sit very close to television sets where, as far as we know, no harmful emissions are likely to damage their eyesight or any other bodily function.

2. *Optical magnification*

Before discussing some of these devices their limitations should be understood. Increasing magnification by whatever means — optical or electronic — has disadvantages. It may be less than helpful to a patient with already restricted visual fields, for example in advanced glaucoma. Even in age-related maculopathy where increasing the retinal image size has its widest application, the greater the magnification, the smaller the visual field, the shorter the working distance and the more limited the depth of focus. The small visual field makes fluent reading laborious when only a few words can be appreciated at one time, and it may be difficult to find the beginning of the next line of print; the reduced depth of focus makes the placing of the reading matter extremely critical.

Moreover, as the magnification is increased so must the lighting, which should be ample and properly directed on the fixation area. In general therefore the lowest magnification compatible with useful vision should be employed. If they are to be helpful these aids to vision must be adapted to each particular case and the disadvantages in their use should be carefully explained to the patient, who usually requires much sympathetic encouragement. It is to be remembered that the periphery of the retina around the fovea is employed to interpret the enlarged images and it is psychologically difficult except after considerable practice in eccentric viewing, carried out with perseverance. Finally, most of the degenerative conditions are progressive, and as the vision deteriorates adjustments to the optical system may be necessary until in many cases they prove insufficient and have to be abandoned.

Simple magnifiers

The simplest device as far as near work is concerned is to employ an ordinary magnifying glass held in the hand near the object of attention. This is merely a biconvex lens. By definition its effective magnification is measured as if for an object 25 cm away from the eye and at the first focal plane of the lens. This equates with approximately one-quarter of its dioptric power: thus a +16 D lens will magnify about ×4 diameters. The main trouble with such an expedient is the distortion of the image which is produced, a defect which can be diminished by using an aplanatic system of lenses such as exemplified in the familiar ophthalmic loupe. The classical magnifying glass is circular, but a rather more useful form of such a lens is rectangular (Fig. 26.2), of such a length that it covers an average line of print and thus often requires only to be moved down the page and not across it as well. A further expedient is a sphero-cylindrical lens with the axis of the cylinder horizontal so that it magnifies preferentially in the vertical direction.

The flexibility of the hand-magnifier derives, however, from the control by the patient over its position in relation to the eye or the object of regard. When such a simple device is used for reading it is sometimes advisable to sacrifice this flexibility and to mount it on a stand so that the object–lens distance is kept fixed, higher magnifications then being practicable. The optical advantage of a *stand magnifier* is the relative constancy of the size of the retinal image if the object is very close to the anterior focal point of

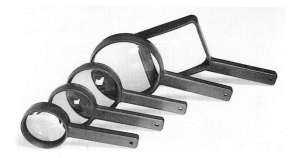

Fig. 26.2 A selection of reading magnifying glasses (Keeler).

the magnifier, although in most cases it is significantly within the focal distance. The eye may be positioned either close to the lens, giving a large field, or some distance away. The further the subject is away from the hand or stand magnifier, the more likely is it that useful binocular vision will be possible.

There are many other variants of the hand-held and stand magnifiers. An additional or optional feature in some stand and hand-held varieties is the incorporation of illumination into the devices, this being particularly helpful if the working distance is short. A further simple device combines an anglepoise light with a simple magnifier. This, like a similar device held round the neck and resting on the chest, retains some flexibility, leaving the hands free for such activities as sewing and knitting. Their lightness and optical properties have been improved by fashioning them in plastic and taking advantage of aspherical surfaces, thereby increasing the useful field. Another single-lens magnifier is the 'paperweight' plano-convex glass (Fig. 26.3); binocular magnifiers such as the head-band loupe require the incorporation of base-in prisms.

Combinations of lenses are also extensively used in magnifiers (Fig. 26.4). Focusable stand

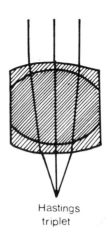

Fig. 26.4 Lens combinations as magnifier.

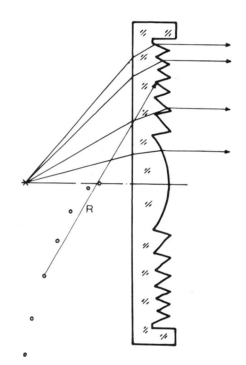

Fig. 26.5 Fresnel lens.

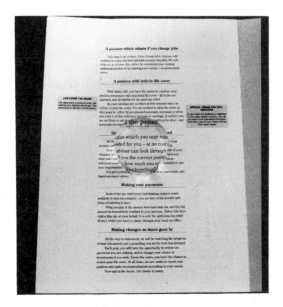

Fig. 26.3 Paperweight magnifier.

magnifiers of doublet design up to +53 D in power are available, with which the patient does not need to wear his spectacle correction.

Stepped lenses, such as were introduced for lighthouses by Fresnel in 1822, can be used as magnifiers (Fig. 26.5). One type is essentially a plastic sheet with concentric ridges on its surface forming a series of prisms of increasing power from the axis to the periphery and has the great advantage of eliminating the thickness and marked aberration that would be unavoidable in a single large lens with a continuous surface.

Spectacle-borne visual aids

Most of the visual aids just reviewed are employed with only a minor degree of approximation of the object to the eye during close work. In those devices worn in spectacle frames, apart from telescopic spectacles, a considerable degree of approximation is usually necessary, and much encouragement is often required to induce the patient to read with the print 'at the nose'. In most of these *spectacle-borne visual aids* the object is to all intents and purposes placed at the anterior focal point of the device and not, as in the case of hand-held and stand magnifiers, within the anterior focal distance. We have already noted that focusing is critical, and some means of maintaining print in a fixed position such as a 'distance post' is necessary. High-power spherical lenses may be used: a lens of +10 D in this position gives a magnification of 2.5, one of 16.00 D, 4.0, and one of 24.00 D, 6. They have the advantage that the hands are freed from holding a magnifying lens, an important matter if the patient is tremulous.

Single or multiple lens units, both microscopic and telescopic devices, can be built into spectacle frames, and some of these optical arrangements incorporate an illuminating device (Fig. 26.6).

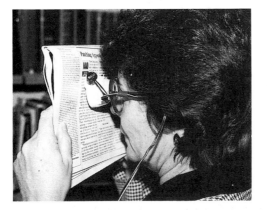

Fig. 26.6 Self-illuminated spectacle-borne magnifier.

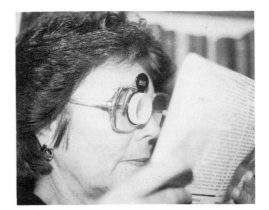

Fig. 26.7 Clip-on magnifier.

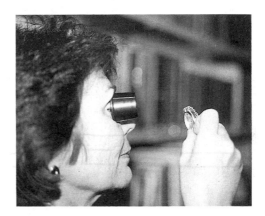

Fig. 26.8 Watchmaker's loupe.

Single lenses may be conventional or best-form convex glasses (Lederer, 1954) occupying a spectacle frame or monocle, or be fitted as a 'clip-on' (Fig. 26.7) over the required correction; jewellers' and watchmakers' loupes can be similarly employed (Fig. 26.8). There are also various aspherical designs offering less aberration peripherally and therefore a larger field — glass 'conoid' lenses (Volk) up to +100 D and plastic lenses (Aolite and Igard) up to +48 D.

Bifocal arrangements are quite feasible and additions may be fused, ground or cemented on; powers up to 32 D are practicable and even higher in some cases; the distance portion may merely be a cut-out.

Multiple lens systems, doublets with or without an air space or triplets (such as the Hastings) can also be used as spectacle magnifiers (see Fig. 26.4). Powers up to +80 D are possible with doublets, and these can also be built in to form a bifocal correction. Modern compound reading spectacles (such as the Bier–Hamblin type) make use of plastic materials and have aspherical surfaces.

Binocular corrections are not usually practicable with high-powered spectacle magnifiers so that a frosted glass is worn before the fellow eye. With relatively lower corrections up to an addition of approximately +10 D in bifocals, or slightly more in a single vision lens, a binocular correction is possible. In such cases insetting of the segments or, in single vision lenses, nasal decentration as well as high base-in prisms may be necessary. A typical binocular 3× magnifier

might consist of a +12 D lens with a 14 Δ base-in prism, for each eye. A binocular correction offers a larger field and a greater depth of focus.

Some of these disadvantages can be overcome by the use of a combination of lenses in a *telescopic* (or *Galilean*) *system* (Fig. 26.9). In this the object glass is a convex lens which converges the incident rays, and the eye-piece, which is a concave lens placed so that the two are separated by the difference between their focal lengths, gives them the necessary divergence for distinct and magnified vision. Figure 26.10 shows the basis of the optical system. A cylindrical correction can be incorporated, and fittings can be adjusted to suit distant and near vision. A Galilean system is the most suitable to employ since, with the use of only two simple lenses, it gives an erect image with a large exit pupil, so that compactness and lightness in weight are readily achieved. Moreover, the combination of a positive and negative lens secures a moderately flat field relatively free from astigmatism. If the available field is to be large, great care must be taken in their design to lessen the effect of peripheral aberrations. It is to be remembered, also, that different lenses must always be prescribed for reading and for distant vision. This is necessary for two reasons. Because of the magnification, approximately +10.0 D of accommodation is required to focus objects at 25 cm (instead of the normal +4.0 D) if the correcting lenses are placed behind the spectacles.

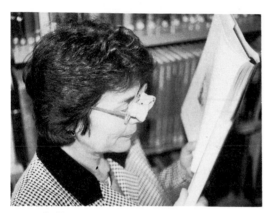

Fig. 26.9 Galilean spectacles.

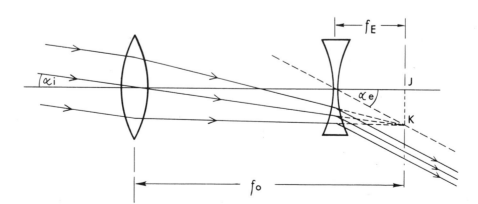

Fig. 26.10 The Galilean system.

f_o is the focal length of the objective, f_E that of the eye-piece. The magnification is given by $\dfrac{\alpha_e}{\alpha_i}$.

Moreover, the patient must look axially through the system, and this necessitates a different pupillary distance and a different angling for the two distances. If efficiently made, such an optical system may be of great value, but it must be remembered that, although it is often the only alternative to virtual blindness, it is cumbersome, weighty and expensive, and suffers from the defect of all magnifying optical instruments that it reduces the field of vision in proportion to the degree of magnification obtained. So great are the difficulties of this restriction that a high spherical correction is often more acceptable to some patients for reading. In others the fact that print need not be held so close and the possibility of binocular corrections decide them in favour of a telescopic device. Modern versions of these make extensive use of plastics both for housing and for lenses, leading to a significant reduction in their weight.

Several such systems are available, the two lenses being fixed the requisite distance apart at the ends of a cylindrical tube which can be hooked onto or be fixed into one aperture of the spectacle frame, the other being usually occluded by an opaque disc. As a rule a strong convex lens of about +20.00 D sphere with a spherical or aspherical curvature is fixed to the front end of the tube and a concave lens (of about −20.00 D to −40.00 D sphere) is mounted at the rear end, the most suitable power being determined by trial and error; the back lens can be modified to incorporate the patient's refractive error. With an auxiliary lens of −3.00 D sphere the combination can be used for distant vision; alternatively the correction may be made for distant vision (which, of course, entails a very restricted field), to which the reading addition can be affixed in an auxiliary cap. Either or both of these may be so incorporated in a spectacle lens in bifocal fashion. Thus both a distance and reading telescope may be inserted in one lens of a uniocular correction, the reading portion being much the larger; such a combination may be of great value to a partially sighted child in the classroom. In all cases the best combination must be determined for each particular patient, and extreme care must be taken in the fitting and centring of the appliance, particularly if an attempt is made to attain binocularity.

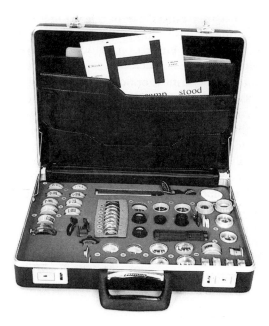

Fig. 26.11 The Keeler LVA trial set.

In the most extensive and effective appliances which have been elaborated, the Keeler LVA (low visual acuity) scheme, the binocular telescopes incorporate a specially angled bar to vary the interpupillary distance. The Keeler range comprises means for the assessment of the most effective magnification, its practical verification by trial units and dispensing sets from which the actual units to be used are provided (Fig. 26.11), perhaps initially on loan.

Some specially designed *contact lenses* allow both normal and magnified vision. The magnified vision is subserved by a small axial concave area on the anterior surface of the contact lens in combination with a convex spectacle lens; when the spectacles are removed normal vision is obtained through the periphery of the optical zone of the contact lens. A teledioptric system incorporating an intra-ocular lens has been tried.

Other aids to distance and intermediate vision

Most visual aids for distance viewing are based on telescopic systems. Head-borne telescopes offer up to 3× magnification, limited again by restricted field, depth of focus weight as well as by optical aberrations. Small telescopic inserts in conventional lenses have been promulgated as aids to driving, but this is a very tendentious subject.

Hand-held prism monoculars are very helpful, for example in identifying bus numbers or street signs. In some cases magnifications up to seven or eight times are available. Their appearance is usually more acceptable than those of head-borne devices in which it is very difficult to walk about. Several optical tricks can be helpful. Aphakic (not pseudophakic) patients may hold up a +3 D lens at arm's length and get a magnified image by the telescopic system so formed.

Phakic patients can do the same by wearing a −20 D spectacle lens and holding a +5 D lens a few inches from the eye. Reversing a monocular prism telescope may help a subject with a very restricted field to assess his whereabouts.

Telescopic devices either specifically designed or with plus add caps are sometimes used for intermediate vision tasks such as typing and using VDUs.

3. Increasing the size of the object to be viewed

Large-size telephone dials, playing cards and of course large-size-print books are examples of this approach to low vision. The advent of enlarging photocopiers may be of help for reading specific documents.

The other approach to this is to view an externally enlarged image of the object being inspected. This brings us to the field of projection devices and closed-circuit television. Neither of these has been widely accepted, perhaps because they are both cumbersome and expensive, but certainly closed-circuit television offers the possibility of magnification up to 40 times in an undistorted way and the patient can get as close as he wishes to the monitor which may be a small or medium sized screen. The video camera usually has a zoom lens, and recently Sony have brought out a reasonably portable version of this type of visual aid, which amongst other uses may find a particular application in leisure activities and hobbies.

Apart from the undistorted magnification closed-circuit television offers two other advantages. The polarity may be reversed, allowing the print to be offered as white on black, and this contrast may be found helpful by some patients. It is also possible to isolate one line of print, which may make it more intelligible.

Non-magnifying visual aids

Where the transparency of the ocular media is at fault, a *stenopaeic hole* sometimes forms the only expedient by which any degree of useful vision may be obtained. Its optical properties have already been discussed (see p. 36). As an emergency measure, it is sometimes useful. Its main disadvantage is that it provides no visual field, and since the eye cannot move behind it it is of very little advantage to the wearer when walking about. It is useful, however, in reading, when it is best held in the hand following the line of print. When it is required for general purposes, a 'glass' composed of several such openings bored in a sheet of opaque metal, as suggested by Knapp, may prove better than nothing (Fig. 26.12).

It is to be noted that the stenopaeic opening will prove equally useful in any error of refraction, and in the event of a pair of spectacles being lost or broken it will enable a presbyope, for example, to read or write in an emergency. It is interesting that its properties have long been used, usually in the form of a horizontal stenopaeic slit, by the primitive Eskimos as a protective measure from the ultraviolet radiation reflected from the snow.

The use of a *reading slit* cut in dark cardboard or plastic material placed immediately over print with approximate dimensions of 0.5 cm to 1.00 cm by 8 cm to 16 cm so that only one or two lines are visible is also sometimes found helpful by patients with early lens opacities. In such cases reflected light from the page is decreased and the contrast is thereby increased

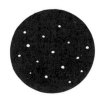

Fig. 26.12 Stenopaeic 'glasses' (after Knapp).

Fig. 26.13 Leinbach's reading slit.

thus allowing greater clarity in reading (Leinbach, 1960) (Fig. 26.13).

THE SUCCESS OF VISUAL AIDS

As every ophthalmologist knows, successful use of low-vision aids is unpredictable and on the whole rather less successful than is desirable. The reasons for this are varied. In some cases there may be a lack of encouragement on the part of the tester; in others there may be poor motivation on the part of the patient, perhaps because the visual aid being used is inappropriate for the patient's condition.

Again, the patient may feel that forcing himself to see may accelerate a deterioration of his condition almost as if he feels that there is a ration of sight which is going to be used up by continued employment of the eyes. He should of course be disabused of such an idea.

It, is also good practice to explain as far as appropriate the nature of the ophthalmic pathology and its likely prognosis. There are still many patients with age-related maculopathy whose poor reading vision with any device convinces them that they are going to go totally blind. This is certainly one area where firm reassurance by the ophthalmologist will be valuable.

Finally a word for the ophthalmologist himself. It will be a matter of personal decision as to how far the general ophthalmologist will take the management of low vision himself. Many will simply refer on to a medical or optometric centre specialising in this field. Others will wish to equip themselves with simple representative devices of the various categories mentioned above, hand-held and spectacle-borne magnifiers and perhaps

a telescopic instrument, if only for demonstration purposes. A small group will find time in their practice for full-blown investigation and ordering of all forms of these devices.

Somehow, perhaps with a grain of truth, it is not unknown for specialists in low vision to voice the idea that once the ophthalmologist feels he can do nothing further in the way of medical or surgical treatment for the patient he wishes to wash his hands of the management completely. There is of course a feeling of frustration in such circumstances, relieved at periodic intervals by short-lived hopes of therapies for senile maculopathy such as widespread laser prevention or treatment of the condition, hopes which are rarely fulfilled. Nevertheless there seems little excuse for the recurring vilification of ophthalmologists for in some way neglecting visual aids as a final management of these unfortunate patients. They are well aware too that to back up the purely optical devices we have been discussing the patient must be introduced to the appropriate social services in their own countries.

In many parts of the world there are agencies both voluntary and statutory to help those who are sight impaired. The list of such agencies is far too long to be included here, and in any case in some of the larger developed countries there are so many that it would be difficult to choose a few or a single one without running the risk of appearing to be in some way politically or socially biased. That having been said, a primary source of information can be obtained from the Royal National Institute for the Blind in the UK. The address is: The Technical Information Section, Royal National Institute for the Blind, 224 Great Portland Street, London W1N 6AA, UK. Telephone number 071 388 1266.

Two invaluable publications from the RNIB are as follows:

Agencies for Visually Disabled People; An International Guide by Ms Gillian Butcher whose assistance in this matter the author is happy to acknowledge, and a forthcoming publication entitled *Equipment for Visually Disabled People, An International Guide* due to be published by the same institution.

Appendices

Appendix I

Table 1 Refractive indices (Fraunhofer line D)

Crown glass, fluor	1.4785
borosilicate	1.5087
hard	1.5155
zinc	1.5149
barium	
light	1.5407
medium	1.5744
dense	1.5881
Flint glass, extra light	1.5290
light barium	1.5515
dense	1.6182
extra dense	1.6469

Table 2 Metre angles (Adapted from Percival, 1928)
The value of the unit metre angle depends on half the inter-ocular distance (IO), which varies commonly from 56 to 64 mm.

Where m denotes half the interocular distance in mm then 1 m.a. = $\sin^{-1}(m/1000)$. The following table gives the values in degrees for some inter-ocular distances.

IO	56 mm	58 mm	60 mm	62 mm	64 mm
1 m.a.	1° 36.27'	1° 39.71'	1° 43.15'	1° 46.59'	1° 50.03'

In the following table are given the values of some of the multiples of the metre angle which corresponds to an inter-ocular distance of 60 mm.

m.a.	Degrees	m.a.	Degrees
1	1° 43.15'	9	15° 39.86'
2	3° 26.39'	10	17° 27.46'
3	5° 9.82'	11	19° 16.13'
4	6° 53.53'	12	21° 6.00'
5	8° 37.62'	13	22° 57.27'
6	10° 22.19'	14	24° 50.08'
7	12° 7.34'	15	26° 44.62'
8	13° 53.19'	16	28° 41.12'

Table 3 Formulae for periscopic lenses (Percival, 1928)
In the formation of these lenses no attention is paid to the images formed on the peripheral parts of the retina; the aim is to make the area of a macular confusion circle less than that of a macular cone (the radius of which is 0.001 mm), when the eye is turned 30 degrees from the primary position to view an object through an eccentric part of the lens.

Convex periscopic lenses
Solid angle of 60°; refractive index = 1.523

D	For distance (D)		For 30 cm (D)	
	Anterior surface	Ocular surface	Anterior surface	Ocular surface
+ 1	+ 7.449	−6.5	+ 4.977	−4.00
+ 2	+ 8.417	−6.5	+ 6.206	−4.25
+ 3	+ 9.371	−6.5	+ 7.175	−4.25
+ 4	+10.560	−6.75	+ 8.138	−4.25
+ 5	+11.490	−6.75	+ 9.088	−4.25
+ 6	+12.641	−7.00	+10.264	−4.50
+ 7	+13.536	−7.00	+11.421	−4.75
+ 8	+14.413	−7.00	+13.022	−5.50
+ 9	+15.270	−7.00	+13.668	−5.25
+10	+16.105	−7.00	+14.299	−5.00
+11	+16.697	−6.75	+15.140	−5.00
+12	+17.488	−6.75	+15.956	−5.00
+13	+17.826	−6.25	+16.532	−4.75
+14	+18.152	−5.75	+17.090	−4.50

Concave periscopic lenses
Solid angle of 60°; refractive index = 1.523

D	For distance (D)		For 30 cm (D)	
	Anterior surface	Ocular surface	Anterior surface	Ocular surface
− 1	+6.25	− 7.25	+4.25	− 5.25
− 2	+5.75	− 7.75	+3.75	− 5.75
− 3	+5.00	− 8.00	+3.25	− 6.25
− 4	+4.75	− 8.75	+2.50	− 6.50
− 5	+4.25	− 9.25	+2.00	− 7.00
− 6	+3.75	− 9.75	+1.50	− 7.50
− 7	+3.25	−10.25	+1.00	− 8.00
− 8	+2.75	−10.75	+0.50	− 8.50
− 9	+2.25	−11.25	Plane	− 9.00
−10	+2.00	−12.00	−0.50	− 9.50
−11	+1.50	−12.50	−1.00	−10.00
−12	+1.25	−13.25	−1.25	−10.75
−13	+1.00	−14.00	−1.75	−11.25
−14	+0.75	−14.75	−2.00	−12.00
−15	+0.50	−15.50	−2.00	−13.00
−16	+0.25	−16.25	—	—
−17	Plane	−17.00	—	—
−20	Plane	−20.00	—	—

Table 4 Standard tapered multicurve trial set of 23 corneal contact lenses (Nissel)

Specification
Back optic zone diameter 6.60 mm
First back peripheral diameter 7.50 mm
Second back peripheral diameter 8.50 mm
Total diameter 9.50 mm
Trial lenses −2.00 D ± 0.12 D
Blended transitions
Lenses engraved 1 to 23

No.	Radius	First peripheral radius	Second peripheral radius	Third peripheral radius
1	7.20	7.70	8.20	8.70
2	7.25	7.75	8.25	8.75
3	7.30	7.80	8.30	8.80
4	7.35	7.85	8.35	8.85
5	7.40	7.90	8.40	8.90
6	7.45	7.95	8.45	8.95
7	7.50	8.00	8.50	9.00
8	7.55	8.05	8.55	9.05
9	7.60	8.10	8.60	9.10
10	7.65	8.15	8.65	9.15
11	7.70	8.20	8.70	9.20
12	7.75	8.25	8.75	9.25
13	7.80	8.30	8.80	9.30
14	7.85	8.35	8.85	9.35
15	7.90	8.40	8.90	9.40
16	7.95	8.45	8.95	9.45
17	8.00	8.50	9.00	9.50
18	8.05	8.55	9.05	9.55
19	8.10	8.60	9.10	9.60
20	8.15	8.65	9.15	9.65
21	8.20	8.70	9.20	9.70
22	8.25	8.75	9.25	9.75
23	8.30	8.80	9.30	9.80

Table 5 Spectacle and ocular refraction: effectivity corrections in hypermetropia (A. G. Bennett)

Spectacle refraction	Effectivity correction when vertex distance is				
	8 mm	10 mm	12 mm	14 mm	16 mm
D	D	D	D	D	D
+ 2.00	+0.03	+0.04	+0.05	+0.06	+0.07
+ 2.50	+0.05	+0.06	+0.08	+0.09	+0.10
+ 3.00	+0.10	+0.13	+0.11	+0.13	+0.15
+ 3.50	+0.10	+0.13	+0.15	+0.18	+0.21
+ 4.00	+0.13	+0.17	+0.20	+0.24	+0.27
+ 4.50	+0.17	+0.21	+0.26	+0.30	+0.35
+ 5.00	+0.21	+0.26	+0.32	+0.38	+0.43
+ 5.50	+0.25	+0.32	+0.39	+0.46	+0.53
+ 6.00	+0.30	+0.38	+0.47	+0.55	+0.64
+ 6.50	+0.36	+0.45	+0.55	+0.65	+0.76
+ 7.00	+0.42	+0.53	+0.64	+0.76	+0.88
+ 7.50	+0.48	+0.61	+0.74	+0.88	+1.02
+ 8.00	+0.55	+0.70	+0.85	+1.01	+1.17
+ 8.50	+0.62	+0.79	+0.97	+1.15	+1.34
+ 9.00	+0.70	+0.89	+1.09	+1.30	+1.51
+ 9.50	+0.78	+0.99	+1.22	+1.46	+1.70
+10.00	+0.87	+1.11	+1.36	+1.63	+1.90
+10.50	+0.96	+1.23	+1.51	+1.81	+2.12
+11.00	+1.06	+1.36	+1.67	+2.00	+2.35
+11.50	+1.16	+1.49	+1.84	+2.21	+2.59
+12.00	+1.27	+1.64	+2.02	+2.42	+2.85
+12.50	+1.30	+1.79	+2.21	+2.65	+3.13
+13.00	+1.51	+1.94	+2.40	+2.89	+3.42
+13.50	+1.64	+2.11	+2.61	+3.15	+3.72
+14.00	+1.77	+2.28	+2.83	+3.41	+4.04
+14.50	+1.90	+2.46	+3.06	+3.70	+4.38
+15.00	+2.04	+2.65	+3.29	+3.99	+4.74
+15.50	+2.19	+2.84	+3.54	+4.29	+5.11
+16.00	+2.35	+3.05	+3.80	+4.62	+5.51
+16.50	+2.51	+3.26	+4.07	+4.95	+5.92
+17.00	+2.68	+3.48	+4.36	+5.31	+6.35
+17.50	+2.85	+3.71	+4.65	+5.68	+6.81
+18.00	+3.03	+3.96	+4.96	+6.06	+7.28

Above corrections to be added.
Example: spectacle refraction +13.50 D, vertex distance 14 mm.
Ocular refraction = +13.50 + 3.15 = +16.65 D.

Table 5 continued. Spectacle and ocular refraction: effectivity corrections in myopia (A. G. Bennett)

Spectacle refraction	Effectivity correction when vertex distance is				
	8 mm	10 mm	12 mm	14 mm	16 mm
D	D	D	D	D	D
− 2.00	+0.03	+0.04	+0.05	+0.05	+0.06
− 2.50	+0.05	+0.06	+0.07	+0.08	+0.10
− 3.00	+0.07	+0.09	+0.10	+0.12	+0.14
− 3.50	+0.10	+0.12	+0.14	+0.16	+0.19
− 4.00	+0.12	+0.15	+0.18	+0.21	+0.24
− 4.50	+0.16	+0.19	+0.23	+0.27	+0.30
− 5.00	+0.19	+0.24	+0.28	+0.33	+0.37
− 5.50	+0.23	+0.29	+0.34	+0.39	+0.44
− 6.00	+0.27	+0.34	+0.40	+0.47	+0.53
− 6.50	+0.32	+0.39	+0.47	+0.54	+0.61
− 7.00	+0.37	+0.46	+0.54	+0.62	+0.70
− 7.50	+0.42	+0.52	+0.62	+0.71	+0.80
− 8.00	+0.48	+0.59	+0.70	+0.81	+0.91
− 8.50	+0.54	+0.66	+0.78	+0.90	+1.01
− 9.00	+0.60	+0.74	+0.88	+1.01	+1.13
− 9.50	+0.67	+0.83	+0.97	+1.12	+1.26
−10.00	+0.74	+0.91	+1.07	+1.23	+1.38
−10.50	+0.81	+1.00	+1.18	+1.35	+1.51
−11.00	+0.89	+1.09	+1.28	+1.47	+1.65
−11.50	+0.97	+1.19	+1.39	+1.60	+1.79
−12.00	+1.05	+1.29	+1.51	+1.73	+1.93
−12.50	+1.14	+1.39	+1.63	+1.86	+2.08
−13.00	+1.22	+1.50	+1.75	+2.00	+2.24
−13.50	+1.32	+1.61	+1.88	+2.15	+2.40
−14.00	+1.41	+1.72	+2.01	+2.29	+2.56
−14.50	+1.51	+1.84	+2.15	+2.45	+2.73
−15.00	+1.61	+1.96	+2.29	+2.60	+2.90
−15.50	+1.71	+2.08	+2.43	+2.76	+3.08
−16.00	+1.82	+2.21	+2.58	+2.93	+3.26
−16.50	+1.93	+2.34	+2.73	+3.10	+3.45
−17.00	+2.04	+2.47	+2.88	+3.27	+3.64
−17.50	+2.15	+2.61	+3.04	+3.41	+3.83
−18.00	+2.26	+2.75	+3.20	+3.62	+4.02
−18.50	+2.38	+2.89	+3.36	+3.80	+4.22
−19.00	+2.51	+3.03	+3.53	+3.99	+4.43
−19.50	+2.63	+3.18	+3.70	+4.18	+4.64
−20.00	+2.76	+3.33	+3.87	+4.37	+4.85

Above corrections to be added algebraically.

Example: spectacle refraction −5.25 D, vertex distance 12 mm.

Ocular refraction = −5.25 + 0.31 = −4.94 D.

Appendix II

The chemistry of contact lenses is complex, and the following classification is based on the work of John Parker BSc for the Association of Contact Lens Manufacturers.

Rigid lens materials, being largely hydrophobic, are classified as Focons and are characterised by the group number followed in brackets by their Dk value. Some commoner names for the most popular materials are in parentheses (Table 1).

Non-rigid lens materials are almost entirely hydrophilic, and, following the initial American practice of using the suffix Filcon for the polymer names, the materials are known as Filcons. As is seen from the following table they are in five groups, and except for group 5 each is subdivided into two subgroups (a) and (b) according to the absence or presence of significant ionisable material. Group 5 materials, the silicon rubber elastomers, are classified as Filcons but are in fact very hydrophobic. Except for this group a material will be further classified by a number in brackets indicating its water (strictly speaking saline) content. For group 5 the number is usually 200 and indicates its Dk (oxygen permeability) value (Table 2).

As pointed out in the main text, a reference source for contact lens products will be found to be invaluable. A good example in the UK is the *Contact Lens Yearbook* published annually by the Medical & Scientific Publishing Co. In the US many similar guides such as that by Soper & Kastl are available.

Table 1 Focons

Group 1a
Essentially pure polymethylmethacrylate (PMMA) (99.0%). Dk essentially zero.

Group 1b
Co-polymers of PMMA with not more than 10% throughout of other monomers that may alter hardness, wettability and stability. Dk essentially zero.

Group 2a
Essentially pure CAB (90%). Dk range typically of 2 to 8.

Group 2b
Co-polymers or mixtures of CAB and other monomers.

Group 3
Co-polymers of one or more alkylmethacrylates with one or more siloxanylmethacrylates, plus other water-active monomers and cross-linking agents. Typical Dk of more than 6. Boston I = Focon 3 (12).

Group 4
Hard lens materials formed from polysiloxanes (very uncommon now).

Group 5
Co-polymers of one or more alkylmethacrylates and/or siloxanylmethacrylates, plus other water-active monomers, cross-linking agents, and at least 5% by weight of a fluoroalkylmethacrylate or other fluorine-containing monomers. Typical Dk of more than 20. Boston Equalens material = Focon 5 (71).

Table 2 Filcons

Group 1a
Essentially pure 2-hydroxyethylmethacrylate, containing not more than 0.2% by weight of any ionisable chemical (e.g. methacrylic acid). Polymacon, Phemfilcon = Filcon 1a (38).

Group 1b
Essentially pure 2-hydroxyethylmethacrylate, containing more than 0.2% by weight of any ionisable chemical.

Group 2a
A co-polymer of 2-hydroxyethylmethacrylate and/or other hydroxyalkylmethacrylates, dihydroxyalkylmethacrylates and alkylmethacrylates, but not more than 0.2% by weight of any ionisable chemicals. CSI lens material = Filcon 2a (38).

Group 2b
As described in group 2a, but containing more than 0.2% by weight of any ionisable chemicals.

Group 3a
A co-polymer of 2-hydroxyethylmethacrylate with an N-vinyl lactam and/or an alkylacrylamide but containing not more than 0.2% by weight of any ionisable chemicals.

Group 3b
As described in group 3a, but containing more than 0.2% by weight of any ionisable chemicals. Permalens = Filcon 3b (71).

Group 4a
A co-polymer of alkylmethacrylate and N-vinyl lactam and/or an alkylacrylamide, but containing not more than 0.2% weight of any ionisable chemicals. Sauflon, Lido-filcon A = Filcon 4a(79).

Group 4b
As described in group 4a, but containing more than 0.2% by weight of any ionisable chemicals. (Note that group 4 Filcons do not contain HEMA, and are of the high water content materials.)

Group 5
Soft lens materials formed from polysiloxanes.

Table 3 Basic contact lens polymer chemistry

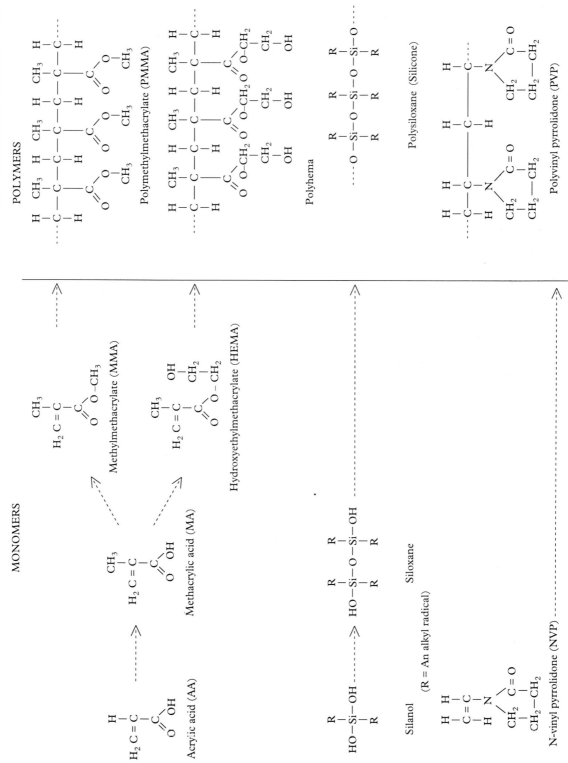

Index

Aberration
  chromatic, 32, 184
  peripheral, 35
  spherical, 33, 72, 170, 204
Acanthamoeba histolytica, corneal
    ulceration, 256
Accommodation, 85
  age variation, 86, 91
  amplitude, 87
  anisometropia, 88
  anomalies, 95
  aphakia, 71
  astigmatism, 88
  availability, 89
  binocular, 135
  convergence and, 4, 133, 134
    ratio, 134
  determination, 186
  elimination, 184
  emmetropia, 88
  excessive, 50, 55, 95
  fatigue, 89
  Helmholtz theory, 86
  hypermetropia, 47, 88, 92
  ill-sustained, 97
  inertia, 98
  insufficiency, 96
    exercises for, 97
  mechanism, 85
  myopia, 88
  near point determination, 186
  paralysis, 98
  phenomena, 89
  physical, 87
  physiological, 87
  presbyopia, 86, 87, 91
  range, 87
  relative, 133, 187
  rules, 186
  spasm, 96, 169
Adie's myotonic pupil, 98
Albinism, 264
Allyl diglycol carbonate lenses
    (CR39), 200, 231
Amblyopia
  ex anopsia, 105, 127
  strabismic, 273
Amblyoscope, 116

Ametropia, 37, 41, 76, 220
  see also Hypermetropia; Myopia, *etc*
Angle
  alpha, 34, 49, 58
  deviation and, 14
  gamma, 35
  kappa, 35
  metre, 132
    table, 285
  refractive, 13
  visual, 32
Aniridia, 264
Aniseikonia, 71, 76, 109
  clinical investigation, 111
  symptoms, 110
  treatment, 113
Anisocycloplegia, 100
Anisometropia, 37, 76, 105, 219
  accommodation, 88
  contact lenses, 107, 234
  treatment, 106
Aphakia, 38, 46, 71, 207, 219
  accommodation, 71
  contact lenses, 72, 234, 263
  disadvantages, 71
  image enlargement, 71
  treatment, 72
  uniocular, 107
  vision in, 71
Arc eye, 231
Arden contrast sensitivity plates, 152,
    153
Asthenopia, 5, 67
  accommodative, 50, 52, 87, 95,
    170
  see also Eye-strain
Astigmatism, 37, 65
  accommodation, 88
  acquired, 65
  aetiology, 65
  aphakia, 68, 72, 78
  asthenopia, 67
  bi-oblique, 37, 66
  clinical features, 67
  compound, 67
  contact lenses, 259
  corneal, 65, 69
  curvature, 65

  direct, 65, 67
  eye-strain, 67
  historical aspects, 65
  hypermetropic, 37, 49, 81
    compound, 67
    simple, 66
  image surfaces, 205
  index, 38, 65
  indirect, 67
  inverse, 65
  irregular, 37, 66, 68
    contact lenses, 261
    treatment, 69
  lenticular, 68
  meridian, 165
  mixed, 37, 67
  myopic, 37, 77
    compound, 67
    simple, 66
  oblique, 35, 66
    pencils of light, 204
  optical condition, 66
  pseudophakia surgery, 77
  regular, 21, 37, 66
  residual, hard contact lenses, 259
  simple, 66
  surgery, 68, 70
  symptoms, 67
  treatment, 68, 69
  types, 66
Atropine, 51, 91, 99, 101, 127
  see also Cycloplegia
Autokeratometer, 240
Automated refraction, 177
Axial length, measurement, 39
Axis
  fixation, 35
  optic, 34
  principal, 17
  secondary, 17
  visual, 34

Back optic zone, 243
  diameter, 243
  radius, 243
Back vertex power, 27, 28, 161, 185
Base line, 131

Belgard's lenscorometer, 185
Bell's palsy, 232
Benoxinate, 244
Benzalkonium chloride, 246, 254, 257
Bifocal contact lenses
    annular, 261
    diffractive, 262
    segment, 261
    types, 261
Bifocal lenses, 221
    designs, 224
    fused, 222
    optical function, 222
    solid (one-piece), 222
    split, 221
    visual function, 223
Binkhorst formula, biometry, 73
Binocular accommodation, 135
Binocular vision see Vision, binocular
Biometry, 73
    regression formulae, 73
    theoretical formulae, 73
Bistropamide, 100
Blepharitis, eye-strain, 5
Blepharospasm, 122
Blinking, abnormal, hard contact
        lenses, 249
Brücke's muscle, 87
Buphthalmos, myopia, 53, 80

Cambridge chart, 153
Canon autorefractor, 177
Cardinal points, 25
Cataract
    hypermaturity, 108
    Morgagnian state, 108
    postoperative astigmatism, 77
    postoperative refraction stability, 78
    refractive changes, 38, 53, 80
    retinoscopy, 171
    surgery see Aphakia and
        Pseudophakia
Catford drum, 150
Cellulose acetate butyrate (CAB), 238
Centre
    of curvature, 16
    geometrical, 211
    optical, 18, 211
    of rotation, 34
Chlorhexidine, 257
Choroiditis, refractive changes, 80
Chromatic aberration, 32, 184
    magnification difference, 33
Ciliary muscle
    contraction mechanism, 87
    failure, 50
    spasm, 50, 59, 96
    weakness, 4, 96
Circles of diffusion (confusion), 22,
        35
Cocaine, 100
Colenbrander-Hoffer formula,
        biometry, 74
Coma, retinal, 35

Computers, and lens design, 208
Concave lenses see Lens/lenses
        (optical)
Concomitant strabismus see
        Heterotropia
Conical cornea see Keratoconus
Conjunctivitis
    eye-strain, 5
    giant papillary (GPC), 256, 257
Contact lenses, 233
    anisometropia, 107, 234
    aphakia, 263
    astigmatism, 259
    chemistry, 291
    complications of wear
        hard, 248
        scleral, 268
        soft, 255
    design
        hard, 242
        scleral, 266
        soft, 251
    disposable, 264
    extended wear, 258
    fitting
        hard, 242
        scleral, 266
        soft, 251
    gas-permeable, 233, 237
    and the generalist, 268
    hydrogel, 238
    hygiene, 246, 254
    hypermetropia, 234
    indications for, 234
    keratoconus, 262
    keratometry, 239
    materials, 237, Appendix II
    Meibomitis and, 258
    myopia, 61, 234
    optical applications, 183
    overwearing syndrome, 250, 255
    presbyopia, 261
    rigid, 233
    spoilage, 256
    therapeutic, 264
    tight lens syndrome, 259
    visual aids, 280
    see also Bifocal contact lenses;
        Corneal contact lenses; Scleral
        contact lenses
Contrast sensitivity, testing, 152
Convergence, 118, 131
    accommodation, 4, 133, 134
        ratio, 134
    amplitude, 132
    anomalies, 137
    deficiency, 192
    excess, 139
    far point, 131
    fatigue, 136
    insufficiency, 137
    line of, 20
    measurement, 132, 189
    near point, 131, 187
    negative, 132, 133

positive, 132, 133
    range, 131
    reflex, 131
    relative, 135, 187
    voluntary, 131
Convex lenses see Lens/lenses
        (optical)
Cornea
    astigmatism, 65, 69
    conical see Keratoconus
    contact lenses see Corneal contact
        lenses
    convergence/axial length
        correlation, 40
    curvature see Keratometry
    disease, refractive changes, 80
    oedema, and contact lenses, 250,
        255, 257
    plana, 46
    reflections, 189
    refraction and, 29
    shape alterations, for myopia, 62
    transplantation, contact lenses, 264
Corneal contact lenses
    aphakia, 72, 234, 263
    astigmatism, 259
    bifocal, 261
    choice, hard/soft, 236
    clinical history, 235
    clinical indications/
        contra-indications, 234
    curvature radius, 241
    extended-wear, 258
        complications, 259, 265
        follow up, 258
    eye curvature, 239
    filcons, 291, 292, 293
    focons, 291, 292, 293
    hard, 233
        corneal proximity/fluorescein
            patterns, 245
        design and parameters, 242
        edge lift, 245, 246
        fitting procedure, 243
        fluorescein patterns, 245
        follow-up and problems, 248
        hygiene, 246
        insertion/removal teaching, 247,
            248
        intolerance and discomfort, 249
        materials, 237
        mobility, 244
        ordering, 246
        over-wearing syndrome, 250
        pain, 250
        patient's management, 246
        poor vision, 250
        signs without symptoms, 248
        spectacle blur, 251
        storage/cleansing solutions, 246
        trial lens, 244
    keratoconus, 262
    lenticular form, 263
    materials, 237
    measurement and inspection, 241

Corneal contact lenses (cont'd)
  multicurve, table, 287
  ophthalmological findings, 235
  and optic error, 234
  overall diameter, 241
  parameter determination, 239
  power, 241
  presbyopia, 261
  single-cut, 263
  soft, 233
    acute complications, 255
    bandage, 265
    chronic inflammation/discomfort, 257
    cleaning/storage solutions, 254
    design and parameters, 251
    fitting procedure, 252
    follow-up and problems, 255
    giant papillary conjunctivitis, 257
    hygiene, 254
    insertion/removal teaching, 253, 256
    lens spoilage, 256
    materials, 238
    ordering, 253
    over-wearing syndrome, 255
    patient's management, 253
    poor vision, 256
    signs without symptoms, 255
    thiomersal toxicity, 257
  tear renewal, 237
  therapeutic uses, 264
  thickness, 242
  tinted, 265
Corneal diameter, contact lenses, 241
Cover test, 189
CR39, 200, 231
Crescent
  myopic, 56, 57, 58
  supertraction, 57, 58
Crookes's glass, 231
Cross-cylinders, 182
Crutch spectacles, 228
Curvature
  centre, 16
  radius, 16
Cyclogyl, 51, 100, 170
Cyclopentolate, 51, 100, 170
Cyclophoria, 120, 121, 122
Cycloplegia, 99
  retinoscopy, 168
Cycloplegics, 50, 99
  see also various compounds
Cylinders
  concave, 21
  convex, 20
  crossed, 182
  notation, 23
  transposition, 208

Decentring of eye, 34, 65
Deorsum vergens, 127
Dermatitis, contact, 203

Deviation
  angle, 14
  minimal, 13
  vertical, 118, 127
Diabetes
  myopia, 53, 55, 80
  refractive changes, 80
Diabetic retinopathy, visual aids, 273
Dimple veiling, 249
Dioptre
  notation, vergence, 22
  prism, 14
Diplopia, 117, 155
  eye-strain, 5
Divergence, 118, 132
  excess, 192
Divers' spectacles, 228
Dk value, contact lenses, gas permeability, 237
Drugs, and refractive changes, 79
Duane's accommodation card/rule, 186
Dunlop test, 140
Duochrome test, 184
Dyslexia, 139

E test, visual acuity, 149
Ectasias, 53
Effectivity of lenses, 209, 288
Eikonometer, space, 111
Elderly, visual aids, 273
Emmetropia, 37, 40, 88, 91
  adolescence, 51
  ophthalmoscopy, 172, 175
  retinoscopy, 155
End point of retinoscopy, 155
Epikeratophakia, 78
  myopia, 63
Epitheliopathy, microcystic, 250, 257
Esophoria, 120, 123, 192
Esotropia, 127
Excimer laser
  hypermetropia, 52
  myopia, 63
Exophoria, 120, 123, 192
  prisms and, 120
Exotropia, 127
Extorsion, 121, 188
Eye movements, examination, 189
Eye-strain, 4, 87
  astigmatism, 67
  hypermetropia, 50
  myopia, 59
  and ophthalmic disease aetiology, 5
  presbyopia, 92
  spectacle placebo effect, 7
  symptoms
    ocular, 5
    referred, 5
    visual, 4
  and visual display units (VDUs), 7
  and visual task nature, 7

Fan, astigmatic, 182, 183
Far point, 58
  accommodation and, 87
  convergence and, 131
Fatigue, visual acuity effects, 4
Filcons, 291, 292, 293
Fishing spectacles, 227
Fixation axis, 35
Fixation point, 34
Focal distance, 18
Focal interval, 22, 66
Focal length, 18, 209
Focal line, 21, 66
  meridional, 205
  radial, 205
  sagittal, 205
  tangential, 205
Focal surface
  meridional, 205
  radial, 205
  sagittal, 205
  tangential, 205
Focimeter, 185, 216, 241
Focons, 291, 292, 293
Focus, 18
  conjugate, 18
  principal, 18
    first, 26
    second, 25
Forced preferential looking (FPL), 150
Förster-Fuchs fleck, 56, 57
Frames
  spectacle, 200, 201, 202
  trial, 160
Franklin bifocal lens, 221
Fresnel lens, 275
Frisby test, 117, 118
Fundus, in myopia, 56, 57
Fusion, 116

Galilean spectacles, 279
Geneva lens measure, 215
Glass
  Crookes's, 231
  gold-plated, 231
  high lights, 200
  magnifying, 276
  photochromic, 230
  spectacle, types of, 199, 200
  tinted, 228
  Triplex, 231
Glasses see Spectacles
Glaucoma, 273
  closed-angle, 48
  refractive changes, 53, 80
Goggles, 231
Goldmann applanation tonometer, 75

Haag-Streit keratometer, 239
Haemianopic spectacles, 228
Haptic lenses see Contact lenses

Headache, 4, 5, 92
  heterophoria, 122
  mechanism, 6
Hering-Hillebrand horopter
    deviation, 110
Heterophoria, 3, 115, 119
  causes, 119
  orthoptic exercises, 122
  prisms in, 122
  symptoms, 121
  tests, 189, 190
  treatment, 122
  varieties, 119
Heterotropia, 115, 125
  and anisometropia, 106
  optical errors, 125
  orthoptic exercises, 128
  treatment, 127
  varieties, 127
  vision in, 126
Homatropine, 100
Hydroxyethylmethacrylate (HEMA),
    238
Hyoscine hydrobromide, 100
Hyoscyamine sulphate, 100
Hyperesophoria, 120
Hyperexophoria, 120
Hypermetropia, 37, 45, 80
  absolute, 47
  accommodation, 47, 88, 91
    excessive, 50
  acquired, 48
  aetiology, 45
  age variation, 46, 48, 79
  axial, 37
  clinical features, 49
  contact lenses, 234
  curvature, 37, 46
  cyclopegia, 169
  effectivity corrections, table,
      288
  eye-strain, 50
  facultative, 47
  historical aspects, 45
  index, 38, 46
  latent, 47, 51, 52
  manifest, 47, 51
  microphthalmos, 41, 45, 49
  ophthalmoscopy, 172, 175
  optical condition, 46
  pathology, clinical, 48
  retinal appearances, 49
  retinoscopy, 157
  strabismus, 4, 49, 50
  surgery, 52
  symptoms, 49, 143
  total, 47, 51
  treatment, 50
  vision blurring, 49
Hyperopia see Hypermetropia
Hyperphoria, 120, 121
Hypertropia, 127
Hypometropia see Myopia
Hypotropia, 127

Image, 18
  astigmatic surfaces, 205
  concave lenses, 19
  convex lenses, 18
  inequality see Aniseikonia
  retinal, 31
    aphakia, 71
    distortion, 35, 218
    formation, 31
  suppression, 126
  virtual, 18, 19, 20
Index of refraction see Refractive
    index
Infra-red rays, protection, 228, 229,
    230
Intorsion, 121
Intra-ocular distances, ultrasonic
    measurement, 39
Iridocyclitis, 96
Iritis, refractive changes, 80

Javal-Schiotz keratometer, 239

K, corneal lens fitting, 243, 245
Katral lens, 207
Keratectomy, photoreactive (PRK),
    63
Keratitis
  infective, corneal soft lenses, 255
  superior limbic (Theodore), 257
Keratoconjuctivitis, thiomersal, 257
Keratoconus, 53, 68
  contact lens, 262
  retinoscopy, 172
Keratometer
  Haag-Streit, 239
  Javal-Schiotz, 239
  Terry, 77
  Wesseley's, 185
Keratometry, 75, 178
  corneal contact lenses, 239
  intraoperative, 77
Keratomileusis, 62, 68, 70, 108
Keratopathy
  bullous, 265
  toxic, 257
Keratoscope, 69
Keratotomy, radial (RK), 62

Lagophthalmos, 232
Landolt's broken ring test, 148
Laser
  Excimer, 52, 63
  Holmium, 52
Laser surgery
  hypermetropia, 52, 63
  myopia, 63
Lasers, subjective refraction, 185
Leinbach's reading slit, 281, 282
Lens (crystalline)
  absence see Aphakia

accommodation and, 86
astigmatism, 65
displacement, 37, 65, 79
obliquity, 37
refraction and, 29
removal in myopia, 63
Lens/lenses (optical)
  achromatic, 33
  aplanatic, 34
  astigmatic, 21
  centring, 211
  concave, 15, 19
  contact see Contact lenses
  convex, 15, 17, 18
  cylindrical, 20
    concave, 21
    convex, 20
    measurement/detection, 24
    notation, 23
  decentring, 34, 211
  detection, 23
  equivalence, 27, 28
  implantation in myopia, 63
  iseikonic, 107, 113
  measurement, 23, 215
  meniscus, 34, 206
  neutralising, 164, 215
  notation, 22
  periscopic, 34, 206
    formula table, 286
  principal axis, 17
  refraction and, 14
  secondary axis, 17
  spectacle see Spectacle lenses
  spherical, 15
    aberration, 33
    measurement/detection, 23
  sphero-cylindrical combinations,
      165
  stepped (Fresnel), 275
  thick, 27
Lenscorometer, Belgard's, 185
Lenticonus, 53, 69, 70
  false, 38
Lenticulus, intra-ocular (IOL), 72
  power, predictability limits, 74
Light
  diffraction, 32
  dispersion, 32
  wavelength, and refraction, 12
  see also Refraction

McCollough effect, 7
Macropsia, 96, 98
Maddox
  groove, 190
  rods, 122, 190
  tangent scale, 190, 191
  V test, 183
  wing test, 191
Magnification
  chromatic differences, 33
  and lighting, 276

Magnification (cont'd)
  optical, 276
  visual aids, 275
Magnifiers
  paperweight (plano-convex), 277
  simple, 276
  spectacle-borne, 278
  stand, 276
Meibomian cysts, 258
Meibomitis, chronic, 258
Metre angle, 132
  Table, 285
Microphthalmos, hypermetropia, 41,
  45, 49
Micropsia, 98
Monocle, 189, 202
Monoyer's visual acuity scale, 147
Müller's muscle, 87
Multifocal lenses, 225
Muscle balance see Heterophoria
Mydriacyl, 100
Mydriatics, 99
Myodioptre, 87
Myopia, 37, 53, 207
  accommodation and, 88
  adjuvant factors, 55
  aetiology, 53
  artificial, 50, 51, 95, 169
  axial, 37, 41, 53, 54
  clinical features, 58
  clinical types, 56
  complications, 57, 59
  contact lenses, 61, 234
  curvature, 37, 53
  diabetes, 53, 55, 80
  effectivity corrections, table, 288
  endocrine aspects, 54
  epikeratophakia, 63
  eye-strain, 59
  hereditary/ethnic aspects, 54, 55,
    60
  historical aspects, 53
  index, 38, 53
  intermediate, 54
  ophthalmoscopy, 56, 173, 175
  optical condition, 58
  optical correction, 60
  pathological, 54, 56
  pathology, clinical, 56
  physiological, 54
  prematurity and, 55
  prognosis, 59
  progress of, 55
  progressive, 54
  prophylaxis, 60
  retinal changes, 54, 56
  retinoscopy, 157
  simple, 54
  surgery, 62
  symptoms, 58
  treatment, 60
  visual hygiene, 61

Near point
  accommodation and, 88, 186
  convergence and, 131, 187
Neurotic temperament, eye-strain, 6
Nodal points, 26, 58
Nose glasses, 202
Notation, standard, 23

Oculomotor anomalies, dyslexia, 140
Ogle and Ames space eikonometer,
  111
Omnifocal lens, 226
Ophthalmetron, 177
Ophthalmological examination,
  refraction and, 143
Ophthalmoscopy
  direct, 174
  indirect, 172
  refraction and, 172
Optic atrophy, 273
Optical defects of eye, 32
  pathological, 36
  physiological, 32
Optical density, 12
Optical systems, 24
  of eye, 29
  homocentric, 25
Optical unit, 162
Opticlude, 128
Optometry, objective, 176
Orthophoria, 115
Orthoptic exercises, 122, 129, 138
Over-wearing syndrome
  hard contact lenses, 250
  soft contact lenses, 255

Pain, ocular, eye-strain, 5
Palpebral aperture width, 241
Pelli-Robson letter sensitivity chart,
  152, 153
Perception, simultaneous, 116
Perspex, 231, 233, 237
Pfund's gold-plated glass, 238
Phorometers, 192
Photo Refractive Keratectomy
  (PRK), 63
Photochromic glass, 230
Photokeratoscopy, 240
Photophobia, and hard contact
  lenses, 250
Photophthalmia, 229
Pilocarpine, 96
Pin-hole aperture, 36, 281
Pin-hole test, 145
Pince-nez, 302
Placido's disc, 69
Plane, principal (equivalent)
  first, 26
  second, 25
Plastic lenses, 200, 231
Point
  fixation, 34

neutral, 155
nodal, 26, 58
principal (equivalent)
  first, 26
  second, 25
of reversal, 155
see also Far point; Near point
Polaroid spectacles, 230
Polymethylmethacrylate (PMMA),
  231, 233, 237
Polyquat, 254
Presbyopia, 3, 81, 86, 87, 91
  contact lenses, 261
  monocles/lorgnettes, 189
  spectacle lenses, 220
  symptoms, 92
  treatment, 92
Prince's rule, 186
Principal planes, 25, 26
Principal points, 25, 26
Prismosphere, 212
Prisms
  abducting, 132, 133
  adducting, 132
  adverse, heterophoria, 122
  convergence measurement, 132
  detection of, 14
  dioptre, 14
  Fresnel design, 123
  measurement, 14
  nomenclature, 14
  refraction and, 13
  relieving, 123, 139
  rotating, 14
Projection
  false, 126
  visual acuity and, 148
Protective spectacles, 228, 230
Pseudocyclophoria, 121
Pseudomyopia, 50, 51, 95, 169
Pseudopapillitis, hypermetropia, 49
Pseudophakia, 72
  calculation, 73
  optical problems, management,
    76
  reading vision, 76
Pseudostrabismus, 189
Pseudomonas pyocanea, 255
Ptosis spectacles, 228
Punctum proximum see Near point
Punctum remotum see Far point
Pupil size
  for contact lenses, 241
  stenopaeic apertures, 36
Pupillary line, 35

Radial keratotomy (RK), 62
Radius of curvature, 16
Reading
  ability, 139
  difficulties, 6, 137
  slit (Leinbach), 281, 282
  and visual aids, 273

Reading (*cont'd*)
see also Dyslexia; Special learning
   difficulty
Recumbent spectacles, 227
Reduced eye, 30
Refraction (of eye), 29
  automated, 177
  binocular correction, 185
  changes, 79
    age and, 79
    cataract, 80
    cataract surgery, 77
    choroiditis, 80
    corneal disease, 80
    diabetes, 80
    and drugs, 79
    glaucoma, 80
    iritis, 80
    lens dislocation, 79
    pathological, 79
    physiological, 79
    scleritis, 80
    surgical prevention, 64
    toxic states, 79
    trauma, 79
  clinical importance, 3
  dynamic, 88
    changes, 79
  errors of, 3
    degree, 38
    heterophoria, 127
    nature and incidence, 38
    pathological, 41
    simple, 41
    surgery for, 52, 62, 68, 78
    types, 37
    see also Hypermetropia; Myopia,
      etc
  examination, 195
    automated, 177
      final calculation, 167
      objective, 155
        keratometry, 178
        ophthalmoscopy, 172
        refractometry, 176
        retinoscopy, 155
      pupillary variations, 170
      subjective, 181
        lasers, 185
  lens, 29
  nature of, 11
  ophthalmological examination
    (general), 143
  psychological factors, 3
  static, 88
  total, 41
Refraction (of light)
  angle, 12, 13
  curved surfaces, 14
  glass plate, 11, 12
  lenses, 14
    astigmatic, 21
    combined, 24
    concave, 15, 19
    convex, 15, 17, 18

    cylindrical, 20, 21, 23
    spherical, 15, 23
  prisms, 13
Refractive index, 12
  anomalies, 38
  glass, table, 285
Refractive surfaces
  anomalies, 37
  curved, 14
Refractometer, 176
  Rodenstock, 176, 177
Refractometry, 176
Resolving power, of eye, 32
Retina
  obliquity, 37
  shot-silk, 49
Retinal changes
  hypermetropia, 49
  myopia, 54, 56
Retinal image *see* Image, retinal
Retinopathy, diabetic, 273
Retinoscopes, 158
  luminous, 159
  reflecting, 159
  streak, 160
Retinoscopy, 155
  cycloplegia, 168
  difficulties, 168, 170
  dynamic, 187
  emmetropia, 155
  end point, 155
  fogging, 168
  hypermetropia, 157
  methods, 158
  myopia, 157
  neutral point, 155
  optics, 155
  practice, 163
  results recording, 167
  shadows, 158, 165
  sphero-cylindrical combinations,
    165
  streak, 167
Reversal, point of, 155
Rotation of eye, and optical errors,
  203
Rotoid lens, 207

Scheerer and Betsch curve, refractive
  errors, 38, 39
Schematic eye, 30
Scissor-shadows, 171
Scleral contact lenses, 233, 265
  fitting, 266
  fluorescein pattern, 267
  modification, 267
  moulding shell, 266
  types, 266
  wear complications, 268
Scleritis, refractive changes, 80
Scopolamine, 100
Scotoma, 59, 72
  'roving ring', 219, 220
Shell, scleral lens moulding, 266

Sheridan-Gardiner test, 149
Shielded spectacles, 228
Shot-silk retina, 49
Siloxanyl methacrylate co-polymers,
  238
Simultaneous macular perception, 116
Snellen's test types, 146, 150
Snell's law, 12
Specific learning disability, 140
Spectacle frames, 200
  fitting, 202
  materials, 201
Spectacle lenses, 199
  aberrations, 204
  antireflective, 220
  aspherical, 207
  asymmetrical, 208
  base surface, 206
  best-form, 206
  bifocal, 221
  case-hardened, 231
  centring, 211
  combinations, 221
  combining surface, 206
  decentring, 211
  determination, near work and, 188
  dispensing errors, 220
  distant vision, 185
  distortion and, 218
  effectivity, 209, 288, 289
  eye rotation and, 203
  form, 203
  gradient, 229
  industrial safety, 230
  intolerance to, 218
  isochromatic, 228
  Katral, 207
  lenticular, 207
  manufacture, 199
  mirrored, 229
  multifocal, 225
    hard/soft, 227
  near vision, 188, 221
  neutralisation, 215
  neutralising, 164
  orthoscopic, 215
  photochromic glass, 230
  plano, 208
  plastic, 200
  polaroid, 230
  position, eye relationships, 209
  prescription, 195
    errors, 220
  progressive addition (PALS), 225
  protractor for, 216
  refraction
    hypermetropia, table, 288
    myopia, table, 289
  rotoid, 207
  size and shape, 203
  splintering, 231
  symmetrical, 208
  tilting, 217
  tinted, 228, 229
  toric, 207, 209

Spectacles lenses (cont'd)
  toughened, 231
  transposition, 209
  trifocal, 225
  varifocal, 226
  verification, 215
  Welsh four drop, 207
Spectacles
  anisometropic, 107
  crutch, 228
  divers', 228
  fishing, 227
  Galilean, 279
  hemianopic, 228
  manufacture, 199
  over-the-counter, 94
  placebo effect, 7
  polaroid, 230
  protective, 228, 230
  ptosis, 228
  recumbent, 227
  sports, 227, 231
  stenopaeic, 281
  telescopic, 279
Sphere
  real, 203, 204
  of sharp definition, 204
  transposition, 208
  virtual, 203, 204
Sports spectacles, 227, 231
Squint see Strabismus
SRK formula, biometry, 73
Staphyloma, posterior, 56, 57
Stenopaeic apertures, 36
  pupillary size, 36
Stenopaeic spectacles, 281
Stereoscope, 116
Stereoscopic vision, tests for, 116
Strabismus, 115
  apparent see Heterotropia
  concomitant see Heterotropia
  convergent, 4, 50, 59
  deorsum-vergens, 127
  latent see Heterophoria
  manifest, 189
  paralytic, 125
  sursum-vergens, 127
Sturm's conoid, 21, 22
Sunglasses, 229
Sursum vergence, 118, 127
Synoptophore, 116

Telescopes, head-borne, 280
Telescopic spectacles, 279
Television, closed-circuit, visual aid, 281
Teller acuity cards, 150

Test lenses, 161
Test types, 147
  E test, 149
  Faculty of Ophthalmologists, 151
  Keeler, 147
  Landolt's, 148, 183
  Snellen's, 146, 150
Tests
  Duochrome, 184
  Stereopsis
    Frisby, 117, 118
    TNO, 118
    Wirt, 118
  Worth's ivory ball, 150
Theodore's superior limbic keratitis, 257
Thermokeratoplasty, 52
Thin lens formula, 23
Thiomersal, 246, 254, 257
Tight lens syndrome, 259
Tinted lens, 228
TNO test, 118
Topogometer, 240
Torticollis, ocular, 143
Trauma, refractive changes, 79
Trial frames, 160
Trifocal lenses, 225
Trigeminal neuralgia, 232
Triplex glass, 231
Tron's frequency curves, 39
Tuition, non-visual, 61

Ultifo lens, 226
Ultra-violet rays, protection from, 228, 229
Ultrasonic measurement, intra-ocular distances, 39

Varilux lens, 226
VDU see Visual display units
Veiling
  dimple, 249
  and hard contact lenses, 249
Vergence
  deorsum, 127
  dioptric notation, 222
  power, 118, 192
  sursum, 127
Vertex power, 216
  back, 27, 28, 161, 185
Vertexometer, parallax (Zeiss), 185
Vertigo, 122
Visible doubling principle, 239
Vision
  alternating, 105
  binocular, 115
    anisometropia, 105

anomalies, 105, 106, 125
  correction, 185
  grades of, 116
  muscular anomalies, 119, 125, 137
  muscular co-ordination, 115, 131
  optical defects, 105, 109
distant
  spectacles, 185
  testing, 181
failure, 3
low, management, 274
near
  spectacles, 188, 221
  testing, 150, 186
  visual aids, 273
Visual acuity, 144, 145
  absolute, 147
  corrected, 147
  and projection, 148
  relative, 147
  testing, 145, 147
  unaided, 147
Visual aids, 273
  clinical assessment for, 273
  contact lenses, 280
  efficacy, 282
  Keeler system, 274
  low vision, 274
  magnification/magnifiers, 275
  non-magnifying, 281
  object size increase, 281
  patients, 273
  reading-slit, 281
  RNIB publications, 282
  Sloan system, 274
  spectacle-borne, 278
Visual angle, 32
Visual axis, 34
Visual display units (VDUs), 7
  bifocals, 224
Visual field, limitation, aphakia, 72
Visual hygiene, myopia, 61
Visual point
  distance, 223
  near, 223

Watchmaker's loupe, 278
Weiss's reflex streak, 56, 57
Welsh four drop lens, 207
Wesseley's keratometer, 185
Wirt test, 118
Worth's ivory ball test, 150

Zeiss parallax vertexometer, 185
Zone, neutral, 158